Pathology of the Lung

European Respiratory Monograph 39
March 2007

Editor in Chief
K. Larsson

This book is one in a series of European Respiratory Monographs. Each individual issue provides a comprehensive overview of one specific clinical area of respiratory health, communicating information about the most advanced techniques and systems needed to investigate it. It provides factual and useful scientific detail, drawing on specific case studies and looking into the diagnosis and management of individual patients. Previously published titles in this series are listed at the back of this book with details of how they can be purchased.

Pathology of the Lung

Edited by
W. Timens and H.H. Popper

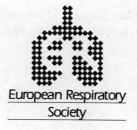

European Respiratory
Society

Published by European Respiratory Society Journals Ltd ©2007
March 2007
Hardback ISBN: 978-1-904097-47-1
Paperback ISBN: 978-1-904097-51-8
ISSN: 1025-448x
Printed by The Charlesworth Group, Wakefield, UK

Business matters (enquiries, advertisement bookings) should be addressed to: European Respiratory
Society Journals Ltd, Publications Office, Suite 2.4, Hutton's Building, 146 West Street, Sheffield,
S1 4ES, UK. Fax: 44 114 2780501.

The European Respiratory Monograph

Number 39　　　　　　　　　　　　　　　　　　　　　　　　　　March 2007

CONTENTS

The Guest Editors

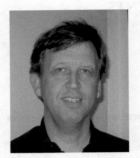

W. Timens

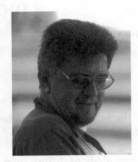

H.H. Popper

Wim Timens studied Medicine at the University of Groningen (Groningen, the Netherlands) and received his MD in 1983. After a short period as a research fellow, he followed the residency training programme at the Dept of Pathology, University Hospital Groningen, and was registered as a pathologist in 1990. In 1988, he received a PhD with his thesis on "Structure and function of the human spleen". In 1990, Wim worked as a post-doc at the Cross-Cancer Institute (Edmonton, Canada), and later that year joined the faculty of the Dept of Pathology, University Hospital Groningen. In 1992, he was appointed as an Associate Professor in this department, and in 1994 as a full Professor in Pathology.

Although he started his career in haematopathology and immunopathology, areas in which he also started his research interests, Wim soon became very interested in and challenged by pulmonary pathology. Over the last 16 years, he has dedicated his diagnostic pathology work to the whole area of pulmonary diseases. He has worked on different research themes involving lung pathology, and has been involved in and leads many research projects, most with external funding and almost invariably in close collaboration with the Dept of Pulmonology and several other disciplines. Within the research themes, there is a strong focus on the pathogenesis of obstructive lung diseases, which is a main research area in the University Medical Center Groningen. He is a Co-Chair of the Groningen Research Institute on Asthma and COPD (GRIAC) and has been a member of the Scientific Board of the Netherlands Asthma Foundation for many years.

Helmut H. Popper studied Medicine at the University of Graz, Medical Faculty (Graz, Austria) and received his MD in 1973. From 1973, he worked as an Assistant at the Institute of Pharmacology, University of Graz, but moved to the Pathology Dept in 1975. In 1984, Helmut finished his training with board certification in Pathology and became Associate Prof. of Pathology with residency at the Institute of Pathology. In 1986, he was appointed Head of the Laboratory of Environmental Pathology and in 1991 was certified for Cytopathology, becoming Prof. of Pathology in 1992. In 1999, Helmut received further certification for Human Genetics and was appointed as Head of the Laboratories for Molecular Cytogenetics and Environmental & Respiratory Tract Pathology in 2000. In 1988 and 1989, he spent some time at the Lovelace Inhalation Toxicology Research Institute, Albuquerque (NM, USA), to learn methods in inhalation toxicology and research. His main focus is genetics in lung diseases with a special interest in lung cancer and sarcoidosis.

From 1999–2003 he served as Chair of the Pulmonary Pathology Working Group of the European Society of Pathology, and again from 2005–2007. Since 2001, Helmut has stood as Chair of an EU project on rare pulmonary diseases, and organised the establishment of the European case collection on rare pulmonary diseases. He is currently Co-Chair for the Latin American–European Pulmonary Pathology Working Group. He is also a member of the Editorial Board of *Virchows Archiv*, and an Associate Editor of *Archives of Pathology & Laboratory Medicine*.

Preface

In order to better understand clinical issues in pulmonary medicine, it has become obvious that knowledge about structural changes in the lungs has to be improved. The lungs constitute the largest contact area of the human body with the environment and surroundings. In addition, the lungs serve as a capillary filter of venous blood, involving heavy exposure to the external and internal environment. This poses a unique situation in which both exposure to external agents and "endogenous" changes have to be considered when evaluating pathological changes of the lungs. Therefore, a close collaboration between pathologists and clinicians is of great importance in diagnosing and treating all disorders displaying alteration of lung structure. It is, therefore, a pleasure to introduce the current issue of the *European Respiratory Monograph*, which is dedicated to lung pathology. The Monograph covers the pathology of neoplastic diseases, infections, obstructive and interstitial lung diseases, and pulmonary manifestations of systemic diseases, with all the chapters written by distinguished experts. It is my firm belief that this Monograph will serve as a tool for clinicians to better understand lung pathology. It will also be useful to clinicians who meet patients with pulmonary diseases. As it is a comprehensive update of the pathological field I am assured that pathologists and scientists within the field, will also find this Monograph helpful.

K. Larsson
Editor in Chief

Eur Respir Mon, 2007, 39, vii. Printed in UK - all rights reserved. Copyright ERS Journals Ltd 2007; European Respiratory Monograph; ISSN 1025-448x.

INTRODUCTION

W. Timens*, H.H. Popper[#]

*Dept of Pathology, University Medical Center Groningen, University of Groningen, Groningen, the Netherlands. Fax: 31 503632510; E-mail: w.timens@path.azg.nl [#]Dept of Pathology, Laboratories for Molecular Cytogenetics, Environmental and Respiratory Pathology, Medical University of Graz, Austria. Fax: 43 31638583646; E-mail: Helmut.popper@meduni-graz.at

Pathology is a discipline that, in interaction with clinicians active in pulmonary medicine, plays an important role in the diagnosis and, in recent years, also in the evaluation of therapy. No less important, the core research in pathology has always been aimed at understanding disease mechanisms. With respect to understanding and diagnosing diseases of the lung, an important challenge and difficulty is that this unique organ has an open connection with the outside world. This results in a large variation in disease presentation, with a mix of hallmarks of underlying disease with environmental effects, such as from smoke, pollution or occupational exposures. With respect to pulmonary diseases with the resulting complex presentation, pathology has its own role, which, in a multidisciplinary approach, can contribute to a better understanding of pathogenesis.

The present Monograph is aimed at clinicians active in pulmonary medicine and at pathologists with an active interest in pulmonary pathology. This Monograph does not cover a truly thematic subject, but rather new trends and advances in a discipline with an active interaction with pulmonary medicine. The Guest Editors have chosen different areas of pulmonary pathology to focus on and have asked experts within those fields to contribute, adding to new views and perspectives. Therefore, several chapters have been co-written by a pathologist and a physician. It was the Guest Editors' aim to obtain an interesting blend of state-of-the-art work, which is relevant for both pulmonary physicians and pathologists based in daily clinical work, as well as colleagues with an interest in recent research advances in pulmonology.

As this Monograph exemplifies the long-standing fruitful collaboration between pathology and different areas of pulmonary medicine, it is hoped that it may also serve in sustaining this interaction and collaboration.

Eur Respir Mon, 2007, 39, viii. Printed in UK - all rights reserved. Copyright ERS Journals Ltd 2007; European Respiratory Monograph; ISSN 1025-448x.

CHAPTER 1

Cystic lesions of the lung in children: classification and controversies

J.T. Stocker*, A.N. Husain[#]

*Dept of Pathology, Uniformed Services University of the Health Sciences, Bethesda, MD, and [#]Dept of Pathology, University of Chicago, Chicago, IL, USA.

Correspondence: J.T. Stocker, Dept of Pathology, Uniformed Services University of the Health Sciences, 4301 Jones Bridge Road, Bethesda, MD 20814-4799, USA. Fax: 1 3012951640; E-mail: jstocker @usuhs.mil

Cystic diseases of the lung cover a broad spectrum of lesions, ranging from clearly congenital lesions to lesions acquired through a variety of aetiologies (infection, barotrauma, neoplasia, infarction, *etc.*; table 1). Although not truly cystic or even pulmonary, a number of both congenital and acquired diseases may be confused both clinically and radiographically with the morphological cystic diseases of the lung. (table 2). A selected few are discussed briefly later in the present chapter.

The organisation and classification of congenital cystic lung diseases began in the mid 1990s with the report by CH'IN and TANG [1] describing a malformation of the lung in an infant born to a mother with polyhydramnios. The solid-appearing lung lesion was composed of gland-like alveoli, all lined with cuboidal epithelium. They called the abnormality congenital adenomatoid malformation. Over the following 30 yrs, various authors described other malformations of the lobes of the lung, some of which resembled the lesion described by CH'IN and TANG [1] and others of which were cystic and composed of bronchioles and other acinar structures in various combinations. This collection of lesions became known as congenital cystic adenomatoid malformation (CCAM).

Table 1. – Cystic lesions

CPAM type 1
CPAM type 2
CPAM type 4
Peripheral cysts
Following infarction
Down's syndrome
Associated with idiopathic spontaneous pneumothorax
Intralobar sequestration
Extralobar sequestration with CPAM type 2
Interstitial pulmonary emphysema
Acute
Persistent
Congenital pulmonary lymphangiectasia
Pleuropulmonary blastoma
Type I (purely cystic)
Type II (cystic/solid)
Infectious/parasitic cysts
Necrotising pneumonia with abscess formation
Hydatid cysts

CPAM: congenital pulmonary airway malformation.

Eur Respir Mon, 2007, 39, 1–20. Printed in UK - all rights reserved. Copyright ERS Journals Ltd 2007; European Respiratory Monograph; ISSN 1025-448x.

Table 2. – Pseudocystic or pseudopulmonary lesions

CPAM type 0
CPAM type 3
Infantile lobar emphysema
Congenital diaphragmatic hernia
Long-standing "healed" bronchopulmonary dysplasia
Bronchogenic cyst
Pneumothorax
Pneumomediastinum
Pneumopericardium
Respiratory syncytial virus pneumonia (with air-trapping)
Bronchiectasis, as with cystic fibrosis
Lymphangioma/vascular malformation

CPAM: congenital pulmonary airway malformation.

In 1977, STOCKER, *et al.* [2] described 35 cases of CCAM and divided them into three groups based on clinical and pathological features. Type 1, the most frequently occurring, were lesions that presented in the first hours to days of life and consisted of large cysts composed of walls lined with respiratory epithelium interspersed with tuft-like collections of mucogenic cells. Type 2 were composed of back-to-back bronchiolar-like structures and were associated with other anomalies, which are often severe (*e.g.* bilateral renal agenesis), in almost 50% of cases. Type 3 were the true adenomatoid lesion of CH'IN and TANG [1] which were often so large as to result in compression and hypoplasia of the other lobes of the lung.

Basis for new and expanded classification of congenital pulmonary airway malformation

During the period following the publication of the classification of CCAM, >250 cases of cystic and noncystic malformations of the lung were reviewed, and it was determined that there were a significant number of cases within this set that were different enough clinically, radiographically and morphologically (tables 3 and 4) to encompass two other groups of lesion, leading to the proposal of a new classification incorporating five types [3, 4]. In addition, the morphological appearance of the five types suggested differing sites of origin of the lesions within the developing tracheobronchial tree (fig. 1).

The expanded classification also included a new term to replace CCAM. STOCKER [4] suggested renaming this group of malformations congenital pulmonary airway malformation (CPAM), since only one of the types (type 3) is adenomatoid and only three (types 1, 2 and 4) are cystic.

The first lesion in this new classification, called CPAM type 0, is a rarely occurring malformation originally described, by RUTLEDGE and JENSEN [5], as acinar dysplasia. The lesion consists of abnormally formed bronchial structures surrounded by loose vascular mesenchyme. There is little development beyond the bronchial stage and the lesion is incompatible with life.

CPAM type 4, the other new type, consists of multiple large cysts lined only with type 1 and 2 alveolar cells over a wall composed of loose-to-dense mesenchyme containing multiple large-to-small vessels. Children with CPAM type 4 vary in age at presentation from 1 day to 4 yrs, with ~25% presenting in the first week of life, 45% between 1 week and 6 months, and the remaining 30% between 15 months and 4 yrs. Most children display various degrees of respiratory distress, including sudden respiratory distress

Table 3. – Clinical features of congenital pulmonary airway malformation (CPAM)

	Type 0	Type 1	Type 2	Type 3	Type 4
In utero ultrasound	Small lungs	1st trimester cystic mass that shrinks in 2nd–3rd trimester	Normal-to-ill-defined-mass	Progressively enlarging mass	Normal-to-cystic mass, as with CPAM type 1
Age at presentation	Birth	Birth to adolescence	Birth	*In utero* to birth	Birth to 4 yrs
Symptoms	Stillbirth; severe RD	Minimal-to-severe RD	None-to-mild RD	Stillbirth; severe RD	None to RD to pneumothorax
Associated anomalies	Rare	Rare	50%, including renal agenesis	Pulmonary hypoplasia of uninvolved lung	Rare
Treatment	None	Resect lobe(s)	Depends on other abnormalities	Resect lobe(s)	Resect lobe(s)
Outcome	Incompatible with life	Excellent following surgery	Depends on severity of other abnormalities	Poor: depends on severity of pulmonary hypoplasia	Excellent following surgery

RD: respiratory distress.

accompanying a tension pneumothorax in ~15% of cases. CPAM type 4 in older children may be asymptomatic and discovered incidentally on routine examination. There is an almost equal male to female ratio and no racial predilection. Other anomalies are rarely seen. Two brothers, one aged 6 weeks and the other 17 months, both exhibited CPAM type 4 lesions.

The CPAM type 4 lesion can be found in any lobe (right lung more than left lung) and may involve more than one lobe in ~20% of cases. Bilateral involvement has been seen in a 6-month-old male and a 3-yr-old female. Resection is usually curative, even with bilateral involvement. The lesions vary greatly in size, with mortality related to very large lesions in young infants. In two infants who died on the first day of life (the only deaths among 23 cases), the involved lobes equalled or exceeded the expected weight of the entire lung. Cysts also vary greatly in size, with some cysts exceeding 10 cm in diameter in older children. [3]

The differential diagnosis of CPAM type 4 includes the other forms of CPAM (whose features are summarised below) and the purely cystic form of pleuropulmonary blastoma (PPB), which may also be seen in young infants [6]. Cystic PPB is characterised by multiple large cysts lined with cuboidal-to-ciliated columnar epithelium overlying a wall that, in areas, displays a well-formed cambium layer associated with the embryonal rhabdomyo-sarcoma component of PPB. Significant discussion has taken place in the literature in the past 8–10 yrs as regards the relationship of CPAM type 4 to cystic PPB (see below).

Clinical and morphological features of the five types of CPAM

CPAM type 0

CPAM type 0 was originally termed acinar dysgenesis (agenesis) by RUTLEDGE and JENSEN [5], and appears to correlate with failure of development of the lung beyond the tracheobronchial origin (fig. 1). CPAM type 0 is the least frequently occurring of the CPAM lesions, with fewer than 12 cases described in the literature [7, 8].

Clinically, infants present with cyanosis and severe respiratory distress at birth and survive only a few hours unless treated with extracorporeal membrane oxygenation, but

Table 4. – Pathology of congenital pulmonary airway malformation (CPAM)

	Type 0	Type 1	Type 2	Type 3	Type 4
Relative frequency %	<2	>65	10–15	<5	10–15
Lesion weight g	20–40	15–50	3–15	20–90	15–100 (age dependent)
Size of largest cysts cm#	0.5	10	2.5	1.5 (if liveborn)	15 (in older patients)
Epithelial (mucosal) lining of cysts	CPTC, tracheal like	CPTC, bronchial like	Tall columnar, bronchiolar like	Cuboidal	Type 1 and 2 alveolar lining cells
Mucogenic cells	All cases	35–40% along epithelial lining	Absent	Absent	Absent
Composition of wall beneath mucosa	Resembles peribronchial tissue of hilum	Thick submucosal muscular band	Thin peribronchiolar tissue	Alveolar septal-like tissue	Thin-to-thick mesenchymal tissue
Cartilage plates	All cases	5–10% of cases	Absent	Absent	Rare
Vasculature	Prominent arteries and veins	Pulmonary arteries resembling those of bronchovascular bundle	Small arteries and arterioles	Only rare thin-walled venous structures	Large thick-walled arteries to delicate alveolar septal capillaries

CPTC: ciliated pseudostratified tall columnar. #: maximum diameter.

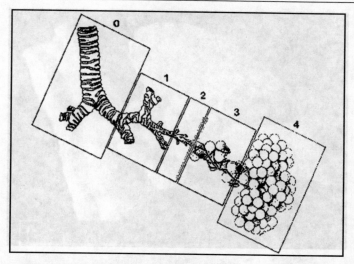

Fig. 1. – Schematic drawing of tracheobronchial tree illustrating the possible site of origin of the five types (0–4) of congenital pulmonary airway malformation based on the histological features of each type.

are then unable to survive after removal of that support. In the few cases reported, an association with cardiovascular abnormalities and dermal hypoplasia has been noted.

Grossly, the lungs are small, with a total weight of <50% of that expected based on gestational age. The lungs are firm and show a diffusely granular surface (fig. 2). Microscopically, the tissue consists entirely of bronchial-like structures with muscle, glands and numerous cartilage plates. More distal components, such as proximal bronchioles, are only rarely seen. The intervening tissue is prominent and consists of loose-to-dense mesenchymal cells and collagen, along with thick-walled arteries, large thin-walled vascular channels, collections of amorphic basophilic debris and foci of extramedullary haematopoiesis.

CPAM type 1

CPAM type 1 is composed of medium and large cysts that appear to be primarily of bronchial and bronchiolar origin. It is the most frequently occurring type (60–70% of cases), and, although seen primarily in the first month of life, may also be first diagnosed in older children and, rarely, young adults [4].

Clinically, most patients present with increasing respiratory distress shortly after birth, but older patients may present with cough, fever or chest pain. The severity of symptoms in newborn children is related to the size of the lesion as a whole and to the size and expansion of individual cysts. The lesion may present *in utero* as a solid thoracic mass during the first trimester, but, in most instances, will collapse during the second or third trimester to allow normal growth of the uninvolved lobes of the lung. The lesion then re-expands after birth as the cysts fill with air. Radiographically, air-filled or air/fluid-filled cysts are apparent in one or more lobes, with compression of adjacent lung, flattening of the diaphragm and shift of the mediastinum.

Grossly, cysts are usually limited to one lobe (95%), but are rarely multiple or bilateral (fig. 3). The present authors have seen one case in which all lobes were affected. The cysts

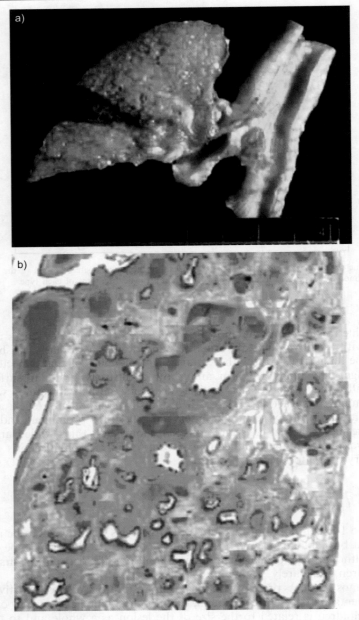

Fig. 2. – Congenital pulmonary airway malformation type 0. a) Grossly, the lung is firm with a finely nodular surface, reflecting the presence of bronchial structures throughout the lesion. b) The lesion is composed of bronchovascular islands surrounded by loose fibrovascular connective tissue (haematoxylin and eosin stain).

range 1–10 cm in size, are thin-walled when distended and lined with a smooth membrane with vascular structures visible beneath the surface.

Microscopically, the cysts are lined with ciliated pseudostratified columnar epithelium in polypoid folds with interspersed segments of mucogenic cells in ∼35% of cases (fig. 4).

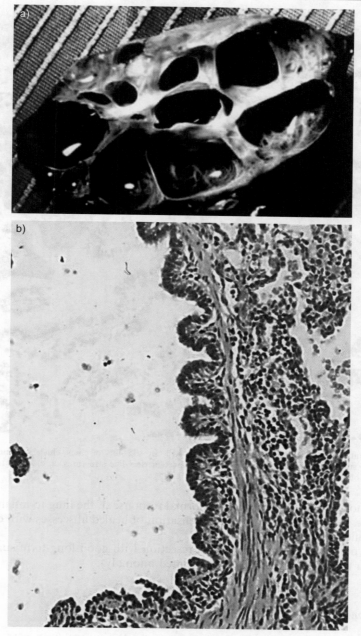

Fig. 3. – Congenital pulmonary airway malformation type 1. a) Grossly, the lesion is composed of multiple interconnecting cysts. b) The cysts are lined with respiratory epithelium (ciliated pseudostratified tall columnar epithelium) overlying a wall composed of bands of smooth muscle and vascular connective tissue (haematoxylin and eosin stain).

The cyst walls are composed of fibromuscular tissue and occasional cartilage islands. Adjacent parenchyma contains smaller cysts resembling bronchioles. In the presence of chronic inflammation (lymphoid aggregates, fibrosis, macrophages, *etc.*), the diagnosis of

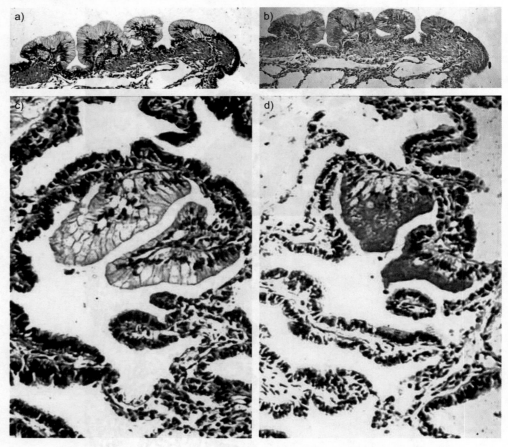

Fig. 4. – Congenital pulmonary airway malformation type 1. In ~35–40% of cases, clusters of mucogenic cells: a, b) lie along the surface of the cysts; or c, d) fill small alveolar duct-like structures. a, c) haematoxylin and eosin stain; b) alcian blue; and d) mucicarmine.

CPAM cannot be made because of the normal response of the lung to inflammation and abscesses, *i.e.* repair by fibrosis and epithelisation of healed abscesses with columnar-to-pseudostratified columnar epithelium.

CPAM type 1 is amenable to surgical resection with good long-term survival (in the absence of a rarely occurring severe associated anomaly).

CPAM type 2

CPAM type 2 is composed of cysts 0.5–2.0 cm in diameter that resemble bronchioles.

The clinical picture is often dictated by the occurrence, in ~50% of cases, of other severe anomalies (sirenomelia, renal agenesis/dysgenesis, diaphragmatic hernia and cardiovascular). When an isolated lesion, it may be seen in the first month of life as mild-to-severe respiratory distress. Radiographically, the lesion may be difficult to visualise as most lesions exhibit cysts of only 0.5–1.0 cm in diameter.

Grossly, the lesions are smaller than other CPAM lesions and blend with the adjacent

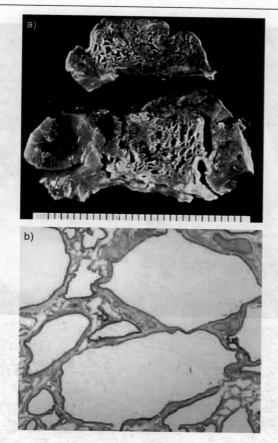

Fig. 5. – Congenital pulmonary airway malformation type 2. a) Small cysts (0.5–1.5 cm) blend with normal parenchyma. b) Microscopically, these cysts consist of back-to-back bronchiolar-like structures lined with simple columnar-to-cuboidal epithelial cells (haematoxylin and eosin stain).

normal parenchyma (fig. 5). They are composed of multiple small cysts (0.5–1.0 cm diameter) lined with a smooth membrane [3, 9].

Microscopically, the lesion is composed of back-to-back dilated bronchioles separated by irregular alveolar duct-like structures. Small arteries, arterioles and venules are interspersed among the bronchioles. CPAM type 2 may be seen in 50% of extralobar sequestrations [10].

Surgical resection in isolated lesions, including those associated with extralobar sequestration, is frequently successful. In cases with other severe anomalies, survival is dependent upon the severity of the anomalies and the ability to successfully treat them.

CPAM type 3

CPAM type 3, the original congenital adenomatoid malformation described in 1949 by CH'IN and TANG [1], is composed of gland-like structures resembling terminal/respiratory bronchioles and alveolar ducts.

Clinically, the lesion occurs almost exclusively in males, is associated with maternal polyhydramnios in nearly 80% of cases and may lead to death *in utero*. Live-born infants

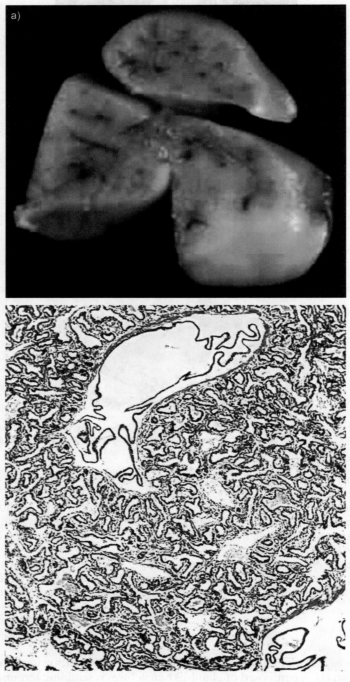

Fig. 6. – Congenital pulmonary airway malformation type 3. a) The lesion is a solid mass resembling atelectatic parenchyma. Only rarely are small "cysts" seen, probably representing dilated bronchioles. b) The lesion consists entirely of small bronchiole- and alveolar duct-like structures lined with cuboidal epithelium. Note the virtual absence of arterial structures (haematoxylin and eosin stain).

show early severe respiratory distress due to associated pulmonary hypoplasia of the uninvolved lung.

Grossly, the lesion is large, somewhat firm and bulky, and involves an entire lobe or even an entire lung, producing mediastinal shift and compression of the adjacent lung, accounting for its hypoplasia (fig. 6). However, if aerated, the lesion may display randomly scattered thin-walled cysts of 0.5–1.5 cm in diameter.

Microscopically, the entire lesion is composed of randomly scattered bronchiolar/ alveolar duct-like structures lined with low cuboidal epithelium and surrounded by alveoli, also lined with cuboidal epithelium. Arteries and even arterioles are notably absent from the lesion.

Survival is possible with resection of the lobe or lung if hypoplasia of the remaining lung is mild enough (*i.e.* ≥ 30–40% of the expected weight remains) to permit adequate oxygenation.

CPAM type 4

CPAM type 4 is composed of large cysts with no readily discernible lining and thus resembles distal acinar structures, *i.e.* alveolar saccules/alveoli.

Clinically, the lesion may be seen in infants or young children (age range birth to 4 yrs), and they may present with mild respiratory distress, sudden respiratory distress due to tension pneumothorax, pneumonia or, on occasion, an incidental finding with no symptoms. Radiographically, the large air-filled cysts are readily identified, along with mediastinal shift and an occasional pneumothorax [4].

Grossly, large thin-walled cysts, often 8–10 cm in diameter in older infants and young children, are present at the periphery of the lobe (fig. 7). Their internal surface appears to be a smooth membrane, and vessels can often be seen beneath the surface. In newborns, the cysts are much smaller (0.3–2.0 cm).

Microscopically, both small and large cysts are lined with flattened epithelial cells (type 2 alveolar lining cells) over most of the wall, with only rare areas in which low cuboidal epithelium may be present. The character of the lining cells can be determined with the use of surfactant and other immunohistochemical stains associated with alveolar lining cells (fig. 8). A capillary bed of varying density is present beneath the epithelial lining and may have a few lymphocytes and macrophages scattered throughout it.

The walls of the larger cysts may be 0.1–0.3 cm thick and are composed of loose mesenchymal tissue containing prominent arteries and arterioles. These large arteries may display a multilayered muscular media far thicker than that seen in normal peripheral acinar vessels (fig. 9). Dense connective tissue may be present in older patients in some cases.

The loose mesenchyme must not be confused with similar tissue seen in the cystic type of PPB (see below), in which mononuclear cells (rhabdomyoblasts) may be present in areas beneath strips of cuboidal/columnar epithelium. For this reason, multiple sections of cyst walls should be taken when examining a suspected case of CPAM type 4 in order to exclude the diagnosis of purely cystic PPB. With resection of the involved lobe, the survival of children with CPAM type 4 is excellent.

CPAM type 1 and bronchioloalveolar carcinoma

Bronchioloalveolar carcinoma (adenocarcinoma; BAC) is the most common form of bronchogenic carcinoma in children (fig. 10), although the lesion as a whole is most frequently seen in the elderly [11, 12], and may rarely be familial [13]. It occurs with cough, pneumonia and chest pain, but, if peripheral, may be asymptomatic. Initial

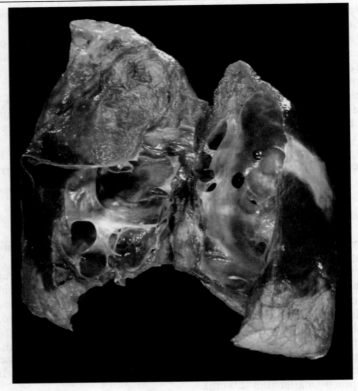

Fig. 7. – Congenital pulmonary airway malformation type 4. Cut section of the lung displaying multiple large cysts with thin walls traversed by areas of density representing vessels in the walls.

symptoms may be related to disseminated disease, such as bone pain or weight. As a subtype of adenocarcinoma, BAC exhibits an excellent prognosis when <2 cm in diameter at the time of diagnosis. Indeed, there is almost 100% 5-yr survival under these circumstances [14].

Does CPAM type 1 with mucinous foci predispose to BAC?

In recent years, the question of the association of CPAM type 1 with BAC has been raised on the basis of case reports of BAC having occurred in older children who, as infants, had had CPAM type 1 partially or completely resected. The first such report, in 1991, was that of BENJAMIN and CAHILL [15], followed in 1995 by that of RIBET *et al.* [16]. In 1998, OTA *et al.* [17], having previously noted gastric mucins in mucinous BAC, studied 12 out of 26 cases of CPAM type 1 containing mucous cells and found mucins similar to those of the mucinous BACs. This association has been supported by the finding of similar genetic abnormalities (including gains in chromosomes 2 and 4) in both CPAM type 1 goblet cells and the cells of BAC [18]. Most recently, IOACHIMESCU and MEHTA [14] described the 15-yr course of the development of a BAC (diagnosis at age 6 yrs, along with CPAM type 1), which subsequently developed into an invasive adenocarcinoma. They emphasised the unique feature of a lesion that may exhibit lack of growth for years before becoming an aggressive lesion and suggest the interim phase of atypical adenomatous hyperplasia between the CPAM-1 and BAC before it becomes an invasive adenocarcinoma.

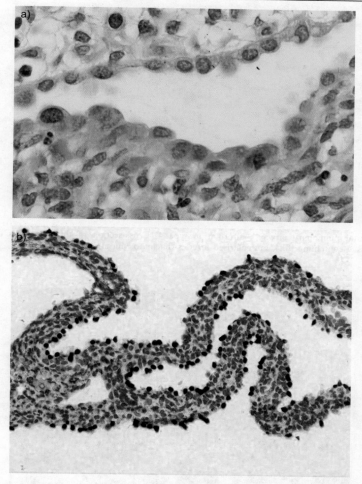

Fig. 8. – Congenital pulmonary airway malformation type 4. a) The cysts are lined with cells with round nuclei and scant cytoplasm (haematoxylin and eosin stain). b) These lining cells are marked intensely with thyroid transcription factor (TTF), indicating that they are alveolar lining type 2 cells (TTF immunohistochemical stain).

CPAM type 4 and PPB

PPB is a rare primary pulmonary tumour in children, with ~75 cases reported in the literature [19]. There is an equal sexual incidence and the vast majority occur during the first 4 yrs of life, although cases have been seen in older children and in an adult aged 36 yrs. Presenting symptoms include respiratory distress, nonproductive cough, fever, chest pain or a combination of symptoms of days' to weeks' duration [6].

Conditions associated with PPB are seen in nearly 25% of patients, and include a positive family history of childhood neoplasms, including PPBs, in siblings, cousins and other close relatives. Other associations in PPB patients include medulloblastoma, ovarian teratoma, Hodgkin's lymphoma, leukaemia, thyroid dysplasia and neoplasia, malignant germ cell tumour and nephroblastic lesions.

Imaging studies may show a solid (62%) or cystic (38%) lesion that may be

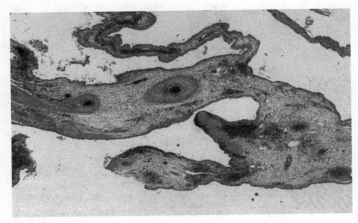

Fig. 9. – Congenital pulmonary airway malformation type 4. Cross-section of the cyst walls displaying thick mesenchymal tissue containing thick muscularised arteries (haematoxylin and eosin stain).

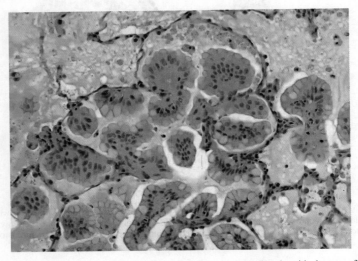

Fig. 10. – Bronchioloalveolar carcinoma. Alveoli are filled with mucin and polypoid clusters of mucogenic cells. The nuclei of the cells retain their basal orientation. Note the absence of any apparent invasion (haematoxylin and eosin stain).

mediastinally or pleurally based, as well as intrapulmonary. Tumours are classified as type I (cystic; 14% of cases), type II (cystic and solid; 48% of cases) and type III (solid; 38% of cases).

The multilobated masses measure 8–23 cm in diameter and weigh up to 1,100 g. Microscopically, the cystic areas are composed of small-to-large cysts lined with respiratory-type epithelium overlying a loose-to-dense fibrous stroma that, in areas, is composed of primitive small cells in a cambium-like arrangement beneath the epithelium (fig. 11). The solid areas of types II and III PPB consist of blastematous islands of loose mesenchyme blending into fibrosarcoma-like foci, nodules of benign appearing to overtly

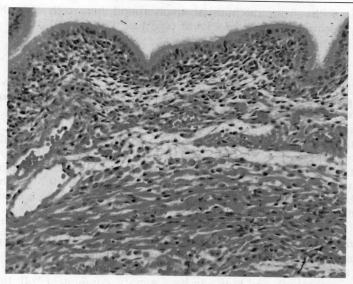

Fig. 11. – Pleuropulmonary blastoma. Ciliated columnar epithelium overlies a dense layer of small round blue cells (rhabdomyoblasts on immunohistochemical staining), which, in deeper layers, become fewer in number and mixed with oval and strap-like cells and, eventually, densely eosinophilic skeletal muscle-like cells (haematoxylin and eosin stain).

malignant cartilage, rhabdomyoblasts and areas of large bizarre pleomorphic multi-nucleate mesenchymal cells.

Immunohistochemical staining is variable from one tissue type to another. Trisomy 2 and 8 have been noted in cytogenetic studies of the tumours. Most recently, ROQUE *et al.* [20] reported the comparative genomic hybridisation of PPB and found several chromosomal imbalances (*e.g.* 1q12–q23), whole chromosome gains of 2 and 7, and loss of genetic material at regions 6q130qter, 10pter–p13, 10q22–qter and 20p13.

Local recurrence may develop in <15% of type I PPBs, but in >45% of type II and III PPBs. Metastatic disease occurs in ~25% of patients (all with type II or III PPB), chiefly to the brain/spinal cord or bone. Patients with pleural or mediastinal involvement fare significantly worse than those without such involvement. In a series of 50 cases reported by PRIEST *et al.* [6], 5-yr survival was 83% for type I and 42% for types II and III.

Can purely cystic pleuropulmonary blastoma arise in a pre-existing CPAM type 4?

Although superficially resembling CPAM type 1 or 4, purely cystic PPB lesions are, in the experience of the present authors and others [21], distinctly different morphologically in that the CPAM type 1 lesion (lined with respiratory epithelium) does not have a loose mesenchymal component in its wall, and the CPAM type 4 lesion (with a loose-to-dense mesenchymal wall) is lined with thinned type 2 alveolar lining cells, not with cuboidal or columnar cells. Small patches of cuboidal and/or columnar epithelium may occasionally be noted along the wall of CPAM type 4 cysts, but these are usually associated with an adjacent component of a normal bronchiolar structure apparently entrapped in the developing lesion. Nevertheless, in the case of CPAM type 1 or 4, great care must be taken to exclude the diagnosis of purely cystic PPB. When in question, immunohisto-chemical stains for rhabdomyoblastoma cells may help in distinguishing the malignant cells of cystic PPBs from the normal small round blue cells (lymphocytes, *etc.*) occasionally present in the walls of CPAM type 1 or 4.

Other cystic and pseudocystic lesions

Peripheral cysts. Peripheral air-containing cysts of the lung can be seen in neonates, infants, young children and teenagers. They occur in association with Down's syndrome, as a result of pulmonary infarction, or in association with idiopathic spontaneous pneumothorax. Occlusion of the pulmonary artery in infants can result in peripheral infarction of the lung, which, with necrosis and organisation, can produce subpleural cysts of varying sizes [22]. In Down's syndrome, it has been suggested that the cysts are an intrinsic feature of the disease that may result from reduced post-natal production of peripheral small air passages and alveoli. The air-filled cysts are 0.2–1.0 cm in diameter and located beneath the pleura. They are formed of vascular fibrous connective tissue walls lined with alveolar lining cells [23].

Sequestrations. Sequestrations are classified as intralobar (often occurring in the older child or young adult and associated with repeated infections, the majority are thought to be acquired) and extralobar (most often occurring in neonates and young children and thought to be congenital), and both can have a cystic component [24]. In many of the former, cystic structures are formed by dilated airways containing mucopurulent material (fig. 12), whereas, in the latter, there is a strong association with CPAM type 2 within the lesion [10, 25, 26].

Congenital pulmonary lymphangiectasia. Congenital pulmonary lymphangiectasia is a rare, usually fatal, disorder involving both lungs and is characterised by distended lymphatics in the bronchovascular bundle, the interlobular septa and the subpleural space. A few cases of unilobar involvement have been described that were radiologically misdiagnosed as infantile (congenital) lobar emphysema [27]. The lymphatics can be identified immunohistochemically using one of the newer markers specific for lymphatic endothelium (D2-40 antibody or lymphatic vessel endothelial hyaluronan receptor 1).

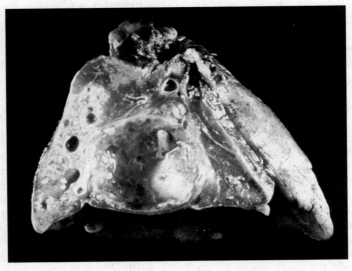

Fig. 12. – Intralobar sequestration. Gross picture of cut surface of resected specimen with a dominant mucus-filled cyst.

Interstitial pulmonary emphysema. Interstitial pulmonary emphysema is the dissection by air around bronchovascular bundles and along interlobular septa as the result of rupture of alveoli, usually in association with mechanical ventilation. It may also be seen in patients dying due to acute asthma, as a result of cardiopulmonary resuscitation, and in association with a variety of infectious diseases. It may be acute or persistent (characterised by a foreign body giant cell reaction to the air) and may be localised to a single lobe or distributed diffusely through all of the lobes [23, 28]. Some of the air may track into lymphatics (but not the pleural lymphatics), raising the differential diagnosis of congenital pulmonary lymphangiectasia, which also involves the pleural lymphatics. Immunohistochemical staining for endothelial cells is helpful in localising the cysts.

Infantile lobar emphysema. Infantile lobar emphysema refers to an overexpansion of a pulmonary lobe occurring in an infant, leading to pulmonary compromise. Pathologically, there is a spectrum of morphological changes, with the two most common patterns being overdistension of normal-appearing lung (classic pattern) and increased complexity of alveoli with increased radial alveolar counts (polyalveolar lobe or hyperplasia of lung; figure 13 shows the classic pattern and a polyalveolar lobe at the same power). These two morphological patterns may occur due to the different timing of an inciting lesion leading to anatomical or functional bronchial abnormality, and the degree of obstruction of the bronchus, with a relatively closed bronchus and fluid retention resulting in hyperplasia. Conversely, a weak bronchial wall without fluid retention would result in relatively normal lung development *in utero*, with the bronchus collapsing only after birth, leading to overdistension of alveoli [29].

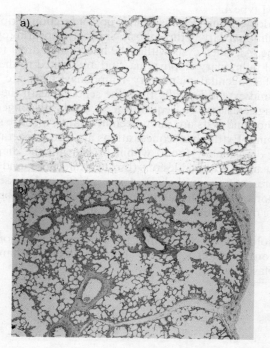

Fig. 13. – Infantile lobar emphysema. a) Classic pattern of overdistension of alveoli, and b) polyalveolar lobe with complex alveolar architecture but relatively normally sized alveoli (haematoxylin and eosin stain).

Bronchogenic cyst. Bronchogenic cysts are thought to arise from abnormal budding of the ventral segment lung buds that give rise to the bronchial tree and lung. One hypothesis is that their position depends upon the timing of the developmental aberration that causes them. If it occurs early, then the cyst is located in the mediastinum (most commonly), but, if it occurs late, then the cyst is located within the lung tissue itself, most often in the lower lobes [30]. Another view is that case reports of intrapulmonary bronchogenic cysts probably represent instances of CPAM type 1 [23], although one series described 10 cases of pathologically verified intrapulmonary bronchogenic cyst [31].

Summary

A new and expanded classification of congenital pulmonary airway malformations (CPAM) of the lung identifies lesions on the basis of the likely site of origin and clinical and pathological features. Within the five types, recent reports have demonstrated an association of CPAM type 1 with bronchioloalveolar carcinoma (BAC), and a degree of confusion in separating CPAM type 4 from the purely cystic form of pleuropulmonary blastoma.

The CPAM type 1 lesion has been noted to contain clusters of mucogenic cells in ~35% of cases, and these clusters are thought to predispose the patient to the development of BAC. The CPAM type 4 lesion, with its large and often thick-walled cysts lined with alveolar lining cells, may be confused with the cysts of type I pleuropulmonary blastoma, although its cyst walls contain subepithelial foci of rhabdomyosarcoma, almost exclusively underlying stretches of cuboidal-to-columnar epithelium, rather than the alveolar cell epithelium of CPAM type 4.

Other cystic or pseudocystic lung lesions include post-infarction peripheral cysts resulting from intrauterine pulmonary artery thrombosis. Similarly appearing cysts have been noted in Down's syndrome. Air-filled cysts within the interstitium are a feature of acute and persistent interstitial pulmonary emphysema, and are limited to the interlobular septa. Fluid-filled cysts of congenital pulmonary lymphangiectasia are present within the interlobular septa, and extend laterally from the septa beneath the pleura. Congenital pulmonary lymphangiectasia is also frequently associated with congenital malformations of the heart. Bronchogenic cysts are rarely seen in infants, and are solid lesions usually separate from the lung. Extralobar sequestrations are also nonaerated lesions separate from the lung and occasionally found within or beneath the diaphragm. Intralobar sequestrations are usually acquired lesions (through infection), and may display air- or fluid-filled cysts, representing re-epithelialised post-infectious abscesses. Finally, one of the most common pulmonary lesions in infants and children, infantile lobar emphysema, is not cystic but simply the overinflation of a segment of lung.

Keywords: Bronchioloalveolar carcinoma, bronchogenic cyst, congenital pulmonary airway malformation, extralobar sequestration, insterstitial pulmonary emphysema, pleuropulmonary blastoma.

References

1. Ch'in KY, Tang MY. Congenital adenomatoid malformation of one lobe of a lung with general anasarca. *Arch Path* 1949; 48: 221–225.

2. Stocker JT, Madewell JE, Drake RM. Congenital cystic adenomatoid malformation of the lung. Classification and morphologic spectrum. *Hum Pathol* 1977; 8: 155–171.

3. Stocker JT. Congenital and developmental diseases. *In*: Dail DH, Hammer S, eds. Pulmonary Pathology. New York, Springer-Verlag, 1994; pp. 155–190.

4. Stocker JT. Congenital pulmonary airway malformation – a new name for and an expanded classification of congenital cystic adenomatoid malformation of the lung. *Histopathology* 2002; 41: Suppl. 2, 424–430.

5. Rutledge JC, Jensen P. Acinar dysplasia: a new form of pulmonary maldevelopment. *Hum Pathol* 1986; 17: 1290–1293.

6. Priest JR, McDermott MB, Bhatia S, Watterson J, Manivel JC, Dehner LP. Pleuropulmonary blastoma: a clinicopathologic study of 50 cases. *Cancer* 1997; 80: 147–161.

7. Gillespie LM, Fenton AC, Wright C. Acinar dysplasia: a rare cause of neonatal respiratory failure. *Acta Paediatr* 2004; 93: 712–713.

8. Davidson LA, Batman P, Fagan DG. Congenital acinar dysplasia: a rare cause of pulmonary hypoplasia. *Histopathology* 1998; 32: 57–59.

9. Stocker JT, Drake RM, Madewell JE. Cystic and congenital lung diseases in the newborn. *Perspect Pediatr Pathol* 1978; 4: 93–154.

10. Conran RM, Stocker JT. Extralobar sequestration with frequently associated congenital cystic adenomatoid malformation, type 2: report of 50 cases. *Pediatr Dev Pathol* 1999; 2: 454–463.

11. Okubo K, Mark EJ, Flieder D, *et al.* Bronchoalveolar carcinoma: clinical, radiologic, and pathologic factors and survival. *J Thorac Cardiovasc Surg* 1999; 118: 702–709.

12. Kantar M, Cetingul N, Veral A, Kansoy S, Ozcan C, Alper H. Rare tumors of the lung in children. *Pediatr Hematol Oncol* 2002; 19: 421–428.

13. Nanki N, Fujita J, Ohtsuki Y, *et al.* Occurrence of bronchioloalveolar cell carcinoma in two brothers: comparison of clinical features and immunohistochemical findings. *Intern Med* 2002; 41: 1002–1006.

14. Ioachimescu OC, Mehta AC. From cystic pulmonary airway malformation, to bronchioloalveolar carcinoma and adenocarcinoma of the lung. *Eur Respir J* 2005; 26: 1181–1187.

15. Benjamin DR, Cahill JL. Bronchioloalveolar carcinoma of the lung and congenital cystic adenomatoid malformation. *Am J Clin Pathol* 1991; 95: 889–892.

16. Ribet ME, Copin MC, Soots JG, Gosselin BH. Bronchioloalveolar carcinoma and congenital cystic adenomatoid malformation. *Ann Thorac Surg* 1995; 60: 1126–1128.

17. Ota H, Langston C, Honda T, Katsuyama T, Genta RM. Histochemical analysis of mucous cells of congenital adenomatoid malformation of the lung: insights into the carcinogenesis of pulmonary adenocarcinoma expressing gastric mucins. *Am J Clin Pathol* 1998; 110: 450–455.

18. Stacher E, Ullmann R, Halbwedl I, *et al.* Atypical goblet cell hyperplasia in congenital cystic adenomatoid malformation as a possible preneoplasia for pulmonary adenocarcinoma in childhood: a genetic analysis. *Hum Pathol* 2004; 35: 565–570.

19. Dehner L, Tazelaar H, Manabe T. Pleuropulmonary blastoma. *In*: TravisW, Brambilla E, Muller-Hermelink K, Harris CC, eds. World Health Classification of Tumours. Pathology and Genetics of Tumours of the Lung, Pleura, Thymus and Heart. Lyon, IARD Press, 2004; pp. 99–100.

20. Roque L, Rodrigues R, Martins C, *et al.* Comparative genomic hybridization analysis of a pleuropulmonary blastoma. *Cancer Genet Cytogenet* 2004; 149: 58–62.

21. Dehner L. Beware of "degenerating" congenital pulmonary cysts. *Pediatr Surg Int* 2005; 21: 123–124.

22. Stocker JT, McGill LC, Orsini EN. Post-infarction peripheral cysts of the lung in pediatric patients: a possible cause of idiopathic spontaneous pneumothorax. *Pediatr Pulmonol* 1985; 1: 7–18.

23. Stocker JT. The respiratory tract. *In*: Stocker JT, Dehner L, eds. Pediatric Pathology. Philadelphia, Lippincott Williams & Wilkins, 2001; pp. 445–518.

24. Stocker JT, Kagan-Hallet K. Extralobar pulmonary sequestration: analysis of 15 cases. *Am J Clin Pathol* 1979; 72: 917–925.

25. Stocker JT. Sequestrations of the lung. *Semin Diagn Pathol* 1986; 3: 106–121.

26. Stocker JT, Malczak HT. A study of pulmonary ligament arteries. Relationship to intralobar pulmonary sequestration. *Chest* 1984; 86: 611–615.

27. Chapdelaine J, Beaunoyer M, St-Vil D, *et al.* an underestimated presentation? *J Pediatr Surg* 2004; 39: 677–680.

28. Stocker JT, Madewell JE. Persistent interstitial pulmonary emphysema: another complication of the respiratory distress syndrome. *Pediatrics* 1977; 59: 847–857.

29. Mani H, Suarez E, Stocker JT. The morphologic spectrum of infantile lobar emphysema: a study of 33 cases. *Paediatr Respir Rev* 2004; 5: Suppl A, S313–S320.

30. Williams HJ, Johnson KJ. Imaging of congenital cystic lung lesions. *Paediatr Respir Rev* 2002; 3: 120–127.

31. Tireli GA, Ozbey H, Temiz A, Salman T, Celik A. Bronchogenic cysts: a rare congenital cystic malformation of the lung. *Surg Today* 2004; 34: 573–576.

CHAPTER 2

Progress in the pathology of diffuse lung disease in infancy: changing concepts and diagnostic challenges

M.K. Dishop, C. Langston

Dept of Pathology, Texas Children's Hospital, Houston, TX, USA.

Correspondence: M.K. Dishop, Dept of Pathology, MC 1-2261, Texas Children's Hospital, 6621 Fannin St, Houston, TX 77030, USA. Fax: 1 8328251032; E-mail: mkdishop@texaschildrenshospital.org

Lung biopsy is commonly performed in children as part of the diagnostic evaluation for diffuse lung disease, in the setting of either acute respiratory decompensation or chronic progressive lung disease [1]. Thoracotomy and video-assisted thoracoscopic surgery are both safe techniques in children and show similar diagnostic yield. Thoracoscopic biopsy has the additional advantages of shorter operating time and decreased duration of hospitalisation [2].

With the increasing frequency of lung biopsy in children, understanding of the classification of paediatric interstitial lung disease has evolved, and a number of reviews on the subject are available [3–7]. Although there is some overlap with adult classification systems, the spectrum of interstitial lung disease in children is clearly different, particularly with regard to the genetic, developmental and growth abnormalities seen with higher incidence in infants and young children [8–11].

The differential diagnosis of diffuse lung disease in children most commonly includes chronic neonatal lung disease due to: 1) prematurity or hypoplasia; 2) infection, particularly in immunocompromised patients; 3) recurrent aspiration, often in the setting of gastro-oesophageal reflux; 4) post-infectious disorders such as obliterative bronchiolitis; 5) vascular changes due to congenital heart disease; and 6) pulmonary haemorrhage syndromes [10]. Other less common considerations include inherited disorders of surfactant metabolism, hypersensitivity pneumonitis, lymphoid hyperplasia and other lymphoproliferative processes, eosinophilic pneumonia, drug reactions, acute interstitial pneumonia, primary pulmonary vascular disorders and pulmonary involvement of systemic disease (table 1).

The European Respiratory Society (ERS) Task Force on chronic interstitial lung disease in immunocompetent children recently examined this spectrum of disease in 185 patients during the period 1997–2002, including clinical features, diagnostic evaluation and outcome data [12]. An updated classification system has also been developed in North America by the Children's Interstitial Lung Disease (chILD) working group, a multidisciplinary group of paediatric pathologists, radiologists, pulmonologists and pulmonary biologists interested in paediatric interstitial lung disease [13]. Based on a pathological review of diagnostic lung biopsy results in both immunocompetent and immunocompromised children, this consensus classification has permitted correlation of histopathology with clinical, imaging and outcome data, and will probably be an important complement to the experience already reported by the ERS Task Force.

Within the spectrum of paediatric interstitial lung disease, diffuse lung disease in infants warrants unique consideration with regard to indications for biopsy and

Eur Respir Mon, 2007, 39, 21–36. Printed in UK - all rights reserved. Copyright ERS Journals Ltd 2007; European Respiratory Monograph; ISSN 1025-448x.

Table 1. – Major causes of diffuse lung disease in infancy

Category	Specific cause
Alveolar growth abnormalities	Chronic neonatal lung disease secondary to prematurity
	Pulmonary hypoplasia
	Chromosomal disorders
	Congenital heart disease, with or without vasculopathy
Infection	Acute injury
	Bronchiolitis/pneumonitis (viral)
	Pneumonia (bacterial, Pneumocystis)
	Granulomatous pneumonitis (fungal, mycobacterial)
	Resolving/remote injury
	Post-viral injury; obliterative/constrictive bronchiolitis
	Diffuse alveolar damage
Aspiration injury	Associated with gastro-oesophageal reflux, laryngotracheal abnormalities
Vascular disorders	Pulmonary arteriopathy
	Associated with congenital heart disease, other secondary causes
	Chronic congestive vasculopathy
	Associated with congenital heart disease, other secondary causes
	Lymphatic disorders (lymphangiectasia, lymphangiomatosis)
	Alveolar capillary dysplasia with misalignment of pulmonary veins
Pulmonary haemorrhage syndromes	Pulmonary capillaritis
	Idiopathic pulmonary haemosiderosis
Pulmonary interstitial glycogenosis	
Neuroendocrine cell hyperplasia of infancy	
Genetic diseases	Surfactant dysfunction disorders
	SP-B, SP-C, ABCA3 mutations, other
	Metabolic/storage diseases
	Niemann–Pick disease, mucopolysaccharidosis, other
	Other
	Cystic fibrosis, primary ciliary dyskinesia, other
Systemic diseases	Immunodeficiency
	Lymphoid hyperplasia and lymphoproliferative processes
	Opportunistic infection
	Autoimmune disease
	Rheumatological disorders (neonatal lupus), ANCA-associated
	capillaritis
	Malignancy
	Leukaemia, Langerhans' cell histiocytosis, other

SP: surfactant protein; ABCA3: adenosine triphosphate-binding cassette subfamily A member 3; ANCA: antineutrophilic cytoplasmic antibody.

differential diagnosis. There are a number of special indications for biopsy in infants, including: 1) failure of a term infant to be weaned from support, including ventilatory support, extracorporeal membrane oxygenation and nitric oxide; 2) late-onset tachypnoea or respiratory failure in a term infant; and 3) recurrence of symptoms in an originally pre-term infant [14, 15]. Lung biopsy may be important not only for specific diagnosis, but also for prognosis and assessment of disease that is unresponsive to available medical therapy, as with alveolar capillary dysplasia with misalignment of pulmonary veins or inherited disorders of surfactant metabolism. In this setting, a biopsy may assist in planning for lung transplantation or end-of-life choices. Of lung biopsy procedures in children, ~20% are performed in infants (aged <1 yr) [10].

The differential diagnosis of diffuse lung disease in infancy includes special diagnostic considerations with particular predilection for this age group [15]. Every infant lung biopsy specimen should be assessed for appropriate alveolar architecture in order to exclude abnormalities of pre-natal or post-natal lung growth, specifically chronic neonatal lung disease due to prematurity, pulmonary hypoplasia and some chromosomal disorders, such as trisomy 21 (Down's syndrome). Attention to the vascular architecture is necessary in order to exclude alveolar capillary dysplasia with misalignment of pulmonary veins and to evaluate chronic haemodynamic alterations of the pulmonary vasculature secondary to congenital heart disease. Recognition of pulmonary alveolar proteinosis (PAP), chronic pneumonitis of infancy (CPI) or desquamative interstitial pneumonia patterns in neonates and infants should suggest further evaluation for surfactant gene mutations.

Since 2000, there have been a number of exciting advances in the understanding of diffuse lung disease in infants, which have changed the approach to diagnosis in this unique population. With the discovery of a third gene responsible for inherited abnormalities of surfactant metabolism in 2004, interest in this area continues to accelerate, along with the number of diagnostic tools available for specific diagnosis. Pulmonary interstitial glycogenosis (PIG) was described in 2002, and, although previously thought to be rare, is being recognised with increasing frequency as a pattern of interstitial disease in the infant lung. Finally, the description of neuroendocrine cell hyperplasia of infancy (NEHI) in 2005 has provided an explanation for the syndrome of persistent tachypnoea of infancy in some babies and young children.

The present update for paediatric pathologists and pulmonologists reviews the changing concepts and current understanding of these three evolving types of infant lung disease: surfactant dysfunction disorders, PIG and NEHI. The clinical, imaging and histopathological characteristics of each are discussed, with emphasis on the role of diagnostic lung biopsy in evaluating the differential diagnosis in infants presenting with similar interstitial lung disease syndromes.

Surfactant dysfunction disorders

Surfactant dysfunction disorders are a group of lung diseases, occurring predominantly in infants and children, which are caused by inherited mutations in genes affecting surfactant metabolism [16–18]. This group now includes mutations in three known genes encoding the following proteins: surfactant protein (SP)-B (*SFTPB*, chromosome 2p12–p11.2); SP-C (*SFTPC*, chromosome 8p21); and, most recently, adenosine triphosphate (ATP)-binding cassette transporter subfamily A member 3 (*ABCA3*, chromosome 16p13.3). Mutations affecting SP-B and ABCA3 genes are inherited in an autosomal recessive fashion, whereas mutations affecting SP-C show an autosomal dominant inheritance pattern, manifesting as chronic lung disease in successive generations [19–21]. The major clinical and pathological features are summarised in table 2. Although mutations in these three genes explain the majority of cases with findings consistent with surfactant dysfunction, a subset of cases with typical clinical and histological features remains unexplained, suggesting the presence of other unrecognised causative genes.

Table 2. – Surfactant dysfunction disorders: summary of typical features of the three mutated genes

	SP-B	ABCA3	SP-C
Inheritance pattern	AR	AR	AD
Typical age at presentation	1 week–3 months	1 week–years	3 months–years
Histological pattern	PAP	PAP, DIP, CPI, NSIP	CPI, DIP, NSIP, PF
Ultrastructural features	Abnormal	Abnormal	Normal
	Composite multivesicular bodies	Dense bodies	
Prognosis	Fatal in infancy	Variable	Variable
		Often fatal in infancy	Longer survival

SP: surfactant protein; ABCA3: adenosine triphosphate-binding cassette subfamily A member 3; AR: autosomal recessive; AD: autosomal dominant; PAP: pulmonary alveolar proteinosis; DIP: desquamative interstitial pneumonia; CPI: chronic pneumonitis of infancy; NSIP: nonspecific interstitial pneumonia; PF: pulmonary fibrosis.

The histological manifestations of surfactant dysfunction disorders in infancy include two major patterns, PAP and CPI. SP-B mutations typically result in a variant PAP pattern with alveolar granular eosinophilic material, prominent alveolar epithelial hyperplasia and little evidence of lobular remodelling (fig. 1a and b) [22–24]. The proteinosis material in this variant PAP histology is typically less abundant and less homogeneous than that seen in acquired forms of PAP, e.g. PAP associated with antibodies directed against granulocyte-macrophage colony-stimulating factor. Affected children typically die during the neonatal period or early infancy. In contrast to infants with SP-B mutations, infants with SP-C mutations typically show a pattern of CPI on lung biopsy, characterised by less proteinosis material and more prominent cholesterol clefts and lobular remodelling (fig. 2) [25, 26]. SP-C mutations have also been recognised in some families as a cause of interstitial pneumonia and pulmonary fibrosis in adults [27, 28]. ABCA3 mutations often result in a variant PAP pattern in infancy (fig. 3a), but may also exhibit a desquamative interstitial pneumonia pattern in some infants and a nonspecific interstitial pneumonia pattern in older infants and children. Although SP-B mutations show relatively uniform clinical manifestations early in infancy, SP-C and ABCA3 mutations appear to cause a wider clinical and histological spectrum, which is probably age-dependent and, in part, mutation-dependent, although detailed genotype–phenotype correlations with large numbers of patients are not currently available.

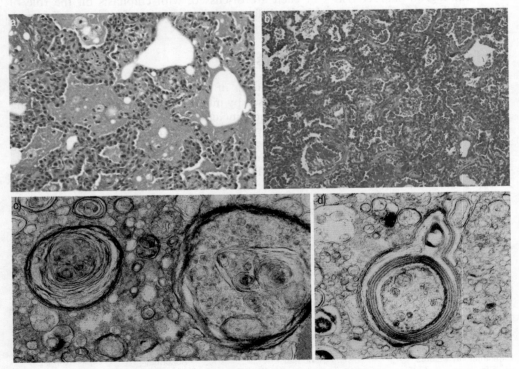

Fig. 1. – Surfactant dysfunction disorders: surfactant protein B mutations. a) Lung biopsy specimen from a 3-month-old female showing a classic pattern of pulmonary alveolar proteinosis, with abundant smooth-to-granular proteinosis material filling alveolar spaces, associated with scattered foamy macrophages (haematoxylin and eosin stain). b) Diffuse uniform type II alveolar epithelial hyperplasia is another important feature of abnormalities of surfactant metabolism. Periodic acid–Schiff stain may be helpful in highlighting the alveolar proteinosis material, as seen in this biopsy specimen from a 5-week-old male. c, d) Electron microscopy, in a 2-week-old male, demonstrating type II alveolar epithelial cells with typical abnormal lamellar body structure, including composite multivesicular and multilamellate bodies (c and d, respectively).

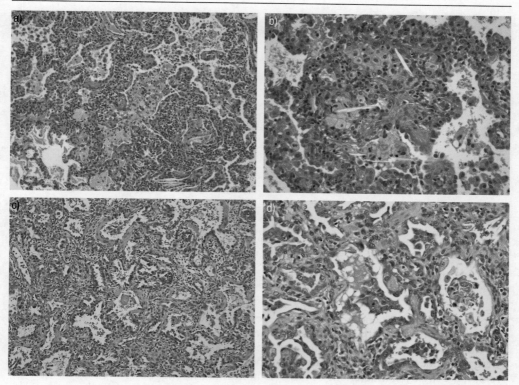

Fig. 2. – Surfactant dysfunction disorders: surfactant protein (SP)-C mutations. SP-C mutations typically result in a pattern of chronic pneumonitis of infancy (a, b). Some cases show particularly abundant foamy macrophages, which often prompts comparison to the desquamative interstitial pneumonia seen in adults, although the pathogenesis is clearly different in infants. Diagnostic clues include the presence of foamy macrophages and cholesterol clefts in the setting of lobular remodelling. Proteinosis material is relatively sparse compared with SP-B and adenosine triphosphate-binding cassette subfamily A member 3 (ABCA3) cases, often forming scattered individual globular aggregates, as seen in this biopsy specimen from an 11-week-old male (c, d). Lobular remodelling with interstitial extension of airway smooth muscle is a prominent feature in this case. Mild interstitial inflammation is also common (haematoxylin and eosin stain).

In many cases, a characteristic constellation of histological features permits the surgical pathologist to recognise congenital surfactant dysfunction disorders. The diagnosis may be supported by use of immunohistochemistry and/or electron microscopy. Immunohistochemistry, using antibodies directed against SP-A, SP-B, pro-SP-B and pro-SP-C, has been applied, although it is not used for routine diagnostic purposes at the Texas Children's Hospital (Houston, TX, USA). Similar immunohisto-chemical staining patterns have been described for both SP-B and ABCA3 deficiency, characterised by robust SP-A and pro-SP-B staining in both alveolar epithelium and intra-alveolar material, weak SP-B staining and robust pro-SP-C staining in alveolar epithelial cells [29]. Patients with SP-B mutations show strong pro-SP-C staining of the alveolar proteinosis material, whereas ABCA3 patients exhibit only alveolar epithelial pro-SP-C staining. In contrast, patients with SP-C deficiency show robust mature SP-B and pro-SP-B staining but deficient pro-SP-C staining [29].

Electron microscopy should be performed in cases suspected of representing surfactant dysfunction disorders in order to document abnormalities associated with SP-B and ABCA3 mutations. Patients with SP-B deficiency typically show deficient mature

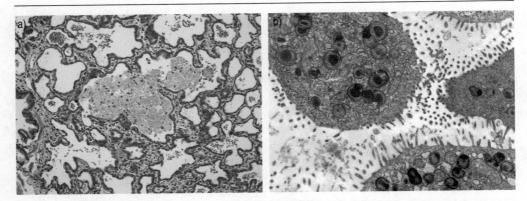

Fig. 3. – Surfactant dysfunction disorders: adenosine triphosphate-binding cassette subfamily A member 3 (ABCA3) mutations. Similar to surfactant protein (SP)-B mutation cases, ABCA3 mutations often result in a pattern of pulmonary alveolar proteinosis in infancy. a) In some cases, the proteinosis material may be coarse, with more cellular debris than typically seen with SP-B mutations, as demonstrated in a 6-day-old female (haematoxylin and eosin stain). Some cases also show more lobular remodelling, similar to infants with SP-C mutations. Older children exhibit variable histology, most often a pattern of nonspecific interstitial pneumonia (not shown). b) Electron microscopy in a 4-week-old female demonstrates typical small poorly formed lamellar bodies, including some with characteristic round dense bodies with a fried-egg appearance.

lamellar bodies with composite multivesicular bodies and multilamellate structures (fig. 1c) [30]. Patients with ABCA3 mutations may have distinctive electron-dense bodies associated with structures resembling small abortive and condensed lamellar bodies [31–33]. These round dense bodies have been described as having a fried-egg appearance, and, if present, are highly characteristic of ABCA3 abnormalities (fig. 3b).

The lamellar bodies in patients with SP-C deficiency are typically normal on ultrastructural examination. Definitive diagnosis of these disorders rests on mutation analysis of the *SPTPB, SFTPC* and/or *ABCA3* genes. This testing is most often performed on a blood sample at the time of the initial diagnostic evaluation, often obtained preceding or concurrent with lung biopsy; however, lung tissue may also be used. In this regard, appropriate triage of lung biopsy tissue is a critical component of the diagnostic process. A protocol for handling paediatric lung biopsy specimens permits appropriate distribution of tissue for ancillary studies, if needed, including electron microscopy and genetic mutation studies [34]. In the setting of infant biopsy procedures, particularly for those with clinical suspicion of a surfactant disorder, priority should be given to retention of tissue in glutaraldehyde for electron microscopy and snap-freezing tissue for possible molecular studies.

In 2004, mutations affecting ABCA3 were described as a cause of fatal surfactant-related lung disease in infants [35]. Since that time, reports of ABCA3 mutations in association with lung disease in older children have also appeared [29]. The *ABCA3* gene encodes one of a family of ATP-binding cassette transporters that often function in lipid transport [36–38]. Human disease is known to be caused by mutations in several other ABC genes, including *ABCA1* (Tangier disease), *ABCB11* (progressive familial intrahepatic cholestasis type 2) and cystic fibrosis transmembrane conductance regulator/*ABCC7* (cystic fibrosis). ABCA3 is found at high levels in the lung, is expressed in type II alveolar epithelial cells, predominantly at the limiting membrane of the lamellar bodies [39], and has been found to be upregulated with glucocorticoid administration in animals, all features which made this gene a strong candidate disease gene for abnormalities of surfactant metabolism. The precise function of ABCA3 in surfactant metabolism is not known; however, similarity to other ABC transporters would suggest a role in phospholipid transport and organisation during lamellar body formation. This concept is supported by the abnormal lamellar bodies noted on ultrastructural examination in patients with mutations in this gene. In some instances, the abnormal dense bodies suggest incorporation of lamellar body material into lysosomes. A variety of mutations in the *ABCA3* gene have been detected, including nonsense and frameshift mutations. Homozygotes or compound heterozygotes typically show severe respiratory disease and death in infancy. A single mutation with reduced but remaining ABCA3 function in heterozygotes may explain the prolonged survival in some cases.

The prognosis for those with surfactant dysfunction disorders varies to some degree with the gene affected. Children with SP-B mutations typically die during the neonatal period, usually in the first weeks and months of life. Similarly, those with ABCA3 mutations often die during the neonatal period, although there are later presentations with chronic lung disease in later childhood. Clinical presentation occurs somewhat later in infancy for those with SP-C mutations and survival is variable. Although some patients manifest with CPI in the first few months of life, others survive to adulthood with chronic lung disease, often manifesting as either nonspecific interstitial pneumonia or idiopathic pulmonary fibrosis. There is currently no effective therapy for the inherited surfactant dysfunction disorders, and patients are managed supportively and with lung transplantation. Administration of surfactant during the neonatal period does not typically result in clinical improvement.

Future advances in this heterogeneous set of diseases will probably come from increased understanding of the biological mechanisms of disease, recognition of other causative genes and genotype–phenotype correlation for further prognosis. The potential for these mutations to act as disease modifiers also merits further investigation, *e.g.* in premature infants with chronic neonatal lung disease or in older children with other forms of concurrent lung injury.

Pulmonary interstitial glycogenosis

PIG was described, in 2002, as a new variant of neonatal interstitial lung disease in seven neonates with tachypnoea, hypoxaemia, diffuse interstitial infiltrates and overinflated lungs on imaging [40]. Lung biopsy specimens obtained between 2 weeks and 4 months of age showed interstitial widening with increased cellularity due to increased numbers of structural cells. These cells had bland ovoid nuclei and were noted to contain periodic acid–Schiff-positive diastase-labile cytoplasmic material, typical of glycogen. Indeed, transmission electron microscopy demonstrated interstitial mesenchymal cells with few organelles and abundant monoparticulate glycogen. Neutral lipid droplets were also noted in some cells, and others showed more prominent rough endoplasmic reticulum, typical of fibroblasts.

A morphologically similar entity had previously been described as cellular interstitial pneumonitis of infancy, and probably represents the same pathological process [41]. Also called infantile cellular interstitial pneumonia or histiocytoid pneumonia, cellular interstitial pneumonitis of infancy was described, in 1992, in five infants (aged between 11 days and 2 yrs), including three term infants and two pre-term infants (33 and 34 weeks' gestation). One of the term infants had a patent ductus arteriosus ligated at the time of lung biopsy. A review of the medical literature found only two subsequent reports of PIG [42, 43]. One describes a term infant with respiratory distress at birth who had a persistent oxygen requirement and imaging abnormalities at 9 weeks of age, prompting lung biopsy [42]. After diagnosis of PIG, the infant was treated with steroids with an initial lack of response but eventual resolution of the oxygen requirement by the age of 10 months. The other describes PIG in monozygotic twins in a pregnancy complicated by twin-to-twin transfusion syndrome, premature delivery at 31 weeks' gestation and respiratory distress syndrome at birth [43]. Recurrent respiratory distress led to lung biopsy in both twins at 8 weeks of age and diagnosis of PIG. The twins were both treated with steroids and showed resolution of symptoms with no evidence of ongoing respiratory disease at 10 months of age.

Diagnosis of PIG is typically made, on lung biopsy, by routine haematoxylin and eosin stain alone, although periodic acid–Schiff stains with and without diastase may be helpful in identifying the glycogen-rich interstitial cells (fig. 4a and b). Since these structural cells may be confused with lymphocytes or histiocytes, immunohistochemistry may be useful in confirming mesenchymal differentiation when necessary (fig. 4c). The proliferated interstitial cells in PIG are positive for vimentin and negative for leukocyte common antigen (CD45), lysozyme and macrophage markers (CD68). These diagnostic features are summarised in table 3.

The incidence of PIG is unknown, but it shows a predilection for young infants, and is not generally seen beyond 6 months of age. PIG is now recognised to be associated with a number of other lung disorders in early infancy, most commonly those affecting alveolar growth (chronic neonatal lung disease, pulmonary hypoplasia and chromosomal disorders) and sometimes with pulmonary arterial vasculopathy. Four out of the

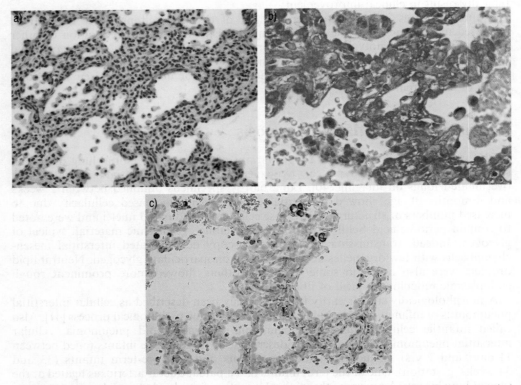

Fig. 4. – Pulmonary interstitial glycogenosis. a) Lung biopsy specimen from a 6-week-old female showing typical histological features of pulmonary interstitial glycogenosis (infantile cellular interstitial pneumonia), specifically interstitial widening by cells with bland ovoid nuclei and indistinct cytoplasm (haematoxylin and eosin stain). b) Periodic acid–Schiff staining demonstrates material consistent with glycogen in the interstitial cells. c) Immunohistochemistry for vimentin gives positive results in the interstitial cells, confirming mesenchymal differentiation. Leukocyte common antigen or macrophage markers may also be helpful in excluding a mononuclear or histiocytic process.

Table 3. – Pulmonary interstitial glycogenosis: diagnostic features

Interstitial widening with increased cellularity
Structural (noninflammatory) cells: vimentin-positive, LCA-negative
Cytoplasmic glycogen: PAS-positive, better demonstrated by electron microscopy
Often associated with other disease processes: alveolar growth abnormalities, congenital heart disease, pulmonary
 hypertension, congenital lung malformations (uncommon), storage disorders (rare)

LCA: leukocyte common antigen; PAS: periodic acid–Schiff.

seven infants initially described were pre-term (25, 29, 33 and 33 weeks' gestation) [40]. The present authors have occasionally seen PIG in the normal, but compressed, lung adjacent to congenital lung malformations, including cystic adenomatoid malformation and congenital lobar overinflation. The present authors have also seen PIG in an infant eventually diagnosed with Hunter's syndrome. Although the interstitial cellularity may be diffuse, many cases show only a patchy distribution, perhaps leading to under-recognition of this process, particularly in cases with superimposed abnormalities.

Although the pathogenesis of PIG is not clear, a number of theories have been proposed. Similar pools of glycogen are not normally seen in pulmonary interstitial cells, either post-natally or at any stage during foetal development. The abundance of glycogen in interstitial cells in PIG is similar to that described in animals in lipofibroblasts, cells which are thought to be precursors of myofibroblasts and to function in surfactant biosynthesis as carriers of lipid to type II alveolar epithelial cells. Although direct evidence is lacking, similar cells almost certainly exist in the human lung. Given the lack of information about this cell type in humans, it has been proposed that PIG represents a developmental disorder involving abnormal differentiation of pulmonary mesenchyme [40].

A genetic determinant of disease was suggested in the report of PIG in identical twins, although prematurity as a risk factor for PIG may be the overriding influence in this case. With increasing recognition of this pattern in association with various forms of lung disease in young infants, the present authors favour the interpretation that PIG is a nonspecific response to lung injury in the rapidly growing infant lung. In other words, rather than a unique disease entity, PIG may be a pathological reaction pattern, similar to reactive alveolar epithelial hyperplasia or diffuse alveolar damage, but one which is restricted to early infancy. Regardless of uncertainty regarding aetiology, recognition of this pattern provides a pathological explanation for the interstitial widening and impaired gas exchange. For example, in cases associated with chronic neonatal lung disease or congenital heart disease, the present authors have seen PIG in biopsy specimens obtained during episodes of clinical exacerbation from baseline function, or in patients for whom the degree of respiratory insufficiency exceeded expectations based upon known clinical factors, such as degree of prematurity.

The prognosis associated with PIG is generally good, but may be dependent upon the severity of any associated disease. Of the seven infants initially described, six had a favourable outcome and one died of complications of extreme prematurity and bronchopulmonary dysplasia [40]. The natural history of PIG is typically that of a self-limiting process with spontaneous symptomatic resolution over time in many cases. Although follow-up biopsy is unusual, the present authors have seen PIG, on lung biopsy, in an 11-week-old female with hypotonia and a suspected mitochondrial disorder; the infant subsequently died at 10 months of age and there was resolution of these histological findings on autopsy. Although not all patients require therapy, steroids may have a role in the acute management of PIG, and have been used successfully in some cases, including four infants showing long-term survival in the initial description of this entity, one of whom also received hydroxychloroquine [40].

Further study is needed to address the questions of cell of origin, pathogenesis and potential triggers, and most effective therapy. The variety of descriptors for this entity has been problematic with respect to uniform pathological description and accessibility of information in the medical literature. The current terminology (PIG, pulmonary interstitial glycogen accumulation disorder, infantile cellular interstitial pneumonia and histiocytoid pneumonia) invites confusion with both metabolic and infectious processes. Although this reflects uncertainty about pathogenesis at this point, terminological revision may be advisable as understanding of this entity evolves.

Neuroendocrine cell hyperplasia of infancy

NEHI is an entity that was first introduced in 2001 and later described more fully, in 2005, as a pathological correlate to the clinical syndrome of persistent tachypnoea of infancy [44, 45]. It was recognised clinically that a subset of patients with signs and symptoms of interstitial lung disease showed surprisingly normal findings on lung biopsy. Fifteen cases were accumulated and examined critically for any subtle unifying abnormalities, leading to the immunohistochemical recognition of increased numbers of neuroendocrine cells in their bronchioles.

Clinically, these patients all presented aged <2 yrs with an interstitial lung disease syndrome including tachypnoea, retractions, crackles and hypoxia. Most of these infants were born at term, with only three pre-term infants (33, 36 and 37 weeks' gestation) in the group. There was no evidence of immune dysfunction, congenital heart disease, genetic disease or other known cause for their respiratory symptoms. Unlike asthma patients, these children did not routinely wheeze or cough, and they were not responsive to bronchodilators or anti-inflammatory therapy. In these children, chest radiography typically shows hyperexpansion (fig. 5a) and interstitial prominence, and chest computed tomography demonstrates minor peribronchial thickening and occasional patchy ground-glass opacities [45]. Some cases have been recognised to exhibit ground-glass opacities most prominently in the central regions of the lung fields, particularly in the right middle lobe and lingula (fig. 5b) [46].

In the initial series, infant pulmonary function testing was performed in four cases, demonstrating evidence of airflow obstruction. Bronchodilators had little effect in these patients, and systemic corticosteroids seemed to reduce the severity of symptoms in some patients but did not resolve symptoms completely. Similar to chronic idiopathic bronchitis of infancy [47] and follicular bronchitis [48], NEHI is considered to be towards the mild end of the spectrum of diffuse lung disease in infancy. Although NEHI patients typically come to medical attention during infancy, symptoms may persist in toddlers and older children. Although there is no effective therapy, symptoms typically improve slowly over time, in some cases resolving altogether. Importantly, there have been no deaths and no cases of respiratory failure associated with NEHI to date.

The diagnosis is suggested pathologically by the striking normality of a biopsy specimen that seems discrepant when considered in the light of the relative severity of the clinical signs and symptoms (fig. 5c). For some biopsy specimens, further examination may reveal subtle airway abnormalities, including a mild nonspecific increase in airway-associated lymphoid tissue, mild reactive epithelial hyperplasia, mildly increased airway smooth muscle and increased numbers of clear cells in the bronchioles. Increased numbers of free alveolar macrophages have also been noted. Diagnosis is confirmed by using immunohistochemistry for neuroendocrine cells, with increases in the percentage of both airways with neuroendocrine cells and neuroendocrine cells relative to total airway cells in individual airway profiles (fig. 5d).

Although a number of antibodies have been applied, bombesin is the one most widely studied. Bombesin-immunoreactive cells are the most common of the neuroendocrine cells in the peripheral airways, and the diagnostic thresholds of the present authors have

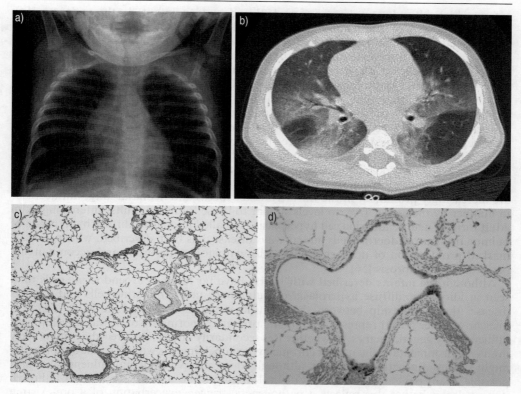

Fig. 5. – Neuroendocrine cell hyperplasia of infancy. A 9-month-old male presented with failure to thrive and chronic tachypnoea. Diagnostic imaging showed a) hyperinflation on chest radiography and b) hazy perihilar ground-glass opacities on chest computed tomography. c) Lung biopsy specimens from the lingula showed only minimal airway-associated lymphoid tissue and focal alveolar duct distension (haematoxylin and eosin stain). d) Bombesin immunohistochemistry demonstrated a high proportion of neuroendocrine cells in individual airways, as well as increased numbers of neuroepithelial bodies (upper right-hand side).

been determined using this antibody. Although objective criteria have not been validated by other groups, for practical purposes the diagnosis is made when four criteria are fulfilled: 1) neuroendocrine cells are present in ≥75% of airways in the biopsy specimen; 2) neuroendocrine cells comprise ≥10% of total airway epithelial cells in at least one bronchiole; 3) increased and/or enlarged neuroepithelial bodies; and 4) other superimposed pathological processes are excluded (table 4). For adequacy, the present authors prefer to evaluate ≥15 airway profiles. The absence of superimposed pathological processes is an important criterion, since neuroendocrine cell hyperplasia *per se* is not a specific finding. There are a number of disorders associated with an increase in the number of airway neuroendocrine cells, including bronchopulmonary dysplasia [49], cystic fibrosis [50], pulmonary hypoplasia secondary to congenital diaphragmatic hernia [51] and panacinar emphysema [52]. Other associations include mechanical ventilation [50], acute lung injury,

Table 4. – Neuroendocrine cell hyperplasia of infancy: diagnostic features

Increased proportion (≥75%) of airways with neuroendocrine cells
Increased proportion (≥10%) of neuroendocrine cells in airway
Large and/or numerous neuroepithelial bodies
Absence of other associated disease processes

extreme high altitude, smoke exposure [53] and sudden infant death syndrome [54]. Increased numbers of neuroendocrine cells have also been described previously in Wilson–Mikity syndrome (pulmonary dysmaturity) [55]. Findings of lymphocytic bronchiolitis, significant airway fibrosis (constrictive or obliterative bronchiolitis) or other interstitial processes would exclude the diagnosis. It is also important to note that NEHI is a clinical, radiographical and pathological diagnosis, and definitive diagnosis should be made only in the appropriate clinical setting and with supportive imaging characteristics.

The pathogenesis of this disorder is poorly understood. The pulmonary neuro-endocrine system is composed of airway epithelial cells and lobular collections (neuroepithelial bodies) that produce bioactive compounds, including bombesin, serotonin and calcitonin. The neuroendocrine cells are oxygen sensitive and are thought to have a role in bronchoconstriction, vasoactivity and immunomodulation, as well as epithelial differentiation and smooth muscle alteration during lung morphogenesis. They are increasingly prominent in the third-trimester foetus and neonatal lung, but decrease in number by the age of 1 yr, to levels similar to those found in adults. Interestingly, an adult form of neuroendocrine cell hyperplasia, so-called idiopathic diffuse hyperplasia of pulmonary neuroendocrine cells and airways disease, has been described, which shows a marked proliferation of neuroendocrine cells, carcinoid tumourlets and accompanying peribronchiolar fibrosis [56].

Although the infants described with NEHI have far fewer neuroendocrine cells than seen in idiopathic diffuse hyperplasia of pulmonary neuroendocrine cells and airways disease, the relationship between these entities remains unclear. Like PIG, it is also unclear whether NEHI represents an innate primary abnormality of airway development influenced by genetic factors, or whether it is secondarily induced by preceding pulmonary injury, environmental influences or chronic hypoxia. Sibling sets with the same abnormality might suggest a genetic component, although common environmental influences are also possible. Many patients have a history of viral illness prior to clinical presentation, although it is unclear whether this reflects a pathogenetic trigger, exacerbation of a pre-existing subclinical developmental process or a completely unrelated event. Since many of these patients were initially recognised in a locale at high altitude (Denver, CO, USA), the potential impact of altitude and hypoxic environment in the induction of neuroendocrine cell hyperplasia has been considered; however, patients with this clinical syndrome and corresponding pathological features on biopsy have now been identified in many regions of the USA and around the world, including both low- and high-altitude regions.

Future questions to be addressed include further characterisation of the imaging features associated with NEHI, determination of the specificity of these features and need for diagnostic lung biopsy, documentation of long-term natural history in known cases, evaluation of serum and urine biomarkers, and investigation of potential therapies.

Future directions

Although these advances in the understanding of paediatric interstitial lung disease have permitted improved recognition and more accurate diagnosis, much work remains to be done in this area. Multi-institutional cooperative groups, such as the ERS Task Force and the chILD working group in North America, provide the opportunity to foster further discussion and application of common terminology for these entities. Accuracy in pathological diagnosis is certainly a prerequisite for meaningful correlation with diagnostic imaging characteristics and clinical syndromes, and will hopefully advance the clinical recognition and management of these syndromes. It is also clear that accurate pathological diagnosis in any given patient is interdependent on knowledge of the clinical setting and imaging characteristics, permitting clinical, radiological and pathological diagnosis.

Summary

The diagnosis of diffuse lung disease in infants remains a challenge for both pulmonologists and pathologists, given the rarity of these disorders and the similarity of clinical presentation in many cases.

Since 2000, advances in diagnosis include the discovery of a new gene affecting surfactant metabolism (adenosine triphosphate (ATP)-binding cassette subfamily A member 3 (*ABCA3*)) and description of two new entitities specifically affecting the infant lung (pulmonary interstitial glycogenosis and neuroendocrine cell hyperplasia of infancy). Mutations in the ATP-binding cassette transporter gene, *ABCA3*, are now recognised as a cause of both respiratory failure in infancy and chronic progressive lung disease in older children and adolescents. Recognition of the histological patterns and ultrastructural abnormalities associated with the inherited surfactant dysfunction disorders should prompt mutation testing of the three known causative genes: surfactant protein (*SFTP*) B and *SFTPC*, and now *ABCA3*.

Pulmonary interstitial glycogenosis (also called infantile cellular interstitial pneumonia) refers to a histological pattern of interstitial widening by glycogen-rich stromal cells seen predominantly in early infancy. This may be an isolated finding, or, more often, is recognised in association with other underlying lung diseases, such as impaired alveolar growth due to prematurity, pulmonary hypoplasia or congenital heart disease. Neuroendocrine cell hyperplasia of infancy is now recognised as a pathological correlate to the syndrome of persistent tachypnoea of infancy. Since lung biopsy specimens from these patients may appear near-normal on initial histological review, application of bombesin immunohistochemistry is necessary in order to identify the increased number of airway neuroendocrine cells needed for diagnosis. Both pulmonary interstitial glycogenosis and neuroendocrine cell hyperplasia of infancy are disorders of unknown aetiology, as it is unclear whether these are manifestations of abnormal lung development, or alternatively reactive phenomena occurring post-natally in response to infection, environmental stimuli or other forms of lung injury.

Keywords: Cellular interstitial pneumonia of infancy, interstitial lung disease, neuroendocrine cell hyperplasia, paediatric, pulmonary interstitial glycogenosis, surfactant.

References

1. Rothenberg SS, Wagner JS, Chang JH, Fan LL. The safety and efficacy of thoracoscopic lung biopsy for diagnosis and treatment in infants and children. *J Pediatr Surg* 1996; 31: 100–103.

2. Fan LL, Kozinetz CA, Wojtczak HA, Chatfield BA, Cohen AH, Rothenberg SS. Diagnostic value of transbronchial, thoracoscopic, and open lung biopsy in immunocompetent children with chronic interstitial lung disease. *J Pediatr* 1997; 131: 565–569.

3. Fan LL, Langston C. Chronic interstitial lung disease in children. *Pediatric Pulmonol* 1993; 16: 184–196.

4. Fan LL, Kozinetz CA, Deterding RR, Brugman SM. Evaluation of a diagnostic approach to pediatric interstitial lung disease. *Pediatrics* 1998; 101: 82–85.

5. Howenstine MS, Eigen H. Current concepts on interstitial lung disease in children. *Curr Opin Pediatr* 1999; 11: 200–204.

6. Clement A, Henrion-Caude A, Fauroux B. The pathogenesis of interstitial lung diseases in children. *Paediatr Respir Rev* 2004; 5: 94–97.

7. Hilman BC, Amaro-Galvez R. Diagnosis of interstitial lung disease in children. *Paediatr Respir Rev* 2004; 5: 101–107.

8. Larray-Cussay LF, Hughes WT, eds. Interstitial Lung Disease in Children. Boca Raton, FL, CRC Press, 1988.

9. Fan LL, Mullen AL, Brugman SM, Inscore SC, Parks DP, White CS. Clinical spectrum of chronic interstitial lung disease in children. *J Pediatr* 1992; 121: 867–872.

10. Langston C, Fan LL. The spectrum of interstitial lung disease in childhood. *Pediatr Pulmonol* 2001; 32: Suppl. 23, 70–71.

11. Fan LL, Deterding RR, Langston C. Pediatric interstitial lung disease revisited. *Pediatr Pulmonol* 2004; 38: 369–378.

12. Clement A, ERS Task Force Committee members. Task force on chronic interstitial lung disease in immunocompetent children. *Eur Respir J* 2004; 24: 686–697.

13. Deutsch GH, Albright E, Chou PM, *et al.* Defining the spectrum of diffuse lung disease in infancy: a working classification of the Pediatric Interstitial Lung Disease Cooperative. *Mod Pathol* 2005; 18: 304 (abstract).

14. Langston C. Pediatric lung biopsy. *In*: Cagle P, ed. Diagnostic Pulmonary Pathology. New York, Marcel Dekker, 2000; pp. 19–47.

15. Langston C, Fan LL. Diffuse interstitial lung disease in infants. *Pediatr Pulmonol* 2001; 32: Suppl. 23, 74–76.

16. Tredano M, de Blic J, Griese M, Fournet JC, Elion J, Bahuau M. Clinical, biological, and genetic heterogeneity of the inborn errors of pulmonary surfactant metabolism. *Clin Chem Lab Med* 2001; 39: 90–108.

17. Cole FS, Hamvas A, Nogee LM. Genetic disorders of neonatal respiratory function. *Pediatr Res* 2001; 50: 157–162.

18. Whitsett JA, Wert SE, Xu Y. Genetic disorders of surfactant homeostasis. *Biol Neonate* 2005; 87: 283–287.

19. Nogee LM, Dunbar AE, Wert SE, Askin F, Hamvas A, Whitsett JA. A mutation in surfactant protein C gene associated with familial interstitial lung disease. *New Engl J Med* 2001; 344: 573–579.

20. Amin RS, Wert SE, Baughman RP, *et al.* Surfactant protein deficiency in familial interstitial lung disease. *J Pediatr* 2001; 139: 85–92.

21. Tredano M, Griese M, Brasch F, *et al.* Mutation in SFTPC in infantile pulmonary alveolar proteinosis with or without fibrosing lung disease. *Am J Med Genet* 2004; 126A: 18–26.

22. Nogee LM, de Mello DE, Dehner LP, Colten HR. Deficiency of pulmonary surfactant protein B in congenital alveolar proteinosis. *N Engl J Med* 1993; 328: 406–410.

23. deMello DD, Lin Z. Pulmonary alveolar proteinosis: a review. *Pediatr Pathol Mol Med* 2001; 20: 413–432.

24. Trapnell BC, Whitsett JA, Nakata K. Mechanisms of disease: pulmonary alveolar proteinosis. *New Engl J Med* 2003; 349: 2527–2539.

25. Katzenstein AA, Gordon LP, Oliphant M, Swender PT. Chronic pneumonitis of infancy: a unique form of interstitial lung disease occurring in early childhood. *Am J Surg Pathol* 1995; 19: 439–447.

26. Cameron HS, Somaschini M, Carrera P, *et al.* A common mutation in the surfactant protein C gene associated with lung disease. *J Pediatr* 2005; 146: 370–375.

27. Chibbar R, Shih F, Baga M, *et al.* Nonspecific interstitial pneumonia and usual interstitial pneumonia with mutation in surfactant protein C in familial pulmonary fibrosis. *Mod Pathol* 2004; 17: 973–980.

28. Lawson WE, Grant SW, Ambrosini V, *et al.* Genetic mutations in surfactant protein C are a rare cause of sporadic cases of IPF. *Thorax* 2004; 59: 977–980.

29. Bullard JE, Wert SE, Whitsett JA, Dean M, Nogee LM. ABCA3 mutations associated with pediatric interstitial lung disease. *Am J Respir Crit Care Med* 2005; 172: 1026–1031.

30. deMello DE, Heyman S, Phyelps DS, *et al.* Ultrastructure of lung in surfactant protein B deficiency. *Am J Respir Cell Mol Biol* 1994; 11: 230–239.

31. Tryka AF, Wert SE, Mazursky JE, Arrington RW, Nogee LM. Absence of lamellar bodies with accumulation of dense bodies characterizes a novel form of congenital surfactant defect. *Pediatr Dev Pathol* 2000; 3: 335–345.

32. Cutz E, Wert SE, Nogee LM, Moore AM. Deficiency of lamellar bodies in alveolar type II cells associated with fatal respiratory disease in a full-term infant. *Am J Respir Crit Care Med* 2000; 161: 608–614.

33. Edwards V, Cutz E, Viero S, Moore AM, Nogee L. Ultrastructure of lamellar bodies in congenital surfactant deficiency. *Ultrastruct Pathol* 2005; 29: 503–509.

34. Langston C, Patterson K, Dishop MK, *et al.* A protocol for the handling of tissue obtained by operative lung biopsy: recommendations of the chILD pathology co-operative group. *Pediatr Dev Pathol* 2006; 9: 173–180.

35. Shulenin S, Nogee LM, Annilo T, Wert SE, Whitsett JA, Dean M. ABCA3 gene mutations in newborns with fatal surfactant deficiency. *New Engl J Med* 2004; 350: 1296–1303.

36. Anon. ATP-binding cassette, subfamily A, member 3; ABCA3. *In*: Online Mendelian Inheritance in Man, OMIM™. MIM Number: 601615. Baltimore, MD, Johns Hopkins University. www.ncbi.nlm.nih.gov/omim/ Date last updated: February, 2 2006. Date last accessed: July 2006.

37. Dean M, Allikmets R. Complete characterization of the human ABC gene family. *J Bioenerg Biomembr* 2001; 33: 475–479.

38. van der Deen M, de Vries EGE, Timens W, Scheper RJ, Timmer-Bosscha H, Postma DS. ATP-binding cassette (ABC) transporters in normal and pathological lung. *Respir Res* 2005; 6: 59–75.

39. Yamano G, Funahashi H, Kawanami O, *et al.* ABCA3 is a lamellar body membrane protein in human lung alveolar type II cells. *FEBS Lett* 2001; 508: 221–225.

40. Canakis AM, Cutz E, Manson D, O'Brodovich H. Pulmonary interstitial glycogenosis: a new variant of neonatal interstitial lung disease. *Am J Respir Crit Care Med* 2002; 165: 1557–1565.

41. Schroeder SA, Shannon DC, Mark EJ. Cellular interstitial pneumonitis in infants. A clinicopathologic study. *Chest* 1992; 101: 1065–1069.

42. Smets K, Dhaene K, Schelstraete P, Meersschaut V, Vanhaesebrouck P. Neonatal pulmonary interstitial glycogen accumulation disorder. *Eur J Pediatr* 2004; 163: 408–409.

43. Onland W, Molenaar JJ, Leguit RJ, *et al.* Pulmonary interstitial glycogenosis in identical twins. *Pediatr Pulmonol* 2005; 40: 362–366.

44. Deterding RR, Fan LL, Morton R, Hay TC, Langston C. Persistent tachypnea of infancy (PTI) – a new entity. *Pediatr Pulmonol* 2001; 32: Suppl. 23, 72–73.

45. Deterding RR, Pye C, Fan LL, Langston C. Persistent tachypnea of infancy is associated with neuroendocrine cell hyperplasia. *Pediatr Pulmonol* 2005; 40: 157–165.

46. Brody AS, Crotty EJ. Neuroendocrine cell hyperplasia of infancy (NEHI), Pediatr Radiol 2006; 36: 1328.

47. Hull J, Chow CW, Robertson CF. Chronic idiopathic bronchiolitis of infancy. *Arch Dis Child* 1997; 77: 512–515.

48. Kinane BT, Mansell AL, Zwerdling RG, Lapey A, Shannon DC. Follicular bronchitis in the pediatric population. *Chest* 1993; 104: 1183–1186.

49. Johnson DE, Anderson WR, Burke BA. Pulmonary neuroendocrine cells in pediatric lung disease: alterations in airway structure in infants with bronchopulmonary dysplasia. *Anat Rec* 1993; 236: 115–119, 172–173.

50. Johnson D, Wobken J, Landrum B. Changes in bombesin, calcitonin and serotonin immunoreactive pulmonary neuroendocrine cells in cystic fibrosis and after prolonged mechanical ventilation. *Am Rev Respir Dis* 1988; 137: 123–131.

51. Asabe K, Tsuji K, Handa N, Kajiwara M, Suita S. Immunohistochemical distribution of bombesin-positive pulmonary neuroendocrine cells in a congenital diaphragmatic hernia. *Surg Today* 1999; 29: 407–412.

52. Alshehri M, Cutz E, Banzhoff A, Canny G. Hyperplasia of pulmonary neuroendocrine cells in a case of childhood pulmonary emphysema. *Chest* 1997; 112: 553–556.

53. Johnson DE, Georgieff MK. Pulmonary neuroendocrine cells. Their secretory products and their potential roles in health and chronic lung disease in infancy. *Am Rev Respir Dis* 1989; 140: 1807–1812.

54. Perrin DG, McDonald TJ, Cutz E. Hyperplasia of bombesin-immunoreactive pulmonary neuroendocrine cells and neuroepithelial bodies in sudden infant death syndrome. *Pediatr Pathol* 1991; 11: 431–447.

55. Gillan JE, Cutz E. Abnormal pulmonary bombesin immunoreactive cells in Wilson–Mikity syndrome (pulmonary dysmaturity) and bronchopulmonary dysplasia. *Pediatr Pathol* 1993; 13: 165–180.

56. Aguayo SM, Miller YE, Waldron JA Jr., *et al.* Idiopathic diffuse hyperplasia of pulmonary neuroendocrine cells and airways disease. *N Engl J Med* 1992; 327: 1285–1288.

CHAPTER 3

The differential diagnosis of pulmonary pre-invasive lesions

K.M. Kerr*, H.H. Popper[#]

*Dept of Pathology, University of Aberdeen School of Medicine, Aberdeen Royal Infirmary, Aberdeen, UK. [#]Dept of Pathology, Laboratories for Molecular Cytogenetics, Environmental and Respiratory Pathology, Medical University of Graz, Graz, Austria.

Correspondence: K.M. Kerr, Dept of Pathology, University of Aberdeen School of Medicine, Aberdeen Royal Infirmary, Foresterhill, Aberdeen, AB25 2ZD, UK. Fax: 44 1224663002; E-mail: k.kerr@abdn.ac.uk

There are a number of localised lesions that are recognised as pre-invasive and with the potential to develop into an invasive malignancy in the lung. In the bronchial tree, most commonly in its proximal branches, a spectrum of lesions grouped together as squamous dysplasia (SD) and carcinoma *in situ* (CIS) is a precursor for invasive bronchogenic carcinoma. In the peripheral parenchymal compartment of the lung, atypical adenomatous hyperplasia (AAH) is now established as a progenitor of localised nonmucinous bronchioloalveolar carcinoma (BAC), which, in turn, is the most likely precursor lesion for pulmonary adenocarcinoma arising in the lung periphery. Although SD/CIS and AAH are the most important of the pre-invasive precursors occurring in the lung, a particular and rare form of pulmonary neuroendocrine cell (PNEC) hyperplasia called diffuse idiopathic PNEC hyperplasia (DIPNECH) is included in the recently published World Health Organization (WHO) classification of pre-invasive lesions of the lung owing to its association with typical carcinoid tumours [1]. There are a number of diseases that are recognised pathological entities in their own right and that confer a risk of development of primary lung cancer. Most of these lesions are diffuse parenchymal fibro-inflammatory diseases, but some, such as congenital cystic adenomatoid malformation, are localised; all are beyond the scope of this chapter, but have been reviewed elsewhere [2].

For each of these three pre-invasive lesions, SD/CIS, AAH and DIPNECH, there are other pathological changes or discrete lesions that may have to be considered in the differential diagnosis (tables 1–3). Some of these alternatives are neoplastic and possibly malignant, whereas others are benign and reactive. As is always the case in differential diagnosis, knowledge of the patient's history and the clinical context in which the lesion occurred is of vital importance in reaching the correct diagnosis. Both SD/CIS and AAH occur relatively frequently, but local clinical practice determines whether the pathologist is likely to see many or few such lesions. SD/CIS may be an incidental finding in standard bronchoscopically derived biopsy specimens. If the pathologist receives samples obtained during so-called autofluorescence bronchoscopy (AFB), rather more are encountered.

Table 1. – Differential diagnoses for squamous dysplasia/carcinoma *in situ*

Basal cell hyperplasia
Squamous metaplasia
Reactive atypia of inflammation, infection and chemo-irradiation
Invasive carcinoma in bronchial biopsy specimens
Endobronchial papillary squamous cell carcinoma

Eur Respir Mon, 2007, 39, 37–62. Printed in UK - all rights reserved. Copyright ERS Journals Ltd 2007; European Respiratory Monograph; ISSN 1025-448x.

Table 2. – Differential diagnosis of atypical adenomatous hyperplasia

Reactive type II pneumocyte proliferations
    Diffuse interstitial lung disease
    Localised fibro-inflammatory lesions
Peribronchiolar metaplasia
Papillary adenoma
Alveolar adenoma
Micronodular pneumocyte hyperplasia
BAC
    Localised nonmucinous BAC
    Multifocal BAC
    BAC as a component of invasive adenocarcinoma

BAC: bronchioloalveolar carcinoma.

Table 3. – Differential diagnosis of diffuse idiopathic pulmonary neuroendocrine cell (PNEC) hyperplasia

PNEC hyperplasia in fibro-inflammatory diseases
Incidental PNEC hyperplasia
Minute meningothelial nodules
Other neuroendocrine neoplasms

AAH is, for all practical purposes, a lesion encountered after sampling the background lung in large pulmonary resection specimens, especially those carried out for primary carcinoma. Of course it is possible that AAH may be found incidentally on wedge biopsy of lung, or even on transbronchial lung biopsy. DIPNECH, as currently defined [3], is an extremely rare lesion, and requires close clinicopathological correlation for diagnosis, which usually involves examination of either a wedge lung biopsy specimen or autopsy material. PNEC hyperplasia occurs in other circumstances and the relevance of this is discussed below.

When pathological material is available as a result of a lung cancer screening programme, pre-invasive lesions are much more likely to be encountered, and may be the primary diagnosis for the case, rather than an additional incidental finding. Screening programmes designed to detect early bronchial neoplasia using sputum cytology and specialised bronchoscopic techniques inevitably discover SD/CIS lesions, whereas spiral computed tomography (CT)-based screening has the power to detect very small peripheral pulmonary parenchymal nodules, including AAH and localised BAC [4].

Clearly the importance of identifying pre-invasive disease in the lung is that, by implication, there is a risk of disease progression, with the development of life-threatening invasive carcinoma. As discussed below, relatively little is known about the rate and risk of progression of SD/CIS and AAH to more advanced disease. In terms of differential diagnosis, it is important to distinguish both neoplastic disease that is already at a more advanced stage and requiring a different and probably more immediate therapeutic approach and reactive conditions that are reversible and carry no risk of progression to malignancy.

SD/CIS

SD and CIS represent a continuous spectrum of changes in a squamous-type epithelium lining the airway, which is considered a precursor of squamous cell carcinoma arising in airway epithelium [5].

Grossly, these lesions are generally invisible to the bronchoscopist using standard white-light bronchoscopy or to the pathologist examining airway mucosa in surgically resected or autopsy lungs. Occasionally, areas of CIS may be visible as granular, pale or flattened patches of opaque mucosa in which the rugal folds and mucosal pits are lost. Although up to 40% of CIS lesions may be seen by an experienced bronchoscopist [6], the use of AFB increases the detection rate for SD/CIS by approximately six times [7]. Although AFB increases sensitivity, it is not very specific, and both inflamed and even normal mucosa may appear positive using this test. It is recognised that SD/CIS is frequently a multifocal disorder, representing a field change in the bronchial mucosa. Although lesions may be widespread in the bronchial tree, individual patches of change are usually small. AFB studies have shown that areas of dysplasia are usually 1–3 mm across, whereas CIS measures 4–12 mm [8]. CIS lesions are especially common on the spurs of airway carinae [9].

The description and criteria for SD/CIS given in the WHO classification are based upon identifying atypia within a full-thickness squamous epithelium [5]. There are four grades of disease: mild, moderate, and severe dysplasia, and CIS. Each of these is distinguished on the basis of cytological and architectural atypia in a manner similar to schemes applied to the uterine cervix and other dysplastic squamous epithelia.

Mild dysplasia is characterised by very minimal nuclear abnormality, expansion of the basal layer of vertically orientated nuclei (basaloid zone) to occupy only the lower third of the epithelium and little or no mitotic activity. This squamous epithelium matures normally and may be minimally thickened and prickle cells are often present (fig. 1a).

In moderate dysplasia, rather more cytological atypia is seen, with evident nuclear angulation and grooving. In a thickened epithelium, the basaloid zone may occupy the lower two-thirds of the epithelium and mitoses are seen confined to the lower third. The epithelium still matures and superficially prickle cells may still be retained (fig. 1b).

Severe dysplasia displays a marked increase in cell size and pleomorphism. Irregular nuclei contain coarse chromatin and nucleoli are frequent. The basaloid zone may extend into the upper third of the epithelium and mitoses are found throughout the lower two-thirds. This markedly thickened epithelium shows only minimal evidence of maturation, with superficial flattening of cells (fig. 1c).

A diagnosis of CIS requires the same high grade cytological features as in severe dysplasia, but replacement of the entire epithelial thickness with a haphazard collection of cells such that an inverted epithelium would look no different. There is no maturation of the epithelium, which may be grossly thickened but may also be thinned (fig. 1d).

These categories are, of course, artificial divisions of a biological continuum, and, as such, not all of the features may be present in a particular lesion and the degree of change often varies in different parts of the bronchial tree and may even vary within a single high-power field. In such a case, it is useful to describe the range of dysplasia present and emphasise the worst case.

It is by no means always the case that dysplasia occurs in the bronchus in the context of a full-thickness squamous-type epithelium. In bronchial biopsy specimens, it is not unusual to see layers of dysplastic epithelial cells overlain by nonatypical differentiated columnar epithelial cells (fig. 2). This appearance poses major problems in interpretation using the published WHO criteria since there is no full-thickness squamous epithelium and the atypical squamous zone is rarely thick enough to allow division into thirds. Occasionally, this appearance is seen at the transition between full-thickness CIS and normal respiratory epithelium, but it is unclear whether this represents lateral spread of CIS, undermining the adjacent normal bronchial lining, or a partial transformation of the epithelium at that point (fig. 3). Another frequent finding is an airway lined by a rather thin layer of variably atypical cells, sometimes with visible squamous features (intercellular bridges), which has a rather ragged surface as if the superficial layers of cells

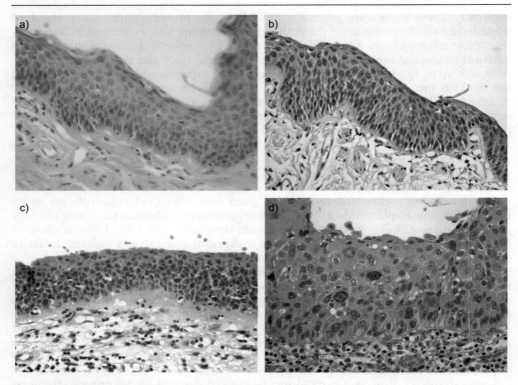

Fig. 1. – a) Mild dysplasia with basal third showing minimal nuclear irregularity. b) In moderate dysplasia, the atypia extends to involve the middle third of the epithelium. c) Cytological atypia is marked in severe dysplasia and mitoses are present mid-epithelium. d) An example of carcinoma *in situ* showing evidence of squamous differentiation, but extreme atypia extends up to the surface (haematoxylin and eosin stain).

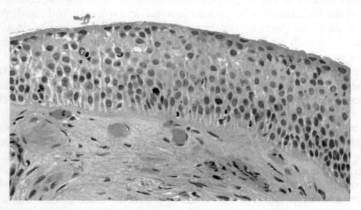

Fig. 2. – Despite mild-to-moderate cytological atypia, mitoses present in the lower third and an easily visible prickle cell layer, columnar cells persist on the surface (haematoxylin and eosin stain).

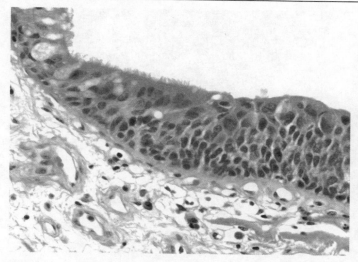

Fig. 3. – Severe dysplasia undermining or overlain by persistent columnar epithelium (haematoxylin and eosin stain).

have been lost. This appearance probably represents dysplasia occurring in an epithelium showing basal cell hyperplasia (BCH; see below) without going through a stage of complete full-thickness squamous metaplasia. Possibly due to trauma related to the bronchoscopic examination, the biopsy procedure or tissue handling in the pathology laboratory, the superficial differentiated layer of respiratory epithelial cells is lost. When faced with this partial dysplastic transformation of the bronchial lining, grading of dysplasia is very difficult since many of the architectural criteria cannot be applied and diagnosis must be based upon cytological appearances. Sometimes, it is impossible to do better than suggest a low- or high-grade dysplasia. Indeed, some published works on bronchial dysplasias have grouped moderate and severe dysplasia together into a single high-grade category [10], and there is some evidence that cases classified as moderate and severe dysplasia are similar in some molecular characteristics [11].

Differential diagnosis: invasive disease

Exophytic and atypical but noninvasive squamous papillary lesions that have been described in the bronchus [12] would seem, at face value, to be acceptable as a form of CIS, but, in the WHO classification, all such atypical endobronchial squamous papillary lesions are classified as squamous cell carcinoma, implying invasion and a relatively poor prognosis.

In small bronchoscopically derived mucosal biopsy specimens, it may be very difficult to distinguish CIS from invasive disease, especially when subepithelial stroma is scanty or absent. There are no cytological differences between CIS and some invasive tumours. As described above, CIS usually consists of large irregular cells showing variable expression of the squamous phenotype and with nuclear and cytoplasmic features indistinguishable from those of standard invasive squamous cell carcinoma. Occasionally, CIS consists of slightly smaller rather basaloid cells with less cytoplasm, and this pattern of CIS has been described in association with invasive basaloid carcinoma [13]. Dissociated fragments of such epithelium may be impossible to distinguish from fragments of invasive tumour. It is worth remembering that CIS occurs in strips lining airways and, thus, tends to have a

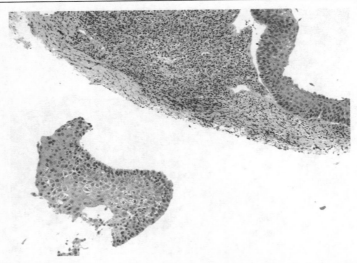

Fig. 4. – Severe dysplasia/carcinoma *in situ* in a bronchial biopsy specimen. Free fragments of atypical squamous epithelium are difficult to categorise in terms of *in situ* or invasive disease in the absence of stroma; this was considered to be *in situ* (haematoxylin and eosin stain).

straight or curvilinear profile, the superficial luminal surface is generally fairly flat in the absence of a papillary lesion and the basement membrane is usually straight or undulating (fig. 4). The presence of basement membrane may itself be a useful pointer to a diagnosis of CIS but cannot be relied upon. The basement membrane in CIS can sometimes be very irregular and thin [14], and may be prominent in some tumours, especially if of basaloid type [13]. Very irregular fragments of tumour, small tumour islands and nodules or large clumps of tumour are more suggestive of invasive disease. Necrosis is not a feature of CIS, and, if any stroma is associated with the epithelium causing diagnostic difficulty, evidence of a dense collagenous stromal response or marked stromal vascularity is again more suggestive of invasive disease. Clearly CIS and invasive disease can coexist in the same biopsy sample, further complicating the issue.

Without definitive evidence of invasion of the bronchial mucosa, care should be exercised before making a diagnosis of invasive carcinoma. In some cases, it is simply not possible to be definitive, and the use of terms such as "at least CIS, possible invasion", *etc.* is perfectly justified. It is important that those who send such biopsy samples for a pathologist's opinion understand the possible limitations of the material being examined. In this situation, knowledge of the radiological findings and, in particular, what the bronchoscopist saw may be of considerable help in reaching the correct diagnosis.

Complex vascularisation of the malignant-looking epithelium would also suggest that it was part of an invasive tumour, but care must be taken not to confuse such an appearance with so-called angiogenic squamous dysplasia (ASD) [15], a noninvasive lesion with an as yet unproven link with tumour development (fig. 5). ASD is characterised by pegs or tufts of basement membrane material invaginating a usually squamous-type epithelium lining an airway, with one or more capillary vessels embedded in the tuft. The apex of the tuft may extend close to the epithelial surface, with only a thin cell layer between it and the airway lumen, and, in some cases, the whole epithelium may have a papillary configuration. Dysplasia is variable in these lesions, although, in the present authors' experience, it is generally mild. It is also worth noting that such vascular tufts may be seen invaginating normal-looking pseudostratified respiratory epithelium, calling into question the assertion that ASD may be evidence of vascularisation of SD as

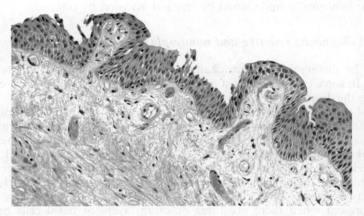

Fig. 5. – Angiogenic squamous dysplasia. Tufts of connective tissue containing several capillary vessels are covered by a thinned mildly atypical squamous epithelium (haematoxylin and eosin stain).

a prelude to invasion. Although the microvascular density of ASD is no higher than that seen in standard forms of SD/CIS, this morphologically distinctive lesion may nonetheless reflect a qualitative change in angiogenesis from that present in SD/CIS. There are conflicting reports regarding the upregulation of vascular endothelial growth factor in ASD [16, 17].

CIS may be mistaken for invasive disease when the intraepithelial changes extend down into bronchial gland ducts and even replace the gland acinar epithelium. Thus small islands of malignant-looking epithelium may appear to be invading the subepithelial tissue; this change may even mimic lymphovascular space invasion. If care is taken to appreciate the location of these small cellular islands close to any cartilage in the section, and the lobulated architecture of the seromucous glands is retained, then the *in situ* nature of the lesion can be discerned (fig. 6). This task is much easier if some of the gland lobules are only partially replaced and some normal seromucous cells remain. It could be argued that such intraepithelial extension of disease

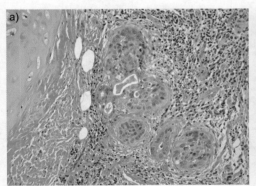
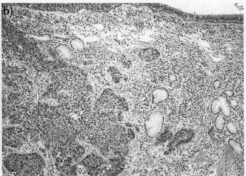

Fig. 6. – a) Carcinoma *in situ* extending into bronchial mucosal glands. The lobulated outline of the glands is preserved. b) Irregular islands of invasive carcinoma infiltrate around uninvolved glands (haematoxylin and eosin stain).

is a form of invasion, and indeed the present authors' experience is that such a pattern of CIS is most often seen when invasive squamous cell carcinoma is present nearby in the bronchial tree, but this argument becomes rather semantic. This pattern of CIS does not fit with what is normally understood by stromal invasion by tumour.

Differential diagnosis: reactive and nondysplastic changes

SD must be distinguished from changes in the airway lining that are reactive or metaplastic. In some circumstances, a degree of cytological atypia may be present, further complicating the distinction.

As alluded to above, it seems likely that SD supervenes in a bronchial epithelium that is already altered by BCH and/or squamous metaplasia. As ever, it is difficult to observe the progression of human lung disease in a longitudinal fashion, but there is animal experimental evidence to support the observational evidence from clinical human lung biopsy material that BCH may be the earliest lesion in the multi-step progression of SD/ CIS [18]. Squamous metaplasia may occur against a background of BCH, whereupon dysplasia may develop.

BCH is present when there are three or more layers of basal cells present in an otherwise normal pseudostratified columnar respiratory-type epithelium (fig. 7). Occasionally this BCH may occupy most of the epithelial thickness, with only a few superficial columnar cells remaining. Care must be taken to observe the very regular small oval nuclei, lack of pleomorphism and fine chromatin pattern in order to distinguish BCH from SD or even CIS. Equally, it can be easy to overdiagnose BCH in normal respiratory epithelium that has simply been cross cut. Signs of oblique transection of adjacent cells, basement membrane and other structures help to avoid this mistake. The basal cell zone usually expresses cytokeratins 5, 6, 8 and 14 particularly well, and may be defined using the anti-cytokeratin antibodies CK5/6 and 34betaE12.

The cells in BCH do not, by definition, show evidence of squamous differentiation, but, not infrequently, intercellular bridges can be found in what would otherwise appear to be BCH. Occasionally, this change is quite marked and the appearance is similar to that seen in so-called immature squamous metaplasia in the uterine cervix. In some cases,

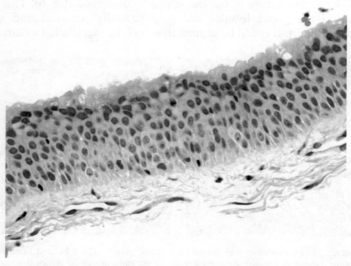

Fig. 7. – Several layers of basal cells are present in basal cell hyperplasia (haematoxylin and eosin stain).

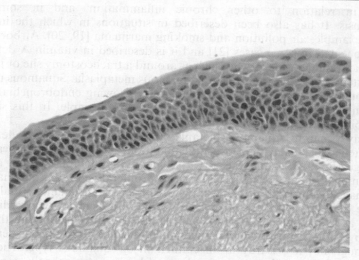

Fig. 8. – Full thickness squamous metaplasia (haematoxylin and eosin stain).

dysplasia occurs in such a setting, although a layer of differentiated columnar cells remains on the surface (figs 2 and 3). This scenario has already been discussed previously. In other cases, the basal layer appears to replace the columnar cells and complete full-thickness squamous metaplasia is seen; of course, this may be shedding rather than replacement of the superficial columnar cells. Thus, full-thickness squamous metaplasia without atypia is not an obligatory precursor of bronchial SD/CIS.

Complete squamous metaplasia without atypia is seen in a number of situations in the bronchus apart from the classic scenario of the tobacco smoker's airway (fig. 8). Squamous metaplasia may be seen in the dilated and chronically inflamed airways in bronchiectasis, lining chronic tuberculous cavities, in the airway draining a chronic lung

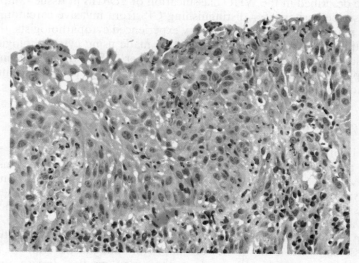

Fig. 9. – Reactive squamous metaplasia with marked inflammation, accounting for the mild nuclear atypia (haematoxylin and eosin stain).

abscess or in relation to other chronic inflammation, and in some cases of pneumoconiosis. It has also been described in situations in which the inhaled air is irritant; for example, air pollution and smoking marijuana [19, 20]. Airborne radiation has been implicated in some cases [21] and it is described in vitamin A deficiency [22]. Direct chronic trauma of the airway, such as around a tracheostomy site or in relation to a bronchial stent, may be responsible for squamous metaplasia. Squamous metaplasia is also quite common in the airway overlying slowly growing endobronchial tumours; a typical carcinoid tumour would be the most common example. In this situation, the squamous epithelium is frequently very thin.

Atypia may occur in squamous metaplasia, but is usually low grade, and, when present, is often associated with marked inflammation, a useful clue to the reactive nature of the change (fig. 9). Beyond the airways, squamous metaplasia may occur in the epithelium lining alveolar walls, especially in the proliferative/organising phase of diffuse alveolar damage (acute respiratory distress syndrome) or in usual interstitial pneumonia. This may be quite atypical, but great care should be taken not to overdiagnose such appearances as squamous cell carcinoma. It is also worth remembering that cytotoxic chemotherapy, radiotherapy and severe viral infections may lead to considerable cellular atypia, although not necessarily in an epithelium of squamous type. The respiratory epithelium may show small groups or individual bizarre atypical cells, especially when there is regenerative hyperplasia following injury and ulceration.

BCH and squamous metaplasia may occur as a prelude to SD/CIS and need to be distinguished from more advanced changes. The same changes may be reactive and carry no risk of progression to SD/CIS. As always, knowledge of the patient's clinical history and the context of the biopsy samples is crucial to reaching the correct diagnosis.

Cytological diagnosis of SD/CIS

Atypical squamous cells may be detected among exfoliated cells derived from bronchoscopic examinations or in sputum samples. There are published criteria describing, in considerable detail, subtle differences in cell-staining characteristics (eosinophilia/orangeophilia and basophilia) and nuclear morphology, the latter very close to those described in the WHO classification of SD/CIS in tissue samples [23]. Tao et al. [24] described criteria for distinguishing CIS from invasive carcinoma. Although these criteria may work in the hands of very experienced cytopathologists, the prevailing view is that this latter distinction is not reliably made using cytopathological material. Cytological squamous atypia may be a useful marker of SD/CIS in screening studies of high-risk populations, but the sensitivity of this technique is probably quite low in this particular situation, probably <50% [25].

Immunohistochemistry in the differential diagnosis of SD/CIS

A diagnosis of SD/CIS does not require immunohistochemistry, and there are no markers that could be considered key to diagnosis. Loss of some cytokeratins is described with progression of SD/CIS, and cytokeratin 10 has been described in one study as a marker of invasion [26], but in another as present in dysplasia but not in metaplasia [27]. The progressive replacement of the respiratory epithelium by an expanding zone of increasingly atypical basal cells is associated with an expansion of the proliferative compartment within the epithelium [28, 29]. Although this presents a potentially valuable tool for assessing SD/CIS, it is of unproven diagnostic value. The use of immunohistochemistry to detect markers that may predict disease progression is discussed later.

Implications of the diagnosis of SD/CIS

There are several potential pitfalls in the diagnosis and grading of SD/CIS, as described previously, and inconsistency of diagnosis among pathologists has been used to explain some of the findings in lung cancer screening studies using AFB [30]. Equally, other work has shown that the WHO classification of SD/CIS may be consistently and reliably applied [31].

The essence of a diagnosis of SD/CIS, as a precursor lesion of invasive bronchogenic carcinoma, is that the lesion carries a risk of progression and that those reactive lesions with which it may be confused do not. It is extremely difficult to quantify the risk of progression, and firm data on this issue are scarce. The necessary longitudinal studies are very difficult in human subjects, owing to the difficulty in detecting, localising and sampling SD/CIS. Fluorescence bronchoscopic studies have contributed greatly to the understanding of this area, but the situation is still anything but clear. Studies have shown that up to 50% of patients with sputum atypia eventually, up to 10 yrs later, develop invasive carcinoma. Studies using bronchoscopic surveillance and repeat bronchial biopsy suggest that the greater the degree of SD, the shorter the time interval and the greater the risk of more advanced disease developing. Relatively few patients have been studied in this way, but, in those patients who had SD/CIS and who subsequently developed invasive carcinoma, the time interval was anywhere between 6 months and 6 yrs [32–34]. Equally, there is evidence that the disease may wax and wane, whereas some SD and even CIS lesions may regress completely [33]. There are also studies suggesting that progression of SD/CIS to invasive disease may be linked to the differential expression of a number of oncogene/tumour suppressor gene products, such as p53, B-cell leukaemia/lymphoma 2 gene product (Bcl-2), Bcl-2-associated X protein, fragile histidine triad, cyclin-dependent kinase inhibitor 2A (P16^{INK4}), and cyclins D1 and E [11, 35–38]. Although these studies are generally interesting, none of these data permit prediction on an individual patient basis.

AAH

AAH is a localised lesion that occurs in the peripheral parenchymal area of the lung, most probably arising from the bronchioloalveolar epithelium, and is considered the probable precursor of most lung adenocarcinomas [39].

Most AAH lesions are macroscopically invisible, and are incidental findings on histological examination of lung tissue. In some instances, lesions may be seen as indistinct white, grey or cream/yellow foci a few millimetres in diameter on the cut surface of the lung. Occasionally, AAH is distinct enough to allow the alveolar spaces to be visualised as small depressions on the lesions' surface. Prior inflation of the lung by perbronchial instillation of fixative and subsequent careful examination, preferably under a good light and while washing the cut surface of the lung with clean water, greatly increases the chance of identifying these lesions grossly. Thus, a significant proportion of gross lesions identified are not AAH, but instead nonspecific inflammatory or fibrotic foci. It is good practice to sample all probable lesions and take some random blocks of parenchymal lung tissue in order to maximise lesion yield. AAH is most likely to be found in the upper lobes and subpleural lung. The presence of diffuse fibrosis, emphysema and pneumonic consolidation prevents lesion identification.

AAH lesions have been found in prospective autopsy studies of noncancer-bearing patients in 2–4% of cases [39], although, given the frequency of diffuse lung pathology at autopsy, these figures could underestimate the true frequency of AAH. However, lesions are most frequently found in lung specimens resected for primary carcinoma, and adenocarcinoma in particular. The reported prevalence of AAH in this setting also varies according to how thinly the lung under examination is sliced and how many tissue blocks are taken for histological examination. AAH lesions are more frequently reported in Japanese than Caucasian populations. In what are reasonably comparable prospective studies, three Japanese groups found a mean prevalence of AAH of 19.8% of all lung cancer resections [40–42], whereas, in two non-Japanese studies, the mean prevalence was 11.2% [43, 44]. From the same five studies, the Japanese cohort had a mean prevalence of 34% for AAH in adenocarcinoma-bearing lungs, whereas the non-Japanese studies averaged 19.4%. The means for squamous-cell-carcinoma-bearing lungs were 17 and 3.1%, respectively.

In many reported instances, AAH is solitary, but, in ~50% of cases, multiple lesions are found, mostly numbering between two and six [2]. In fewer reported cases, larger numbers of AAHs are present. ANAMI et al. [45] reported one exceptional case with 161 AAH lesions, whereas one of the present authors has a case exhibiting 125 lesions. Multiple AAHs are almost always concurrent with BAC or invasive adenocarcinoma, and cases with large numbers of AAH lesions are associated with multiple synchronous primary adenocarcinomas.

AAH is described, in the current WHO classification of lung tumours, as "a localised proliferation of mild-to-moderately atypical cells lining involved alveoli and, sometimes, respiratory bronchioles, resulting in focal lesions in peripheral alveolated lung, usually less than 5 mm in diameter and generally in the absence of underlying interstitial inflammation and fibrosis" [39].

At low magnification, AAH lesions stand out from the surrounding normal lung due to mild alveolar wall thickening as a result of fibrosis (collagen and fibroblasts), not infrequently an interstitial infiltrate of lymphocytes that may occasionally be heavy, and sometimes elastosis (fig. 10). The alveolar architecture may be disturbed by not only enlarged alveolar spaces but also alveoli of reduced size, particularly when fibrosis is prominent. These airspaces often contain alveolar macrophages. Lesions are frequently seen close to or incorporating a respiratory bronchiole.

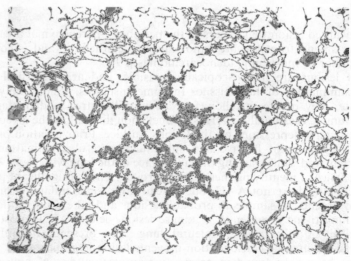

Fig. 10. – Atypical adenomatous hyperplasia standing out from the surrounding normal lung on low-power examination due to the thickened alveolar walls and prominent alveolar lining cells (haematoxylin and eosin stain).

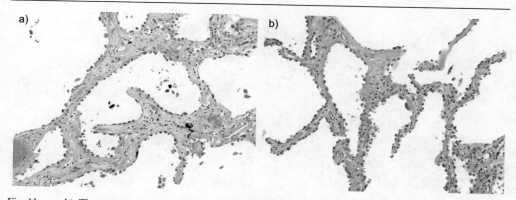

Fig. 11. – a, b) These examples of atypical adenomatous hyperplasia show variable thickening of the alveolar walls and a cuboidal cell lining with large gaps between cells. In b) occasional multinucleate cells are visible (haematoxylin and eosin stain).

The cell population lining the alveoli in AAH is characteristically heterogeneous. As well as normal flat type I pneumocytes, a mixture of round cells and low columnar cells, frequently with apical snouts (so-called peg cells), line the alveoli in AAH, giving it an interrupted appearance (fig. 11). Cell stratification is absent and cell size varies, with occasional giant forms sometimes present. Cell nuclei tend to be round or oval and have a smooth outline. The chromatin is homogeneous and occasionally hyperchromatic. Nuclear inclusions are present in at least a quarter of the cells [46]. Double nuclei are not uncommon, and occasionally the nucleus is situated at the cell apex. Mitotic figures are extremely uncommon. Ultrastructural studies indicate that AAH shows a mixture of cells differentiated towards type II pneumocytes and Clara cells [47]. Ciliated or mucous cells are not found in AAH.

In less-cellular AAH lesions, the edge of the lesion appears to blend into the adjacent normal alveolar lining cells. In more-cellular lesions, if there is a respiratory bronchiole within or adjacent to the lesion, the atypical cell population may be seen extending proximally and lining the airway. Lesions range in size from foci comprising a few alveoli up to rare examples of >15 mm in diameter. When AAH was first included in the WHO classification, it was defined as a lesion of ≤5 mm in diameter, following the assertion of MILLER [44] that any lesion of >5 mm in diameter should be considered carcinoma. It is now recognised that lesions that are still regarded as AAH may measure >5 mm in diameter. There are relatively few published data on lesion size. In one study, 25% of lesions measured <1 mm in diameter, 55% ranged 1–3 mm, 10% 3–5 mm and the remaining 10% were 5–10 mm [40]. In the series of cases collected in the study by KERR [48], approximately two-thirds measured ≤3 mm in diameter, 17% ranged 3–5 mm and 9% were 5–10 mm, whereas 10% measured 10–19 mm. NAKANISHI [46] reported one AAH lesion measuring 24 mm in diameter.

There is no doubt that cellularity and atypia in AAH vary between patients, and, although, in many patients with multiple AAHs, the appearance between each is remarkably similar, in some there is variation. Up to a quarter of lesions are distinctly more cellular than usual (fig. 12) [40, 48]. In these, there is a tendency for more of the cells to be columnar in shape and the nuclei may be larger, but atypia is rarely marked, and the cells are more crowded, with continuous rather than intermittent runs of cells lining alveolar spaces; thus, cell–cell contact appears greater and there is more, often notable, alveolar wall thickening. These more-cellular atypical lesions tend to be larger [44, 48, 49]. However, the concept of grading AAH is not widely accepted and is not recommended in the WHO classification [39]. Nonetheless, there are numerous references in the

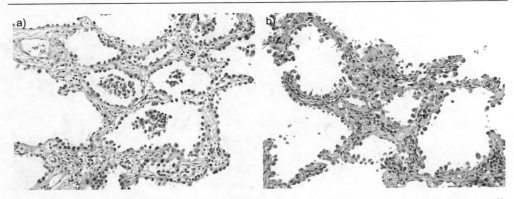

Fig. 12. – a) More-cellular atypical adenomatous hyperplasia (AAH). a) Smaller gaps are visible between cells, which remain cuboidal. Double nuclei are also present. b) Gaps remain between cells, which are more columnar, and there is more nuclear atypia. This is still AAH, but at the high-grade end of the spectrum (haematoxylin and eosin stain).

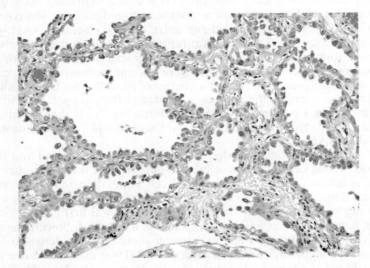

Fig. 13. – A transitional lesion? A matter of opinion. This lesion is much more difficult to separate from bronchioloalveolar carcinoma since there are continuous runs of cells, but no overlapping, stratification or tall columnar cells (haematoxylin and eosin stain).

literature to low- and high-grade AAH, with this latter group of more cellular lesions falling into the high-grade category. Although a number of studies have shown a greater frequency of malignancy-associated molecular changes in the higher-grade forms of AAH, others have shown no difference. There are no established criteria for categorising low- and high-grade AAH. Distinction between the more-cellular and atypical forms of AAH and localised nonmucinous BAC is discussed below (fig. 13).

Differential diagnosis: localised nonmucinous BAC

AAH is considered a precursor lesion of invasive adenocarcinoma arising in the lung parenchyma. It is believed that AAH develops into a lesion that is now defined in the WHO classification of lung tumours as a localised nonmucinous BAC. This lesion retains

Table 4. – Discriminatory features between atypical adenomatous hyperplasia (AAH) and bronchioloalveolar carcinoma (BAC)

Main features[#]	Additional features[¶]
Marked cell stratification	BACs are mostly >10 mm in diameter
High cell density with marked overlapping of nuclei	Cell population more homogeneous in BAC than in AAH
Coarse nuclear chromatin and prominent nucleoli	BAC shows sharp transition to normal lung
True papillae or cells growing in a picket fence-type arrangement	Larger BACs show central collapse of alveolar architecture with increased stroma
Tumour cell height is increased and tends to exceed that of the columnar cells in surrounding terminal bronchioles	

[#]: AAH rarely shows more than one of these, whereas BAC shows three or more; [¶]: may assist discrimination.

an intact alveolar architecture, and, although there may be evidence of collapse or compression of this alveolar structure with increased fibrosis [50], there is, by definition, no evidence of stromal invasion. Thus, this form of BAC could be considered adenocarcinoma *in situ*. It is believed that stromal invasion develops within the collapsed fibrotic areas, which are often central within a BAC lesion, and, when this occurs, the lesion is designated adenocarcinoma. In this way, AAH may be regarded as the adenoma in an adenoma–carcinoma sequence that defines peripheral lung adenocarcinogenesis.

Therefore, AAH and BAC are both lesions exhibiting an intact alveolar architecture lined with a population of atypical bronchioloalveolar cells. It seems likely that there is a continuous progression from AAH to BAC, and that distinction between the two is arbitrary, and yet necessary, at least for consistent classification. The distinction between the most-cellular form of AAH and BAC is a fine one, and is, to some extent, subjective, but criteria have been proposed by KERR and NOGUCHI [4] and incorporated into the WHO classification [51]. Of the five primary features noted in table 4, AAH lesions show no more than one, whereas BAC demonstrates three or more. Lesions that fulfil the criteria for BAC under this scheme are generally larger than AAH lesions, measuring ≥5 mm in diameter, with most measuring >15 mm. As well as being more cellular, crowded and atypical (fig. 14), the cell population in BAC tends to be more homogeneous and lacking the range of cytological appearance seen in AAH. Distinction from the surrounding lung is usually sharp in BAC, and expansion of the alveolar interstitium by collagen is the norm. Lymphocytic infiltrates in BAC are frequently substantial. Pure forms of localised nonmucinous BAC are rare lesions in pulmonary surgical pathological practice, although pathologists who deal with lesions excised after detection during spiral CT-based lung cancer screening programmes see this tumour more often.

Occasionally, at the margin of an invasive adenocarcinoma of mixed type, there may be a BAC component around the edge of a tumour which cytologically meets the criteria

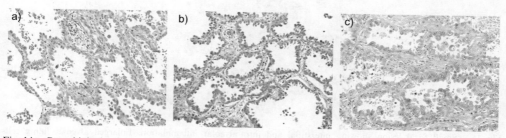

Fig. 14. – Bronchioloalveolar carcinoma (haematoxylin and eosin stain).

mentioned in table 4. In some lesions, however, such a zone of BAC may merge peripherally into alveoli that are lined with a cell population much more reminiscent of AAH. From a biological perspective, this could well represent residual AAH, from which the invasive tumour developed, and it would be perfectly reasonable to include in the report on such a tumour a description of the AAH-like component. To describe this appearance simply as AAH, however, could be misleading.

In the specific context of type I congenital cystic adenomatoid malformation, atypical mucous cells may be found focally lining alveolar walls adjacent to the cyst [52]. These cells have been suspected to be the source of mucinous BAC, which rarely occurs in association with this already rare condition, and there is genetic evidence to support this assertion [53].

Differential diagnosis: reactive changes, benign tumours and other proliferations

Reactive proliferation of type II pneumocytes may potentially be confused with AAH. It is well known that, in many inflammatory and fibrosing conditions affecting the alveolate lung, there may be marked proliferation of the alveolar epithelium, and the reactive nature of such a change is usually obvious when the other associated pathological changes are taken into account (fig. 15). This is also the reason why the WHO definition of AAH contains the statement "generally in the absence of underlying interstitial inflammation and fibrosis" [39].

A diagnosis of AAH cannot be made in the presence of established diffuse interstitial disease such as usual interstitial pneumonia. AAH lesions are discrete focal lesions in the vast majority of cases, and recognition of the lesion is extremely difficult, if not impossible, if the surrounding lung is abnormal. It is not unusual to find lymphocytic infiltrates, sometimes quite marked and even occasionally with germinal centres, in the interstitium of AAH. There may also be accompanying fibrosis. A useful distinction from interstitial pneumonia in such a case is the fact that, in AAH, the inflammation does not extend within alveolar walls beyond the limits of the lesion as defined by the alveolar

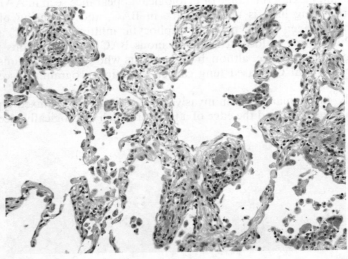

Fig. 15. – Small focal lesion showing interstitial and intra-alveolar inflammation. Enlarged alveolar lining cells are present, but this is reactive and not atypical adenomatous hyperplasia (haematoxylin and eosin stain).

epithelial lining. Sometimes reactive lesions lack much inflammation, but, when the epithelial population lining the alveoli is made up of a homogeneous population of regular cuboidal or low columnar cells with no gaps or peg cells and lacking atypia, a reactive lesion should be diagnosed (fig. 16).

When small localised lesions are found incidentally in the lung surrounding a resected cancer, some demonstrate a mixed inflammatory infiltrate filling alveoli and alveoli lined with runs of columnar epithelial cells. In the presence of alveolar airspace inflammation, a diagnosis of AAH should not be made. AAHs may show numerous macrophages in their airspaces but not active inflammation.

Peribronchiolar metaplasia may account for a localised centriacinar lesion in which alveoli are lined with columnar epithelial cells (fig. 17). These lesions, however, often show quite coarse peribronchiolar fibrosis, and the cell population lining the alveoli is essentially bronchiolar in type and normally shows ciliated cells. The parent bronchiole frequently exhibits a distorted configuration. Although this lesion is regarded as reactive and probably related to previous bronchiolar injury since it is seen as a late sequel to many diseases involving bronchiolitis, one study described atypia in such lesions, but the significance of this is uncertain and there is no good evidence to support any suggestion that peribronchiolar metaplasia is preneoplastic [54].

ULLMANN *et al.* [55] described a lesion that they called bronchiolar columnar cell dysplasia, and supported their contention that this lesion was preneoplastic by using comparative genomic hybridisation to demonstrate chromosomal aberrations in these lesions. This paper remains the only report of this lesion. More recently, WANG *et al.* [56] described nonsquamous lesions, such as basal cell dysplasia, columnar cell dysplasia and bronchial epithelial dysplasia, showing transitional differentiation. More descriptions and experience of these changes are needed before conclusions can be drawn regarding their nature.

Papillary and alveolar adenoma may also enter into the differential diagnosis [1]. Alveolar adenoma is a peripheral well-circumscribed tumour measuring ≤6 cm in diameter. This lesion is made up of spaces of variable size lined with a simple low cuboidal epithelium, but the interstitium shows a variably prominent spindle-cell rich stroma, and sometimes myxoid change. Squamous metaplasia may be seen lining the

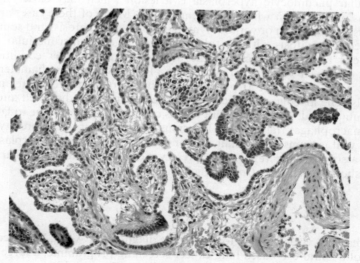

Fig. 16. – Reactive lesion with an unusual papillary configuration. Note the continuous runs of bland cuboidal cells, typical of some reactive lesions (haematoxylin and eosin stain).

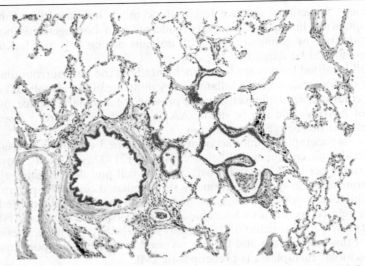

Fig. 17. – Peribronchiolar metaplasia (Lambertosis). This centriacinar lesion shows bronchiolisation of alveoli, airspaces are lined with nonatypical ciliated columnar epithelium (haematoxylin and eosin stain).

larger spaces. These spaces recapitulate alveoli, but do not have the configuration of the native alveoli of the lung as in AAH, and alveolar adenoma is a discrete and well-circumscribed, often lobulated, mass lesion. Papillary adenoma is, again, a circumscribed well-defined neoplasm, often with a granular brown to cream/white cut surface measuring 1–4 cm in diameter. The lesion shows a distinctive papillary architecture, with fibrovascular cores showing chronic inflammation lined with a generally regular population of cuboidal-to-columnar epithelial cells. Ciliated cells may be found. AAH lesions may show occasional epithelial cell tufts but true papillae are not a feature.

Micronodular pneumocyte hyperplasia is a lesion which may closely mimic more-cellular forms of AAH, but which is extremely rare. Many of these cases are associated with tuberous sclerosis with or without lymphangioleiomyomatosis, and some are seen in lymphangioleiomyomatosis without tuberous sclerosis, but micronodular pneumocyte hyperplasia can apparently occur in the absence of these other conditions [57–59]. Lesions tend to be well-demarcated nodules of a few millimetres in diameter made up of enlarged but nonatypical type II pneumocytes lining frequently cellular and thickened alveolar walls. The alveolar architecture may be collapsed or distorted and the lesions may appear quite solid, partly the result of this collapse and partly due to large numbers of airspace macrophages (fig. 18). AAH lesions exhibit larger and more atypical nuclei, and are less well circumscribed than micronodular pneumocyte hyperplasia, with less tendency to a solid architecture due to preservation of the native alveolar framework, which itself shows much less stromal thickening.

Cytology

Cytology has effectively no role to play in the diagnosis of AAH. Very occasionally, in the context of a spiral CT-based lung cancer screening programme, a large AAH lesion may be detected and percutaneous fine-needle aspiration biopsy performed. The cytological material derived from AAH, and even localised BAC, is not diagnostic, since

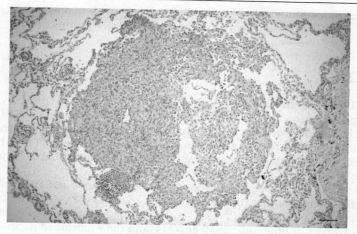

Fig. 18. – Focus of micronodular pneumocyte hyperplasia showing a more solid architecture than that of atypical adenomatous hyperplasia (haematoxylin and eosin stain). Scale bar=100µm.

diagnosis of these lesions depends upon assessment of the alveolar architecture and exclusion of an invasive adenocarcinoma component in the lesion. When faced with a sample showing bronchioloalveolar epithelial cells with atypical cytological features falling short of those required for a diagnosis of adenocarcinoma, use of the term "atypical bronchioloalveolar cell proliferation" is recommended [60].

Immunohistochemistry and other techniques in the differential diagnosis of AAH

Immunohistochemistry has little role to play in the diagnosis of an individual case of AAH. The cell population of AAH has the immunohistological features expected, given the presence of Clara cells and type II pneumocytes. AAH lesions express surfactant apoprotein A [61], whereas a few may express urine protein 1, a Clara cell marker. Urine protein 1 is said to show greater expression in BAC [47]. Thyroid transcription factor 1 is probably a good lineage marker for the epithelium of the terminal respiratory unit and alveoli, and is strongly expressed in AAH [62]. The expression of p53, human epidermal growth factor receptor 2, carcinoembryonic antigen and other oncoproteins increases during the transition from AAH to BAC, but these are not diagnostically useful [48]. It has recently been suggested that the p63 staining found in reactive lesions occurs less frequently in AAH or more advanced disease, but more data are required before this could be relied upon in diagnosis [63]. Cell cycle activity has been measured using antibodies directed against Ki-67 and minichromosome maintenance protein 2 (MCM2), and a progression of staining index was noted, even between low- and high-grade AAH, pure BAC and invasive adenocarcinomas [64, 65]. AAH lesions scored 0.5–2% using Ki-67 and 0.9–2.6% with MCM2, whereas pure BAC lesions tended to have higher mean scores, ~5–6% with Ki-67 and 11.5% with MCM2. Once again, in an individual case, this may be of limited value as a discriminatory test.

Several studies have sought differences between AAH and BAC based upon cell and nuclear size and cytofluorimetrically measured nuclear DNA content [66]. A progressive increase in mean nuclear area and DNA content was variably demonstrated between reactive hyperplasia, AAH, BAC and invasive adenocarcinoma in these studies. These data provide support for the neoplastic nature of AAH and its relationship to BAC, but these techniques are not mainstream enough for diagnostic use, and considerable overlap in individual results was found between the various study groups.

DIPNECH

DIPNECH is an extremely rare lesion [3, 67]. It is characterised by diffuse and widespread proliferation of PNECs, manifested by runs of basal PNECs in airway epithelium, clusters and nodules of airway PNECs, extension of neuroendocrine cells beyond the limits of the affected airway in association with fibrosis (so-called carcinoid tumourlets) and similar lesions measuring >5 mm in diameter that are thus defined as spindle-cell-type carcinoid tumours in the WHO classification [1]. Not all patients with DIPNECH exhibit such peripheral-type carcinoid tumours, but many do, hence its inclusion in the WHO classification as a precursor lesion.

Endobronchiolar nodules of PNECs and carcinoid tumourlets or the associated fibrosis may obstruct or obliterate small airways, and the widespread nature of this lesion leads to significant airflow limitation in patients and a clinical presentation resembling asthma or a diffuse interstitial lung disease (fig. 19). The disease predominates in females. Although the use of immunohistochemistry to demonstrate the neuroendocrine nature of the cells is rarely necessary, neuroendocrine markers such as chromogranin usually highlight foci of hyperplastic PNECs not appreciated on the haematoxylin and eosin-stained sections.

Differential diagnosis

As mentioned previously, the clinical presentation of DIPNECH can resemble bronchial asthma or a diffuse interstitial lung disease. Radiologically, there may be bilateral small nodules of variable size with evidence of air-trapping on CT due to small airways obstruction. Such an appearance has a broad differential diagnosis.

DIPNECH cannot be diagnosed without surgical lung biopsy, and when the above features are found, in the correct clinical context, the diagnosis is secure.

Widespread PNEC hyperplasia may be seen in a range of other circumstances, but any relationship to patients with DIPNECH is currently unclear. PNEC hyperplasia and

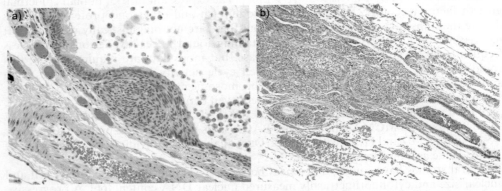

Fig. 19. – Diffuse idiopathic pulmonary neuroendocrine cell hyperplasia. a) Mural nodule of pulmonary neuroendocrine cells protruding into the airway lumen, and b) bronchiole obliterated by the nodule of spindle-shaped neuroendocrine cells, which extend beyond the limits of the airway, a tumourlet (haematoxylin and eosin stain).

carcinoid tumourlets are well-known accompanying features in lungs showing a range of fibro-inflammatory diseases, the most common of which is bronchiectasis [68]. Carcinoid tumours have not been described in such cases. In ~76% of patients with a peripheral spindle cell carcinoid tumour, carcinoid tumourlets and PNEC hyperplasia may be seen in the surrounding lung, in the absence of fibro-inflammatory disease [69]. These patients do not fit with the above description of DIPNECH, but, in this series of cases, some showed measurable airflow limitation that could not be attributed to chronic obstructive pulmonary disease, and the authors speculated that they may have a *forme fruste* of DIPNECH. Similar foci of PNEC hyperplasia and tumourlets may also be found as an incidental finding when examining lung tissue surgically excised for another reason, *e.g.* primary carcinoma (fig. 20).

There are few lesions that could be confused with PNEC hyperplasia and tumourlets. Minute meningothelial nodules are tiny collections of plump spindle cells that occur interstitially, giving a microscopic nodule in the alveolated lung (fig. 21). They are usually solitary incidental findings, are not associated with airways and are of no known clinical significance. If tumourlets become crushed they may be mistaken for lymphoid tissue or even metastatic foci of small cell carcinoma. Immunocytochemistry helps distinguish the former, but distinction from small cell carcinoma may be difficult if the clinical context is appropriate and uncrushed cells are absent. Although tumourlet cells may exhibit hyperchromatic nuclei, they are smaller and more fusiform than those of small cell carcinoma, and lack their characteristic stippled chromatin, apoptosis, mitoses and nuclear moulding.

Conclusion

The present chapter reviews those specific lesions, SD/CIS, AAH and DIPNECH, which are regarded as the precursors of a range of invasive tumours of the lung. The two former lesions are relatively common, but the latter is extremely rare. In the differential

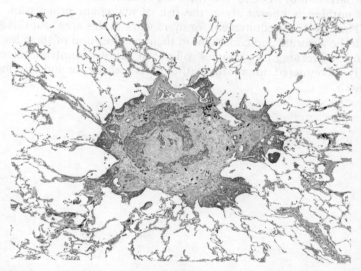

Fig. 20. – Carcinoid tumourlet, one of many in this lung, resected for metastatic adenocarcinoma. The airway is obliterated, the pulmonary arteriole remains at the upper margin of the lesion. There were no symptoms or physiology suggestive of diffuse idiopathic pulmonary neuroendocrine cell hyperplasia and background fibro-inflammatory disease was absent (haematoxylin and eosin stain).

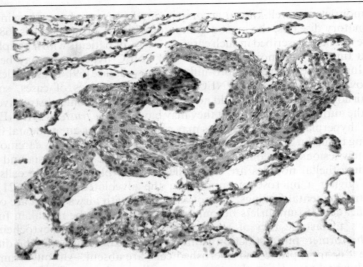

Fig. 21. – A small example of a minute meningothelial nodule. Interstitial clusters of plump spindle cells, typically with clear nuclei, characterise this lesion (haematoxylin and eosin stain).

diagnosis in each case, there are both benign lesions, with no risk of progression to malignancy, and lesions which are neoplastic, some of which are malignant. Some of these differential diagnoses are particularly challenging since published criteria are subjective and may be difficult to apply to the lesion under study. All of these lesions are small and prone to artefacts due to tissue handling.

Recognition of these lesions is important both for the individual patient and for a more general understanding of lesion biology and significance. There are some data on the risk and rate of progression of SD/CIS, but these are of limited value in any individual case. More or less nothing is known about the risk of malignant progression of AAH or DIPNECH. There is still a requirement for more work in this area, but this also requires pathologists to be accurate and consistent in their classification of these lesions. As and when lung cancer screening programmes roll out in various countries, these lesions will be increasingly encountered, improving pathologists' experience and offering opportunities for research.

Summary

Squamous dysplasia (SD)/carcinoma *in situ* (CIS) of the bronchus is a precursor lesion for bronchogenic squamous cell carcinoma. It is found most frequently in tobacco smokers, often associated with invasive carcinoma. It comprises a range of lesions of increasing atypia, with complex criteria for distinguishing mild, moderate and severe dysplasia and CIS based on abnormal cytology and architecture of a squamous-type epithelium. SD/CIS must be distinguished from basal cell hyperplasia and squamous metaplasia, themselves likely precursors of SD/CIS, from reactive atypia seen in a number of situations and from invasive squamous cell carcinoma. Lesions of SD/CIS are small, often incidental, findings in bronchial biopsy specimens, and published criteria are difficult to apply.

Atypical adenomatous hyperplasia (AAH) occurs in alveolated lung. It is the precursor of localised bronchioloalveolar carcinoma, and also of peripheral invasive adenocarcinoma. AAH lesions are small and consist of alveoli lined with atypical bronchioloalveolar cells. They most frequently occur in lung bearing invasive adenocarcinoma. AAH must be distinguished from reactive proliferations of type II pneumocytes associated with diffuse interstitial lung diseases or with localised fibro-inflammatory lesions. Distinction between AAH and bronchioloalveolar carcinoma is both important and challenging, and is based upon the degree of cellular atypia, stratification, crowding and increased cell size. Other differential diagnoses of AAH include micronodular pneumocyte hyperplasia, peribronchiolar metaplasia, and alveolar and papillary adenomas.

Diffuse idiopathic pulmonary neuroendocrine cell (PNEC) hyperplasia is an extremely rare condition, in which proliferation of PNECs forms multiple carcinoid tumourlets and fibrosis of airways leading to airflow limitation. Carcinoid tumours may also develop. Differential diagnoses include other forms of PNEC hyperplasia, either incidental in occurrence or associated with fibro-inflammatory diseases, such as bronchiectasis. The relationship between these other forms of PNEC hyperplasia and carcinoid tumours is unclear.

Keywords: Atypical adenomatous hyperplasia, differential diagnosis, diffuse idiopathic neuroendocrine cell hyperplasia, lung, preneoplasia, squamous dysplasia/carcinoma *in situ*.

References

1. Travis WD, Brambilla E, Muller-Hermelink HK, Harris CC, eds. World Health Organization Classification of Tumours. Pathology and Genetics of Tumours of the Lung, Pleura, Thymus and Heart. Lyon, IARC press, 2004.

2. Kerr KM, AE Fraire. Preinvasive diseases of the lung. *In*: Tomashefski J, Farver C, Cagle P, Fraire A, eds. Dail and Hammer's Pulmonary Pathology. New York, NY, Springer, 2007 (in press).

3. Gosney JR, Travis WD. Diffuse idiopathic pulmonary neuroendocrine cell hyperplasia. *In*: Travis WD, Brambilla E, Muller-Hermelink HK, Harris CC, eds. World Health Organization Classification of Tumours. Pathology and Genetics of Tumours of the Lung, Pleura, Thymus and Heart. Lyon, IARC press, 2004; pp. 76–77.

4. Kerr KM, Noguchi M. Pathology of screen-detected lesions. *In*: Hirsch FR, Bunn PA Jr, Kato H,

Mulshine JL, eds. IASLC Textbook on Prevention and Early Detection of Lung Cancer. London, Martin Dunitz Publishers, 2005; pp. 245–267.

5. Franklin WA, Wistuba II, Geisinger K, *et al.* Squamous dysplasia and carcinoma *in situ*. *In*: Travis WD, Brambilla E, Muller-Hermelink HK, Harris CC, eds. World Health Organization Classification of Tumours. Pathology and Genetics of Tumours of the Lung, Pleura, Thymus and Heart. Lyon, IARC press, 2004; pp. 68–72.

6. Lam S, MacAulay C, LeRiche JC, Palcic B. Detection and localization of early lung cancer by fluorescence bronchoscopy. *Cancer* 2000; 89: 2468–2473.

7. Lam S, Kennedy T, Unger M, *et al.* Localization of bronchial intraepithelial lesions by fluorescence bronchoscopy. *Chest* 1998; 113: 696–702.

8. Lam S, LeRiche JC, Zheng Y, *et al.* Sex-related differences in bronchial epithelial changes associated with tobacco smoking. *J Natl Cancer Inst* 1999; 91: 691–696.

9. Nagamoto N, Saito Y, Sato M, *et al.* Clinicopathological analysis of 19 cases of isolated carcinoma *in situ* of the bronchus. *Am J Surg Pathol* 1993; 17: 1234–1243.

10. Hirsch FR, Prindiville SA, Miller YE, *et al.* Fluorescence *versus* white-light bronchoscopy for detection of preneoplastic lesions: a randomised study. *J Natl Cancer Inst* 2001; 93: 1385–1391.

11. Jeanmart M, Lantuejoul S, Fievet F, *et al.* Value of immunohistochemical markers in preinvasive bronchial lesions in risk assessment of lung cancer. *Clin Cancer Res* 2003; 9: 2195–2203.

12. Spencer H, Dail DH, Arneaud J. Non-invasive bronchial epithelial papillary tumors. *Cancer* 1980; 45: 1486–1497.

13. Brambilla E, Moro D, Veale D, *et al.* Basal cell (basaloid) carcinoma of the lung. A new morphologic and phenotypic entity with separate prognostic significance. *Hum Pathol* 1992; 23: 993–1003.

14. Fisseler-Eckhoff A, Prebeg M, Voss B, Muller KM. Extracellular matrix in preneoplastic lesions and early cancer of the lung. *Pathol Res Pract* 1990; 186: 95–101.

15. Keith RL, Miller YE, Gemmill RM, *et al.* Angiogenic squamous dysplasia in bronchi of individuals at high risk for lung cancer. *Clin Cancer Res* 2000; 6: 1616–1625.

16. Lantuejoul S, Constantin B, Drabkin H, Brambilla C, Roche J, Brambilla E. Expression of VEGF, semaphorin SEMA3F, and their common receptors neuropilins NP1 and NP2 in preinvasive bronchial lesions, lung tumours, and cell lines. *J Pathol* 2003; 200: 336–347.

17. Merrick DT, Haney J, Petrunich S, *et al.* Overexpression of vascular endothelial growth factor and its receptors in bronchial dysplasia demonstrated by quantitative RT-PCR analysis. *Lung Cancer* 2005; 48: 31–45.

18. Nettesheim P, Klein-Szanto AJP, Yarita T. Experimental models for the study of morphogenesis of lung cancer. *In*: Shimosato Y, Melamed MR, Nettesheim P, eds. Morphogenesis of Lung Cancer. Vol. 2. Boca Raton, FL, CRC Press, 1982; pp. 131–166.

19. Calderon-Garciduenas L, Rodriguez-Alcaraz A, Villarreal-Calderon A, Lyght O, Janszen D, Morgan KT. Nasal epithelium as a sentinel for airborne environmental pollution. *Toxicol Sci* 1998; 46: 352–364.

20. Gong H Jr, Fligiel S, Tashkin DP, Barbers RG. Tracheobronchial changes in habitual, heavy smokers of marijuana with and without tobacco. *Am Rev Respir Dis* 1987; 136: 142–149.

21. Saccomanno G, Saunders RP, Archer VE, Auerbach O, Kuschner M, Becklake PA. Cancer of the lung: the cytology of sputum prior to the development of carcinoma. *Acta Cytol* 1965; 9: 413–423.

22. Mayne ST, Redlich CA, Cullen MR. Dietary vitamin A and prevalence of bronchial metaplasia in asbestos-exposed workers. *Am J Clin Nutr* 1998; 68: 630–635.

23. Saccomanno G, Archer VE, Auerbach O, Saunders RP, Brennan LM. Development of carcinoma of the lung as reflected in exfoliated cells. *Cancer* 1974; 33: 256–270.

24. Tao LC, Chamberlain DW, Delarue NC, Pearson FG, Donat EE. Cytologic diagnosis of radiographically occult squamous cell carcinoma of the lung. *Cancer* 1982; 50: 1580–1586.

25. Anon. Early lung cancer detection: summary and conclusions. *Am Rev Respir Dis* 1984; 130: 565–570.

26. Fisseler-Eckhoff A, Rothstein D, Muller KM. Neovascularisation in hyperplastic, metaplastic and potentially preneoplastic lesions of the bronchial mucosa. *Virchows Arch* 1996; 429: 95–100.

27. Pendleton N, Dixon GR, Green JA, Myskow MW. Expression of markers of differentiation in normal bronchial epithelium and bronchial dysplasia. *J Pathol* 1996; 178: 146–150.

28. Khuri FR, Lee JS, Lippman SM, *et al.* Modulation of proliferating cell nuclear antigen in the bronchial epithelium of smokers. *Cancer Epidemiol Biomarkers Prev* 2001; 10: 311–318.

29. Hirano T, Franzen B, Kato H, Ebihara Y, Auer G. Genesis of squamous cell lung carcinoma. Sequential changes of proliferation, DNA ploidy and p53 expression. *Am J Pathol* 1994; 144: 296–302.

30. Venmans BJ, Van der Linden JC, Elbers JRJ, *et al.* Observer variability in histopathological reporting of bronchial biopsy specimens: influence on the results of autofluorescence bronchoscopy in detection of bronchial neoplasia. *J Bronchol* 2000; 7: 210–214.

31. Nicholson AG, Perry LJ, Cury PM, *et al.* Reproducibility of the WHO/IASLC grading system for pre-invasive squamous lesions of the bronchus: a study of inter-observer and intra-observer variation. *Histopathology* 2001; 38: 202–208.

32. Venmans BJ, van Boxem TJ, Smit EF, Postmus PE, Sutedja TG. Outcome of bronchial carcinoma *in situ*. *Chest* 2000; 117: 1572–1576.

33. Bota S, Auliac J-B, Paris C, *et al.* Follow-up of bronchial precancerous lesions and carcinoma *in situ* using fluorescence endoscopy. *Am J Crit Care Med* 2001; 164: 1688–1693.

34. Banerjee AK, Rabbitts PH, George J. Lung cancer. 3: Fluorescence bronchoscopy: clinical dilemmas and research opportunities. *Thorax* 2003; 58: 266–271.

35. Brambilla E, Gazzeri S, Lantuejoul S, *et al.* p53 mutant immunophenotype and deregulation of p53 transcription pathway (Bcl2, Bax and Waf1) in precursor bronchial lesions of lung cancer. *Clin Cancer Res* 1998; 4: 1609–1618.

36. Brambilla E, Gazzeri S, Moro D, Lantuejoul S, Veyrenc S, Brambilla C. Alterations of Rb pathway (Rb-p16^{INK4}-cyclin D1) in preinvasive bronchial lesions. *Clin Cancer Res* 1999; 5: 243–250.

37. Ponticiello A, Barra E, Giani U, Bocchino M, Sanduzzi A. P53 immunohistochemistry can identify bronchial dysplastic lesions proceeding to lung cancer: a prospective study. *Eur Respir J* 2000; 15: 547–552.

38. Sozzi G, Oggionni M, Alasio L, *et al.* Molecular changes track recurrence and progression of bronchial precancerous lesions. *Lung Cancer* 2002; 37: 267–270.

39. Kerr KM, Fraire AE, Pugatch B, Vazquez MF, Kitamura H, Niho S. Atypical adenomatous hyperplasia. *In*: Travis WD, Brambilla E, Muller-Hermelink HK, Harris CC, eds. World Health Organization Classification of Tumours. Pathology and Genetics of Tumours of the Lung, Pleura, Thymus and Heart. Lyon, IARC press, 2004; pp. 73–75.

40. Weng S-Y, Tsuchiya E, Kasuga T, Sugano H. Incidence of atypical bronchioloalveolar cell hyperplasia of the lung: relation to histological subtypes of lung cancer. *Virchows Arch A Pathol Anat Histopathol* 1992; 420: 463–471.

41. Nakahara R, Yokose T, Nagai K, Nishiwaki Y, Ochiai A. Atypical adenomatous hyperplasia of the lung: a clinicopathological study of 118 cases including cases with multiple atypical adenomatous hyperplasia. *Thorax* 2001; 56: 302–305.

42. Koga T, Hashimoto S, Sugio K, *et al.* Lung adenocarcinoma with bronchioloalveolar carcinoma component is frequently associated with foci of high-grade atypical adenomatous hyperplasia. *Am J Clin Pathol* 2002; 117: 464–470.

43. Chapman AD, Kerr KM. The association between atypical adenomatous hyperplasia and primary lung cancer. *Br J Cancer* 2000; 83: 632–636.

44. Miller RR. Bronchioloalveolar cell adenomas. *Am J Surg Pathol* 1990; 14: 904–912.

45. Anami Y, Matsuno Y, Yamada T, *et al.* A case of double primary adenocarcinoma of the lung with multiple atypical adenomatous hyperplasia. *Pathol Int* 1998; 48: 634–640.

46. Nakanishi K. Alveolar epithelial hyperplasia and adenocarcinoma of the lung. *Arch Pathol Lab Med* 1990; 114: 363–368.

47. Kitamura H, Kameda Y, Ito T, *et al.* Cytodifferentiation of atypical adenomatous hyperplasia and bronchioloalveolar lung carcinoma: immunohistochemical and ultrastructural studies. *Virchows Arch* 1997; 431: 415–424.

48. Kerr KM. Morphology and genetics of preinvasive pulmonary disease. *Curr Diagn Pathol* 2004; 10: 259–268.

49. Kitamura H, Kameda Y, Nakamura N, *et al.* Atypical adenomatous hyperplasia and bronchoalveolar lung carcinoma. Analysis by morphometry and the expressions of p53 and carcinoembryonic antigen. *Am J Surg Pathol* 1996; 20: 553–562.

50. Noguchi M, Morokawa A, Kawasaki M, *et al.* Small adenocarcinoma of the lung. Histologic characteristics and prognosis. *Cancer* 1995; 75: 2844–2852.

51. Colby TV, Noguchi M, Henschke C, *et al.* Adenocarcinoma. *In*: Travis WD, Brambilla E, Muller-Hermelink HK, Harris CC, eds. World Health Organization Classification of Tumours. Pathology and Genetics of Tumours of the Lung, Pleura, Thymus and Heart. Lyon, IARC press, 2004; pp. 35–44.

52. Sheffield EA, Addis BJ, Corrin B, McCabe MM. Epithelial hyperplasia and malignant change in congenital lung cysts. *J Clin Pathol* 1987; 40: 612–614.

53. Stacher E, Ullmann R, Halbwedl I, *et al.* Atypical goblet cell hyperplasia in congenital cystic adenomatoid malformation as a possible preneoplasia for pulmonary adenocarcinoma in childhood: a genetic analysis. *Hum Pathol* 2004; 35: 565–570.

54. Jensen-Taubman SM, Steinberg SM, Linnoila RI. Bronchiolization of the alveoli in lung cancer: pathology, patterns of differentiation and oncogene expression. *Int J Cancer* 1998; 75: 489–496.

55. Ullmann R, Bongiovanni M, Halbwedl I, *et al.* Bronchiolar columnar cell dysplasia–genetic analysis of a novel preneoplastic lesion of peripheral lung. *Virchows Arch* 2003; 442: 429–436.

56. Wang GF, Lai MD, Yang RR, *et al.* Histological types and significance of bronchial epithelial dysplasia. *Mod Pathol* 2006; 19: 429–437.

57. Popper HH, Juettner-Smolle FM, Pongratz MG. Micronodular hyperplasia of type II pneumocytes – a new lung lesion associated with tuberous sclerosis. *Histopathol* 1991; 18: 347–354.

58. Lantuejoul S, Ferretti G, Negoescu A, Parent B, Brambilla E. Multifocal alveolar hyperplasia associated with lymphangioleiomyomatosis in tuberous sclerosis. *Histopathology* 1997; 30: 570–575.

59. Muir TE, Leslie KO, Popper H, *et al.* Micronodular pneumocyte hyperplasia. *Am J Surg Pathol* 1998; 22: 465–472.

60. Flieder DB. Screen-detected adenocarcinomas of the lung. Practical points for surgical pathologists. *Am J Clin Pathol* 2003; 119: Suppl. 1, S1–S19.

61. Mori M, Tezuka F, Chiba R, *et al.* Atypical adenomatous hyperplasia and adenocarcinoma of the human lung: their heterology in form and analogy in immunohistochemical characteristics. *Cancer* 1996; 77: 665–674.

62. Stenhouse G, Fyfe N, King G, Chapman A, Kerr KM. Thyroid transcription factor 1 in pulmonary adenocarcinoma. *J Clin Pathol* 2004; 57: 383–387.

63. Sheik HA, Fuhrer K, Cieply K, Yousem S. p63 expression in assessment of bronchioloalveolar proliferations of the lung. *Mod Pathol* 2004; 17: 1134–1140.

64. Kitamura H, Kameda Y, Nakamura N, *et al.* Proliferative potential and p53 overexpression in precursor and early stage lesions of bronchioloalveolar lung carcinoma. *Am J Pathol* 1995; 146: 876–887.

65. Kerr KM, Fyfe N, Chapman AD, Nicolson MC, Coleman N. Cell cycle marker MCM2 in peripheral lung adenocarcinoma and its precursors. *Lung Cancer* 2003; 41: Suppl. 2, S15.

66. Kerr KM. Pulmonary preinvasive neoplasia. *J Clin Pathol* 2001; 54: 257–271.

67. Aguayo SM, Miller YE, Waldron JA, *et al.* Idiopathic diffuse hyperplasia of pulmonary neuroendocrine cells and airway disease. *N Engl J Med* 1992; 327: 1285–1288.

68. Churg A, Warnock ML. Pulmonary tumourlet. A form of peripheral carcinoid. *Cancer* 1976; 37: 1469–1477.

69. Miller RR, Muller NL. Neuroendocrine cell hyperplasia and obliterative bronchiolitis in patients with peripheral carcinoid tumours. *Am J Surg Pathol* 1995; 19: 653–658.

CHAPTER 4

New concepts in pulmonary oncology

R. Pirker*, H.H. Popper#

*Dept of Internal Medicine I, Medical University of Vienna, Vienna, and #Dept of Pathology, Laboratories for Molecular Cytogenetics, Environment and Respiratory Pathology, Medical University of Graz, Graz, Austria.

Correspondence: R. Pirker, Dept of Internal Medicine I, Medical University of Vienna, Währinger Gürtel 18, A-1090 Vienna, Austria. Fax: 43 1404004461; E-mail: robert.pirker@meduniwien.ac.at

Significant progress has been achieved since the early 1990s in the systemic treatment of lung cancer, particularly nonsmall cell lung cancer (NSCLC). Palliative chemotherapy of advanced NSCLC has been recognised as standard treatment since the mid 1990s [1]. Palliation of symptoms can be achieved in ~50% of symptomatic patients, and cisplatin-based protocols lead to an absolute increase in the 1-yr survival rate of ~10% compared with best supportive care alone [1, 2]. Further progress was achieved with the clinical introduction of the third-generation anticancer drugs, vinorelbine, gemcitabine, paclitaxel and docetaxel. Platinum-based doublets with either of the third-generation drugs are now considered standard protocols for the chemotherapy of advanced NSCLC [2, 3]. Three-drug combinations might increase response rates at the expense of increased toxicity without improving survival [4]. According to the American Society of Clinical Oncology guidelines [2], first-line chemotherapy of four cycles is recommended, and six cycles should not be exceeded. Chemotherapy should particularly be withheld after four cycles in those patients who only show stable disease during chemotherapy. Elderly patients and patients with poor performance status also benefit from palliative chemotherapy, but regimens with good tolerability should be preferred for these patients. Important issues to be clarified include the optimal type of platinum (cisplatin or carboplatin), the role of nonplatinum-containing regimens and the role of maintenance therapy in responding patients.

Second-line chemotherapy with either docetaxel or pemetrexed has also been established [5–7]. Docetaxel improves cancer-related symptoms and prolongs survival compared with best supportive care in patients previously treated with platinum-based chemotherapy [5,6]. Pemetrexed shows similar efficacy but improved tolerance compared to docetaxel [7].

Chemotherapy combined with local treatments (surgery, radiotherapy or both) is part of the treatment of stage III NSCLC. In patients receiving definitive chemoradiotherapy, improvement in outcome is attempted by the inclusion of induction chemotherapy, consolidation chemotherapy or surgery.

Another major clinical advance has been the establishment of adjuvant chemotherapy in patients with completely resected NSCLC since the beginning of the 21st Century [8, 9]. Further progress is expected with the characterisation of those patients who benefit from adjuvant chemotherapy. A better understanding of the tumour cell biology resulting in a more aggressive phenotype might help to identify patients with a high risk of recurrence and lead to new treatment strategies.

Topotecan has recently been established as second-line chemotherapy in patients with small cell lung cancer (SCLC). Oral topotecan improved survival in pre-treated patients compared to best supportive care alone [10], and intravenous topotecan resulted in

Eur Respir Mon, 2007, 39, 63–84. Printed in UK - all rights reserved. Copyright ERS Journals Ltd 2007; European Respiratory Monograph; ISSN 1025-448x.

similar survival but improved tolerability in comparison with cyclophosphamide/ doxorubicin/cisplatin [11]. Several anticancer drugs, including irinotecan and oxaliplatin, are currently being evaluated within clinical trials.

Customised chemotherapy is another approach to improving outcome, reducing toxicity and saving costs. One strategy is to evaluate enzymes involved in DNA repair, such as DNA excision repair protein ERCC-1, and use them for guiding chemotherapy [12].

Progress has also been achieved in supportive care measures. In particular, the routine use of erythropoietic proteins in patients with cancer-related anaemia has led to a major improvement in the quality of life for patients with lung cancer [13].

Targeted therapies

Targeted therapy has become an intensive area of research, and several targeted therapies are undergoing clinical evaluation. Targeted therapies include interference with growth factors and their receptors, inhibition of angiogenesis, tumour vaccines and other strategies. These strategies can be used alone or in combination with chemotherapy or radiotherapy.

Growth factors and growth factor receptors

Growth factors and their receptors are involved in the proliferation of tumours cells. Thus blockade of their function, by either neutralising ligands, inhibition of ligand binding or blocking the tyrosine kinase function of the receptor, could improve clinical outcome. The epidermal growth factor (EGF)/EGF receptor (EGFR) and vascular endothelial growth factor (VEGF)/VEGF receptor (VEGFR) systems are the targets that have already been successfully used in the treatment of lung cancer.

EGFR

The rationale for using the EGFR as a target is its frequent expression in NSCLC (40–80%) and the association of EGFR expression with invasion, metastasis and poor prognosis (reviewed in [14]). EGFR-directed tyrosine kinase inhibitors (TKIs) have either been licensed or are undergoing clinical development. Monoclonal antibodies are currently in various stages of clinical development, including phase III trials.

Gefitinib. In initial phase II trials, gefitinib (Iressa®, AstraZeneca, UK; 250 or 500 mg daily) as a single agent improved symptoms in ~40% of patients with advanced NSCLC previously pre-treated with one (Iressa Dose Evaluation in Advanced Lung Cancer (IDEAL)-1) or at least two (IDEAL-2) chemotherapy protocols [15, 16]. Symptom improvement was rapid and associated with tumour response and survival. The response rates were 12 and 19%, respectively, and the disease control rates (complete and partial response plus stable disease) were slightly >50%. Response rates were higher in females, patients with adenocarcinomas, never-smokers and Japanese patients. No differences in activity were seen between the two gefitinib doses, but, because of better tolerability, the 250-mg dose was selected for further study.

Since the IDEAL trials did not include a control arm, a randomised placebo-controlled phase III trial (Iressa Survival Evaluation in Lung Cancer (ISEL)) was subsequently performed on a large patient population (n=1,692) [17]. In order to be eligible, patients with advanced NSCLC had either to be refractory or to progress within 90 days following chemotherapy. This randomised trial failed to show a significant survival benefit for gefitinib (250 mg daily), although a subgroup analysis suggested a benefit for never-smokers and patients of Southeast Asian heritage [17].

Erlotinib. In a randomised placebo-controlled phase III trial enrolling 731 patients previously pre-treated with chemotherapy (488 in erlotinib (Tarceva®, OSI Pharmaceuticals, Inc., Melville, NY, USA) group; 243 in placebo group), erlotinib, at a dose of 150 mg daily, significantly increased survival in comparison with placebo (median 6.7 *versus* 4.7 months; 1-yr survival rate 31 *versus* 22%; hazard ratio 0.7) [18]. Progression-free survival was also increased in the erlotinib group (median 2.2 *versus* 1.8 months). The corresponding response rates were 9 and <1%, respectively. The response rates were higher in never-smokers, females, Japanese patients and patients with adenocarcinomas. The disease control rate (complete and partial response plus stable disease) was 45%. Deterioration of symptoms was delayed in the erlotinib group. Dose reductions were required in 19% of the patients. The major side-effects were skin rash and diarrhoea.

Mutations of the EGFR gene were associated with better prognosis in both the erlotinib and the placebo group, but these mutations did not predict response to erlotinib [18, 19]. Predictors of clinical benefit were never-smokers, adenocarcinomas, females and EGFR overexpression [18, 19]. Skin rash was also associated with better response to erlotinib.

TKIs combined with chemotherapy. In order to determine whether the addition of TKIs improves the outcome of palliative chemotherapy in patients with advanced NSCLC, both gefitinib (Iressa NSCLC Trial Assessing Combination Treatment (INTACT) 1 and 2) and erlotinib (TArceva Lung cancEr iNvesTigation (TALENT) and Tarceva® Responses in Conjunction with Paclitaxel and Carboplatin (TRIBUTE)) were evaluated in combination with either gemcitabine/cisplatin (INTACT 1 and TALENT) or paclitaxel/carboplatin (INTACT 2 and TRIBUTE) [20–23]. None of these randomised trials could demonstrate a survival advantage for chemotherapy plus TKI in comparison to chemotherapy alone. One of the explanations for these rather unexpected findings is that TKI-mediated blockade of cell growth does not permit anticancer drugs to exert their full activity.

Predictors of response. Great attention is currently being given to potential predictors of response to TKIs [24–26]. Initially, retrospective studies on low patient numbers suggested that specific mutations in the EGFR gene determined response to TKIs. Other trials indicated that female sex, adenocarcinoma, Asian heritage, being a never-smoker and EGFR overexpression might predict benefit from TKIs. Thus these parameters might help to select patients for treatment with EGFR-directed TKIs.

Further evaluation of TKIs. TKIs are currently being further evaluated in patients with NSCLC. In the palliative setting, TKIs are being studied as maintenance therapy following first-line chemotherapy, as first-line therapy in specific patient populations (*e.g.* elderly patients and patients with specific EGFR alterations) and as second-line therapy. In patients with completely resected NSCLC, erlotinib following adjuvant chemotherapy will be compared with adjuvant chemotherapy alone. Gefitinib maintenance therapy following chemoradiotherapy for stage III NSCLC not only failed to improve outcome but also might even be detrimental in this particular clinical setting [27]. This finding, together with the negative results of phase III trials of gefitinib in advanced disease, resulted in premature closure of the adjuvant trial with gefitinib.

Monoclonal antibodies against EGFR. Several monoclonal antibodies directed against the EGFR are undergoing clinical development. They include cetuximab (Erbitux®, Merck KGaA, Damstadt, Germany), matuzumab (EMD 72000) and panitumumab (ABX-EGF).

Monoclonal antibodies block EGF binding, lead to internalisation and degradation of the EGFR, and also act *via* immunological mechanisms such as antibody-dependent cellular cytotoxicity.

Cetuximab, the chimeric version of monoclonal antibody M225, is an immunoglobulin (Ig) G1 monoclonal antibody [14]. Cetuximab, in combination with platinum-based regimens, has demonstrated anti-tumour activity in pre-clinical studies [14]. The effect of cetuximab, both as single agent and in combination with chemotherapy or radiotherapy, was investigated in several NSCLC cell lines (squamous and adenocarcinoma) exhibiting high (H226), moderate (A549 and H157) and low (H322) EGFR expression. Cetuximab monotherapy was found to inhibit growth of cells with high EGFR expression. Synergistic/additive effects were seen with cetuximab plus radiotherapy and cetuximab plus chemotherapy in highly/moderately EGFR-expressing cells. On the basis of these promising pre-clinical data, cetuximab is currently being evaluated for use either as single agent or in combination with chemotherapy in advanced NSCLC, and in combination with radiotherapy or chemoradiotherapy in stage III NSCLC.

Several phase II trials of cetuximab in combination with palliative chemotherapy have been performed [28–30]. The randomised phase II trial in previously untreated advanced EGFR-positive NSCLC suggested that cisplatin/vinorelbine plus cetuximab might be superior to chemotherapy alone [28]. The corresponding phase III trial (study of cisplatin/vinorelbine +/- cetuximab as first-line treatment of EGFR expressing advanced NSCLC) in patients with advanced EGFR-positive NSCLC recently completed patient accrual after >1,100 patients had been randomised, and the results of this pivotal trial are expected in 2007.

Panitumumab, a fully human IgG2 monoclonal antibody directed against the EGFR, has shown promising activity in combination with carboplatin/paclitaxel in advanced NSCLC [31].

Human epidermal growth factor receptor 2/human epidermal growth factor receptor 2neu as target

Trials with trastuzumab (Herceptin™) in patients with advanced NSCLC indicate that the clinical usefulness of trastuzumab is limited due to the low frequency of tumours showing high human epidermal growth factor receptor 2 (HER2)/neu expression (the various expression levels are defined in several original articles) [32–34]. In a randomised trial enrolling 103 patients with HER2-positive NSCLC IIIB–IV, patients received cisplatin/gemcitabine with or without trastuzumab (2 $mg \cdot kg^{-1}$ weekly). HER2 positivity was defined using immunohistochemistry (2+, 3+), fluorescence *in situ* hybridisation (FISH) or HER2 serum levels (>15 $ng \cdot mL^{-1}$). HER2 expression of 2+ was observed in 90% of the tumours. No differences were seen between the two groups with regard to response rates (41 *versus* 32%) and time to disease progression (median 7.2 *versus* 6.3 months). Thus the authors concluded that trastuzumab, due to only moderate HER2 overexpression, does not have a major impact on the outcome of palliative chemotherapy in advanced NSCLC.

In another study on 279 patients with NSCLC IIIB/IV, HER2 expression was 1+ in 12%, 2+ in 10% and 3+ in only 5% of the tumours [33]. Therefore, only 21 patients received the planned treatment of gemcitabine/cisplatin plus trastuzumab, and the partial response rate was 40% in this small patient population. Another study found HER2 expression in 64% of 139 screened patients, but 3+ expression in only 9% of the tumours [34]. Patients (n=56) were treated with paclitaxel/carboplatin plus trastuzumab (4 $mg \cdot kg^{-1}$ loading dose and then 2 $mg \cdot kg^{-1}$ weekly). The outcome (response rate 24.5%; median survival 10 months; 1-yr survival rate 42%) was similar to those of other trials with paclitaxel/carboplatin alone. However, patients with 3+ tumours exhibited better outcome, suggesting a benefit of trastuzumab in these patients; however, further clinical evaluation in these patients will be difficult because of their small number.

Angiogenesis inhibitors

Angiogenesis plays a major role in the growth of tumours, and, therefore, inhibition of this process should improve clinical outcome in patients with cancer [35]. Angiogenesis is regulated by VEGFRs expressed on endothelial cells. VEGFR ligands (VEGF-A, -B, -C and -D, and placenta growth factor) bind to the receptor and activate the intracellular kinase activity of specific VEGFRs.

Several angiogenesis inhibitors are undergoing clinical evaluation. One strategy is to block the VEGF/VEGFR pathway, using either monoclonal antibodies (anti-VEGF or anti-VEGFR), ribozymes or VEGFR-directed TKIs. Other inhibitors of angiogenesis include sorafenib, metalloproteinase inhibitors and thalidomide.

Bevacizumab: antibody against VEGF. Bevacizumab is a humanised monoclonal antibody directed against VEGF-A. In a phase II trial, bevacizumab improved the outcome of first-line chemotherapy with paclitaxel/carboplatin in patients with advanced NSCLC [36]. However, fatal bleedings occurred, primarily in patients with centrally located tumours and/or squamous cell carcinomas. Thus the subsequent phase III trials excluded patients with squamous histology, centrally located tumours, brain metastasis and history of bleeding. The first of these phase III trials enrolled 878 chemonaive patients and demonstrated that paclitaxel/carboplatin plus bevacizumab (15 mg·kg^{-1} intravenously every 3 weeks) increased the response rate (35 *versus* 15%), progression-free survival (6.2 *versus* 4.5 months) and survival (median 12.3 *versus* 10.3 months) compared with chemotherapy alone in selected patients with advanced NSCLC [37]. Side-effects of bevacizumab are hypertension, thrombovascular events and bleeding. This favourable result led to carboplatin/paclitaxel plus bevacizumab being the new Eastern Cooperative Oncology Group standard for palliative chemotherapy of advanced NSCLC. The second phase III trial (Avastin in Lung Cancer (AVAiL)) is still ongoing and is evaluating gemcitabine/cisplatin +/- bevacizumab in selected patients with advanced nonsquamous NSCLC.

In light of its activity in advanced NSCLC, bevacizumab in combination with chemotherapy will be evaluated in the adjuvant setting, in patients with stage III NSCLC, as part of first-line chemotherapy in patients with squamous cell NSCLC and in the second-line setting.

Bevacizumab in combination with erlotinib gave promising results in patients with advanced NSCLC [38]. Rationales for this combination are at least additive effects of both drugs in pre-clinical studies and a broader targeted approach.

Low-molecular-weight drugs. ZD6474 is a TKI directed against both the EGFR and VEGFR. In a randomised phase II trial in patients previously treated with chemotherapy, ZD6474 resulted in longer progression-free survival than gefitinib [39]. In a phase II trial in patients with refractory NSCLC, ZD6474 plus docetaxel prolonged the median time to disease progression compared with docetaxel alone [40].

Matrix metalloproteinase inhibitors

Matrix metalloproteinases (MMPs) digest extracellular proteins and are frequently expressed in cancers including lung cancer. Although pre-clinical studies suggested that inhibitors of metalloproteinase could inhibit tumour growth, clinical phase III trials failed to demonstrate a benefit [41–43]. Patients with SCLC responding to first-line chemotherapy did not benefit from maintenance therapy with marimastat but suffered from clinically relevant side-effects [41]. Similarly, prinomastat or BMS-275291 did not improve survival when added to first-line chemotherapy in patients with advanced NSCLC [42, 43]. One explanation for the lack of clinical efficacy of MMP inhibitors is that inhibition of a small number of the many MMPs does not translate into a clinical benefit. Therefore, a better understanding of the biology and clinical relevance of the MMP system is required before further clinical trials with these agents are justified.

Farnesyl transferase inhibitors

Farnesyl transferase is involved in the post-translational modification of several proteins, including Ras proteins, which transduce tyrosine kinase activation to downstream cytoplasmic and nuclear effectors. Activating ras mutations have been observed in ~40% of NSCLCs, and, through constitutive signalling, lead to cell proliferation and inhibition of apoptosis [44, 45]. Inhibition of farnesyl transferase should inhibit ras function and might improve outcome in NSCLC [46]. In a phase III trial, however, the farnesyl transferase inhibitor lonafarnib did not improve the outcome of palliative chemotherapy with carboplatin/paclitaxel in patients with advanced NSCLC [46].

Protein kinase C as target

Aprinocarsen is an antisense oligonucleotide directed against protein kinase C-α. In a phase III trial in 670 patients with previously untreated stage IIIB/IV NSCLC, the addition of aprinocarsen (2 mg·kg^{-1}·day^{-1}, continuous infusion for 14 days) did not improve the outcome of palliative chemotherapy with gemcitabine/cisplatin [47]. Grade 3 and 4 toxicities were significantly increased for thrombocytopenia, epistaxis and thrombosis/embolism in the experimental arm.

Bexarotene

Bexarotene binds to retinoid receptor X and modulates tumour proliferation. In two phase III trials in patients with advanced NSCLC, bexarotene, which was given in combination with chemotherapy and was continued after the chemotherapy, did not improve survival and was associated with a trend towards a shorter progression-free survival [48]. However, patients who developed hypertriglyceridemia during treatment showed a significant improvement in survival.

Tumour vaccines

Tumour vaccines are currently at various stages of clinical development. They are particularly suited for patients with low tumour load, and are useful for maintenance therapy after curative treatment of early NSCLC or locally advanced NSCLC. Several vaccination trials have been performed, but, to date, no consistent benefit has been demonstrated. These trials were performed with Bec2/bacille Calmette–Guérin [49], BLP25 liposome vaccine [50], SRL172 (killed Mycobacterium vaccae) [51], Ras peptides, allogenic vaccination with a B7.1 human leukocyte antigen A gene-modified adeno-carcinoma cell line [52] and autologous dendritic cell vaccines [53]. Although these studies suggest that biologically active vaccines can be obtained for lung cancer patients, these vaccines will have to be evaluated in properly designed and conducted clinical trials. It is believed that vaccines will ultimately be of value as adjuvant or consolidation treatment.

Bec2/bacille Calmette–Guérin. Bec2/bacille Calmette–Guérin is an anti-idiotypic antibody that mimics GD3 ganglioside, which is of neuroectodermal origin and present on the surface of tumour cells. In patients with limited-disease SCLC after a major response to chemotherapy and chest radiation, adjuvant vaccination with Bec2/bacille Calmette–Guérin failed to improve survival in the Survival in an International Phase III Prospective Randomized LD Small Cell Lung Cancer Vaccination Study with Adjuvant BEC2 and BCG (SILVA) trial [49]. Vaccinated patients who developed an immune response showed a trend towards prolonged survival. Therefore, vaccines that lead to a better immune response are required.

BLP25 liposome vaccine. This vaccine was evaluated in a randomised open-label phase II study on 171 patients responding to first-line chemotherapy (65 IIIB; 106 wet IIIB or IV) [50]. BLP25 liposome vaccine was given as eight weekly subcutaneous vaccinations. Overall survival for all patients did not differ between the vaccination group and the control group (median survival 17 *versus* 13 months; p=0.1). However, patients with stage IIIB disease showed improved survival (median survival not reached *versus* 13 months; adjusted hazard ratio 0.524 (95% confidence interval 0.261–1.052); p=0.069). Thus a phase III trial has been initiated in patients with stage III NSCLC.

Gene therapy

The tumour suppressor gene p53 is an interesting candidate for gene therapy in lung cancer for several reasons. p53 mutations frequently occur in NSCLC. In some, but not all, studies these are associated with adverse prognosis. A loss of p53 function may decrease the response to chemotherapy or radiotherapy. Thus transfer of wild-type p53 could restore chemosensitivity. In a phase II trial in selected patients with advanced NSCLC, adenovirus-mediated wild-type p53 gene transfer *via* intratumoral injection was added to palliative chemotherapy [54]. The response rate of lesions treated with chemotherapy plus intratumoral p53 injection did not differ from that for lesions treated with chemotherapy alone. Transgene expression could be detected in 68% of the tumours injected with wild-type p53. However, intratumoral injections will, at best, be of limited value, and further gene therapy trials will depend upon the establishment of vectors that can be administered systemically.

Contribution of pathology to targeted therapy

In contrast to carcinomas of the breast and other organ systems, lung carcinomas have organised their proliferation signalling pathways to be much more complex. One of the results of this complexity is evident from the low response of therapies directed towards blockade of EGFR-1 [55, 56]. In contrast to the high numbers of NSCLCs with upregulated EGFR, demonstrated immunohistochemically, only a minority of these patients respond to anti-EGFR therapy with decreased growth or increased apoptosis of their tumours. It is evident that the majority of these carcinomas have developed alternative signalling pathways, thus circumventing EGFR blockade.

EGFR 1, transforming growth factor-α, insulin-like growth factor-I receptor 1α/β and the Raf/Ras/mitogen-activated protein kinase/extracellular signal-regulated kinase signalling pathway

Normally, EGFR activation causes downstream activation of Raf (Ras family member), Ras oncogene, mitogen-activated protein kinases (MAPKs), extracellular signal-regulated kinase (ERK) and, finally, many different transcription factors, such as Ets oncogene-related transcription factor (Elk) 1, cAMP-response-element-binding protein (CREB), p90S6K3 (a kinase) and eukaryotic translation initiation factor (fig. 1) [57]. Some of these activated transcription factors act on cell cycle molecules, such as cyclins D1–3.

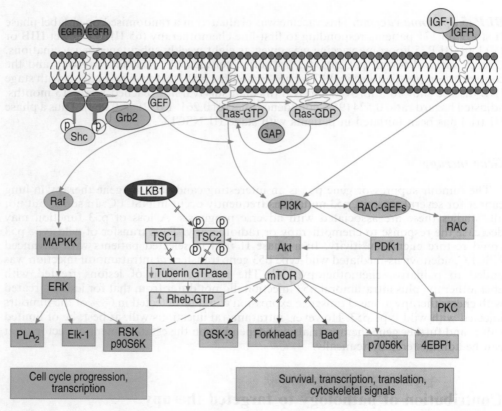

Fig. 1. – Schematic signalling pathway showing the interrelationship of epidermal growth factor (EGF) and insulin-like growth factor (IGF) with the Raf/extracellular signal-regulated kinase (ERK) and phosphatidylinositol-3'-kinase (PI3K)/Akt kinase (Akt) activation cascade. Bars represent inhibition. EGFR: EGF receptor; IGFR: IGF-I receptor; P: phosphate; Shc: Src-homology collagen protein; Grb: growth factor receptor-bound protein; GEF: guanine nucleotide exchange factor; GTP: guanosine triphosphate; GDP: guanosine diphosphate; GAP: GTPase-activating protein; MAPKK: mitogen-activated protein kinase kinase; PLA$_2$: phospholipase A$_2$; Elk: Ets oncogene-related transcription factor; RSK/p90S6K: ribosomal protein S6 kinase (90 kDa), polypeptide 1; LKB1: serine/threonine kinase 11; TSC: tuberous sclerosis complex; Rheb: Ras homologue enriched in brain; mTOR: mammalian target of rapamycin; GSK: glycogen synthase kinase; RAC: receptor-associated coactivator; PDK: phosphoinositide-dependent protein kinase; p70S6K: ribosomal protein S6 kinase (70 kDa), polypeptide 2; PKC: protein kinase C; 4EBP1: eukaryotic translation initiation factor 4E-binding protein 1. ↓: decrease; ↑: increase.

However, other receptor kinases can signal towards the same system. A good example is transforming growth factor (TGF)-α, which can activate Raf and Ras *via* its own TGF-α receptor or can directly associate with EGF (dimer formation), bind to EGFR and activate the same pathway as EGF dimers, or alternatively activate the phosphatidylinositol-3'-kinase/Akt kinase (Akt; PI3K/Akt) cascade, resulting in activation of mammalian target of rapamycin (mTOR) [58]. There is some evidence that the combined activation of EGFR by EGF and TGF-α might be responsible for the unresponsiveness of NSCLC towards anti-EGFR treatment [58, 59]. Insulin-like growth factor (IGF)-I can activate IGF-I receptor 1α and/or β, which can either signal *via* adaptor proteins growth factor receptor-bound protein (Grb) 2 and Son of Sevenless (SOS) towards Raf and further downstream into ERK, or it may activate PI3K/Akt/mTOR [60, 61]. This means that there is another way by which carcinoma cells might circumvent a blockade of the EGFR or obtain another activation/receptor signal for the downstream EGFR pathway.

It is an interesting finding that, unlike the blockade of HER2/neu by antibodies, the inhibition of the EGFR pathway by antibodies directed against the EGFR extracellular domain did not work as efficiently in pulmonary carcinomas as did intracellular receptor kinase inhibition [62–64].

c-Met receptor tyrosine kinase and the signal transducer and activator of transcription 1/3/5 signalling pathway

cMet kinase or hepatocyte growth factor receptor (c-Met), another receptor tyrosine kinase, often upregulated in SCLC and NSCLC, when activated by hepatocyte growth factor (HGF), signals either *via* Grb2/SOS towards Ras/Raf and MAPK/ERK or *via* adaptor protein Gab1 into PI3K/Akt/mTOR, or alternatively *via* the same binding protein Gab1 into adaptor protein Crk and Rap1 guanosine triphosphatase (fig. 2). This means that HGF/c-Met can substitute for the EGFR system and activate both downstream signalling cascades. In addition, c-Met can directly activate another signalling pathway, namely signal transducer and activator of transcription (STAT) 3 and 5, which again results in proliferation [65–67]. Under physiological conditions, this activation is counterbalanced by STAT1, which is also upregulated by c-Met, and, like an autocrine loop, is proposed to downregulate STAT3 and 5, thus limiting their action [68, 69]. In lung cancer, this regulatory loop might be altered. A blockade of just one receptor does not mean that the signalling cascade no longer functions and the carcinomas will stop growing.

v-src Sarcoma viral oncogene homologue (Src), a cytosolic tyrosine kinase, and focal adhesion kinase are often upregulated in different types of lung cancer, and can directly activate ERK as well as STAT3 [70, 71], therefore, forming another activation loop, which circumvents EGFR. If Src associates with Crk, they activate STAT3 and 5 independently of c-Met [70]. The Src/Crk pathway can be activated either by integrin receptors or by VEGF/VEGFR, or by many other activation signals directly within the cytosol [72, 73].

E-cadherin/β-catenin and the Wnt oncogene analogue signalling pathway

The many interconnections of the pathways make the story even more complex. For example, the Wnt oncogene analogue pathway was regarded as an independent signalling system. This is not the case. Akt, often expressed in pulmonary carcinomas, can inhibit glycogen synthase kinase (GSK)-3β [59, 74]. GSK-3β is necessary for the degradation/ ubiquitination of β-catenin. In cases where there is mutation of E-cadherin, or

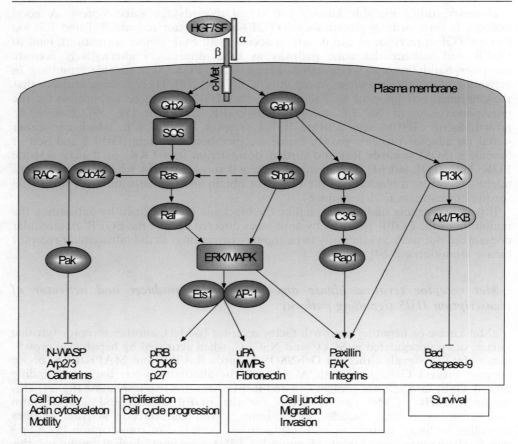

Fig. 2. – Hepatocyte growth factor (HGF) receptor (c-Met) signalling pathway. The importance of the binding proteins that determine the activation of downstream molecules, growth factor receptor-bound protein (Grb) 2 and Gab hypothetical protein (Gab) 1, are seen. Receptor activation itself is the prerequisite; binding protein activation is like a modulator. SOS: Son of Sevenless; RAC: receptor-associated coactivator; Cdc42: cell division cycle 42 (guanosine triphosphate-binding protein); Pak: Pak kinase; N-WASP: neural Wiskott–Aldrich syndrome protein; Arp: ankyrin-like protein; Shp: monohaem class I cytochrome c; ERK: extracellular signal-regulated kinase; MAPK: mitogen-activated protein kinase; Ets: erythroblastosis virus E26 oncogene homologue 1; AP: activator protein; pRB: phosphorylated retinoblastoma protein; CDK: cyclin-dependent kinase; uPA: urokinase-type plasminogen activator; MMP: matrix metalloproteinase; Crk: v-crk sarcoma virus CT10 oncogene homologue; PI3K: phosphatidylinositol-3'-kinase; Akt: Akt kinase; PKB: protein kinase B; FAK: focal adhesion kinase.

alternatively amplification of β-catenin, this results in an accumulation of β-catenin in the cytoplasm, subsequently shifting into the nucleus, where it enhances transcription. If GSK-3β is inhibited by Akt, it is no longer able to degrade β-catenin and so can facilitate its accumulation and finally translocation into the nucleus. β-Catenin and ERK/Elk-1 independently cause the upregulation of myelocytomatosis oncogene and cyclin D1 [75, 76]. However, there are other transcription factors that are activated by the ERK/Elk-1 system. It remains to be clarified whether ERK1/2 randomly activates downstream transcription factors, or only selected ones. Some preliminary data from the Institute of Pathology (Medical University of Graz, Graz, Austria) suggest that there is no random activation but rather selection of specific transcription factors, such as Elk-1 and CREB [77].

Platelet-derived growth factor receptor signalling pathway

Another tyrosine kinase receptor important in lung cancer and mesothelioma growth signalling is platelet-derived growth factor receptor (PDGFR) α/β [78]. PDGFR can activate STATs, especially STAT3 and 5, but can also directly activate PI3K and Akt, or alternatively Src kinase [79]. c-Fos, one of the transcriptions factors often detected in lung cancer, can be upregulated *via* the STAT5 activation [80].

Hypoxia-inducible factor 1 and the VEGF signalling pathway

Hypoxia-inducible factor (HIF)-1 might be an important molecule in almost all cancers [81]. It protects cells from damage due to hypoxia and thus from apoptosis. Normally HIF-1α is induced in the cytoplasm by PI3K, but also by prostaglandin E_2, which associates with HIF-1β in the nucleus and induces VEGF transcription [82]. GSK-3β induces proteasome degradation of HIF-1α. Therefore, inhibition of GSK-3β by Akt could also influence the degradation of HIF-1α and contribute to VEGF upregulation, which might subsequently induce neo-angiogenesis.

CXC chemokine receptor (CXCR) 4 is an important factor associated with metastasis in NSCLC. CXCR4 expression can be upregulated in cell culture by hypoxia and HIF-1α, which itself is regulated by the PI3K/Akt/mTOR signal transduction pathway [83].

PI3K and Akt signalling pathway

The PI3K pathway has been touched upon several times (fig. 3). It is one of the major pathways responsible for the cell cycle, but also for apoptosis, differentiation and protein synthesis regulation. A balance between phosphatase and tensin homologue (PTEN) and PI3K finely tunes its activation [84, 85]. A disturbance of this balance by loss of PTEN function and/or a shift into continuous activation of PI3K by receptor tyrosine kinases results in a multitude of changes at the transcriptional level. There are several transcription factors which are activated by Akt and mTOR causing inhibition of apoptosis [86–88], block cell cycle checkpoint molecules [89], induce progress of the cell cycle and mitosis, and also induce protein synthesis. In addition to the well-known downstream effector molecule mTOR, Akt can also signal *via* other downstream molecules, such as ERK, GSK-3β, nuclear factor-κB and mouse double minute 2 homologue. By inhibiting molecules, such as Bad and forkhead factor forkhead homologue in rhabdomyosarcoma, it also inhibits apoptosis by another means. It is becoming evident that targeting lung cancer cells using specific drugs requires careful selection of target molecules positioned at the crossroads of the interacting signalling pathways for efficient inhibition of cancer cell growth and induction of apoptosis.

Metalloproteinases and inhibitors

Metalloproteinases were regarded as important molecules in cancer cell invasion. Therefore, it was quite surprising that inhibition of metalloproteinases did not improve outcome in cancer patients [41–43]. However, the reasons for this failure became clear when the actions of metalloproteinases were studied in detail. Metalloproteinases are essential during the very early phase of carcinoma development. Cancer cells use these enzymes to digest and remodel matrix proteins for invasion and movement within the matrix.

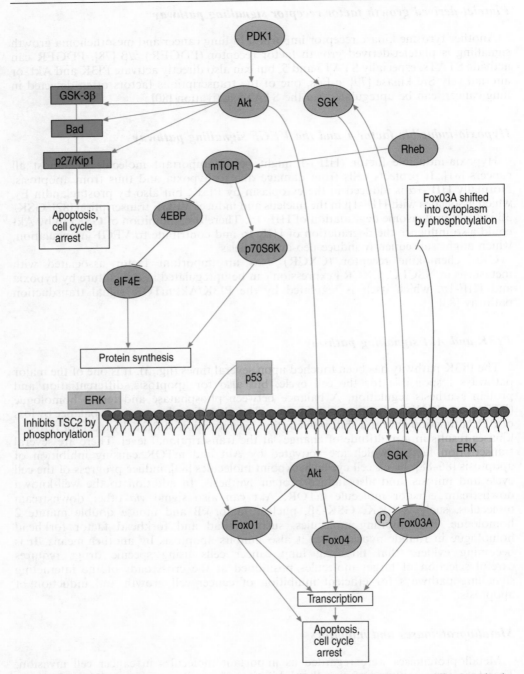

Fig. 3. – The phosphatidylinositol-3'-kinase and Akt kinase pathways and their downstream effector molecules. PDK: phosphoinositide-dependent protein kinase; SGK: serum- and glucocorticoid-induced kinase; GSK: glycogen synthase kinase; Kip1: knotted1-interacting protein; Rheb: Ras homologue enriched in brain; mTOR: mammalian target of rapamycin; 4EBP: eIF4E-binding protein; Fox: forkhead box protein; p70S6K: ribosomal protein S6 kinase (70 kDa), polypeptide 2; eIF: eukaryotic translation initiation factor; ERK: extracellular signal-regulated kinase; TSC: tuberous sclerosis complex.

However, metalloproteinases are also efficient molecules, which can inhibit or modulate immune reactions directed against the carcinoma cells by degradation of chemokines, cleave Fas ligand and, thus, prevent apoptosis, and promote neo-angiogenesis by activating basic fibroblast growth factor, VEGF and TGF-β. Metalloproteinase 7, in addition, upregulates some anti-apoptotic mediators, which makes carcinoma cells more resistant to apoptotic signals. Therefore, further research is warranted before a revival of metalloproteinase inhibitor therapy can be reinvented, most probably in combination with other drugs.

Problems in single-target inhibition, especially in lung cancer, and lessons from the EGFR story

As has been learnt from therapeutic protocols used since the mid 1990s, and especially from EGFR studies, blocking just one growth factor or receptor tyrosine kinase does not abrogate growth signals in lung cancer. Therefore, another therapeutic approach is required. Therapies must be based on a comprehensive analysis of the individual tumour tissue. The most promising approach is analysis of major pathways directly in tumour tissue, in order to define the possible therapeutic targets in each individual case.

Available techniques

Analysis of signalling pathways using immunohistochemistry

Since the beginning of the 21st Century, many antibodies have been produced, directed towards different molecules of the signalling pathways in cancer. Many of these antibodies can be used on formalin-fixed paraffin-embedded tissues, and quite a lot of them can recognise phosphorylated forms of signalling proteins. Figures 4 and 5 show

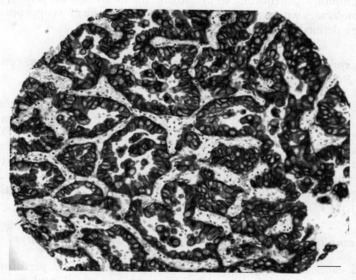

Fig. 4. – Tissue microarray technology. Pulmonary adenocarcinoma stained using antibodies directed against epidermal growth factor receptor. There is intense 3+ staining, confined to the cell membrane and cytoplasm (expression levels defined in [32–34]). Light nuclear counterstain. Scale bar=50 µm.

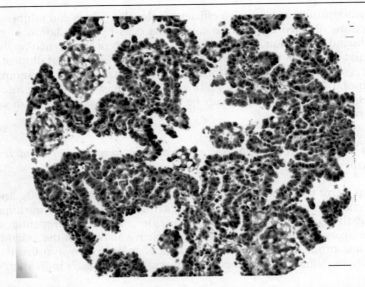

Fig. 5. – Tissue microarray technology. Pulmonary adenocarcinoma stained using antibodies directed against phosphorylated signal transducer and activator of transcription 3. There is 2+ nuclear and cytoplasmic staining (expression levels defined in [32–34]). Light nuclear counterstain. Scale bar=50 µm.

the reaction in pulmonary adenocarcinomas for antibodies directed against EGFR and STAT3, respectively.

With the technique of tissue microarray, studies into the most important molecules of different signalling pathways can be performed on several lung cancer types at once, thus providing the necessary information about the usefulness of an inhibitor therapy. Similarly tumour tissue derived from lung resections or diagnostic biopsy procedures can be studied immunohistochemically to investigate the individual expression/upregulation of signalling molecules within a defined pathway, and thus the most appropriate inhibitor therapy can be defined.

Analysis of expression profiles by fluorescence in situ hybridisation, complementary DNA array, PCR and sequence analysis for small mutations

The failure to respond to anti-EGFR treatment, based on positive immunohisto-chemical staining, has highlighted the importance of additional investigations. Many pathways can be simultaneously analysed using complementary DNA arrays. Amplifications of specific genes can be defined using FISH. It has turned out that mutation of the EGFR gene, evaluated by FISH, is the most reliable test for defining patients who might benefit from EGFR inhibitor therapy [90]. Point mutations of genes known to be involved in the progression of lung cancer or even metastasis can be demonstrated via PCR and sequence analysis.

Analysis of amplicons by comparative genomic hybridisation arrays

In selected cases, an analysis of the whole genome can be performed by array comparative genomic hybridisation. Amplicons can be located, and, in case there are small overrepresented regions, direct PCR sequencing of involved bacterial artificial chromosome clones can be undertaken in order to characterise the genes involved.

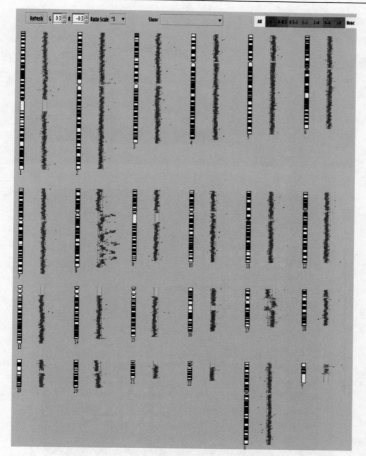

Fig. 6. – Array comparative genomic hybridisation of a pulmonary adenocarcinoma with complex chromosomal aberrations. Since the amplicons are small, such cases can be analysed directly using antibodies directed against the identified genes lying within the amplicons.

However, this should always be confirmed immunohistochemically. Figure 6 shows array comparative genomic hybridisation of an adenocarcinoma with multiple small amplicons on chromosome 8 [91]. In other cases, common regions can be defined for selected tumour types, and this region can be screened more closely for potential oncogenes, to be targeted by inhibitors.

Analysis of proteomes using antibody chip technology

A new technology is proteomics using antibody chips (fig. 7). In this case, antibodies directed against selected members of different pathways are spotted and immobilised on glass slides, and protein extracts from tumour tissue are hybridised to this antibody array. By coupling the antibodies to fluorochromes, the binding reaction can be visualised and thus members of these different pathways found in each given tumour type. Again this test provides the necessary information to the oncologists for an additional treatment with new pathway inhibitors.

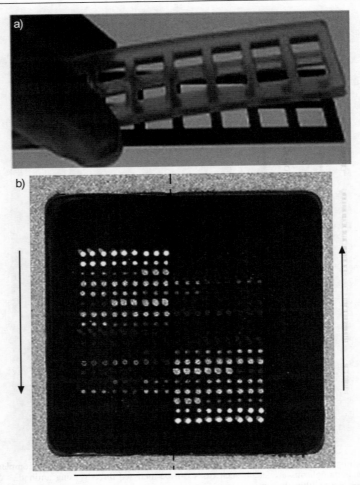

Fig. 7. – Antibody chip produced by Proteomika (courtesy of J.L. Castrillo; Proteomika, Bilbao, Spain). a) Matrix for production of antibody array, and b) antibodies spotted on to a glass slide and hybridised with proteins extracted from an adenocarcinoma. Those spots for which there is a corresponding protein in the tumour extract are highlighted.

Summary

Since the mid 1990s, major progress has been achieved in the systemic therapy of lung cancer. These achievements include new cytotoxic drugs, the establishment of adjuvant chemotherapy in patients with completely resected nonsmall cell lung cancer (NSCLC) and improved supportive care. Of major clinical relevance are new concepts that have become available through the development of targeted therapies.

Targeted therapies have entered clinical practice, or are undergoing clinical evaluation, either as a single treatment modality or in combination with chemotherapy or radiotherapy. Growth factors and their receptors have become important targets. Epidermal growth factor receptor (EGFR) directed tyrosine kinase inhibitors, such as erlotinib, improve symptoms and prolong survival in patients with advanced NSCLC who have previously been treated with chemotherapy. Intensive research on the prediction of response to these agents is ongoing. Cetuximab, in combination with palliative chemotherapy, is being evaluated in phase III trials, and other EGFR-directed monoclonal antibodies are in earlier stages of clinical development. Several dual kinase or multikinase inhibitors are undergoing clinical evaluation in patients with advanced NSCLC.

Inhibition of angiogenesis also holds great promise, and can be achieved by means of various strategies, including blockade of the vascular endothelial growth factor (VEGF)/VEGF receptor pathway. Bevacizumab, an anti-VEGF monoclonal antibody, increases the efficacy of paclitaxel/carboplatin in selected patients with advanced nonsquamous NSCLC. Several other targeted therapies (matrix metalloproteinase inhibitors, farnesyl transferase inhibitors, aprinocarsen and bexarotene) did not improve outcome in selected groups with lung cancer.

Tumour vaccines are at various stages of clinical development, but, to date, no benefit could be demonstrated in phase III trials. Gene therapy has also been attempted, but still requires the development of vectors that can be administered systemically. In order to successfully use targeted therapies, a detailed knowledge of the molecular events involved in tumour growth is necessary. Molecular pathology needs to determine clinically useful targets and provide reliable methods for their determination in patients with lung cancer.

Keywords: Angiogenesis, lung cancer, monoclonal antibodies, targeted therapy, tyrosine kinase inhibitors, vaccination.

References

1. Chemotherapy in non-small cell lung cancer: a meta-analysis using updated data on individual patients from 52 randomised clinical trials. Non-small Cell Lung Cancer Collaborative Group. *BMJ* 1995; 311: 899–909.

2. Pfister DG, Johnson DH, Azzoli CG, *et al.* American Society of Clinical Oncology treatment of unresectable non-small-cell lung cancer guideline: update 2003. *J Clin Oncol* 2004; 22: 330–353.

3. Pirker R. Therapy of advanced non-small-cell lung cancer: take-home-message. *Lung Cancer* 2004; 45: Suppl. 2, S259–S262.

4. Pirker R. Two- *versus* three-drug combinations in the chemotherapy of advanced non-small-cell lung cancer. *Lung Cancer* 2002; 38: Suppl. 3, S53–S55.

5. Fossella F, Pereira JR, von Pawel J, *et al.* Randomized, multinational, phase III study of docetaxel

plus platinum combinations *versus* vinorelbine plus cisplatin for advanced non-small-cell lung cancer: the TAX 326 study group. *J Clin Oncol* 2003; 21: 3016–3024.

6. Shepherd FA, Dancey J, Ramlau R, *et al.* Prospective randomized trial of docetaxel *versus* best supportive care in patients with non-small-cell lung cancer previously treated with platinum-based chemotherapy. *J Clin Oncol* 2000; 18: 2095–2103.

7. Hanna NH, Shepherd FA, Rosell R, *et al.* A phase III trial of pemetrexed *versus* docetaxel in patients with recurrent non-small cell lung cancer who were previously treated with chemotherapy. *Proc ASCO* 2003; 22: 622.

8. Arriagada R, Bergman B, Dunant A, Le Chevalier T, Pignon JP, Vansteenkiste J, on behalf of the International Adjuvant Lung Cancer Trial Collaborative Group. Cisplatin-based adjuvant chemotherapy in patients with completely resected non-small-cell lung cancer. *N Engl J Med* 2004; 350: 351–360.

9. Pisters KM, Le Chevalier T. Adjuvant chemotherapy in completely resected non-small-cell lung cancer. *J Clin Oncol* 2005; 23: 3270–3278.

10. O'Brien MO, Ciuleanu T, Tsekov H, *et al.* Survival benefit of oral topotecan plus supportive care *versus* supportive care alone in relapsed, resistant SCLC. *Lung Cancer* 2005; 49: Suppl. 2, S54.

11. von Pawel J, Schiller JH, Shepherd FA, *et al.* Topotecan *versus* cyclophosphamide, doxorubicin, and vincristine for the treatment of recurrent small-cell lung cancer. *J Clin Oncol* 1999; 17: 658–667.

12. Rosell R, Cobo M, Isla D, *et al.* Applications of genomics in NSCLC. *Lung Cancer* 2005; 50: Suppl. 2, S33–S40.

13. Pirker R, Wiesenberger K, Pohl G, Minar W. Anaemia in lung cancer: clinical impact and management. *Clin Lung Cancer* 2003; 5: 90–97.

14. Mendelsohn J. Targeting the epidermal growth factor receptor for cancer therapy. *J Clin Oncol* 2002; 20: Suppl. 18, 1S–13S.

15. Fukuoka M, Yano S, Giaccone G, *et al.* Multi-institutional randomized phase II trial of gefitinib for previously treated patients with advanced non-small-cell lung cancer. *J Clin Oncol* 2003; 21: 2237–2246.

16. Kris MG, Natale RB, Herbst RS, *et al.* Efficacy of gefitinib, an inhibitor of the epidermal growth factor receptor tyrosine kinase, in symptomatic patients with non-small cell lung cancer: a randomized trial. *JAMA* 2003; 290: 2149–2158.

17. Thatcher N, Chang A, Parikh P, *et al.* Gefitinib plus best supportive care in previously treated patients with refractory advanced non-small-cell lung cancer: results from a randomised, placebo-controlled, multicentre study (Iressa Survival Evaluation in Lung Cancer). *Lancet* 2005; 366: 1527–1537.

18. Shepherd FA, Rodrigues Pereira J, Ciuleanu T, on behalf of the National Cancer Institute of Canada Clinical Trials Group. Erlotinib in previously treated non-small-cell lung cancer. *N Engl J Med* 2005; 353: 123–132.

19. Tsao MS, Sakurada A, Cutz JC, *et al.* Erlotinib in lung cancer – molecular and clinical predictors of outcome. *N Engl J Med* 2005; 353: 133–144.

20. Giaccone G, Herbst RS, Manegold C, *et al.* Gefitinib in combination with gemcitabine and cisplatin in advanced non-small-cell lung cancer: a phase III trial – INTACT 1. *J Clin Oncol* 2004; 22: 777–784.

21. Herbst RS, Giaccone G, Schiller JH, *et al.* Gefitinib in combination with paclitaxel and carboplatin in advanced non-small-cell lung cancer: a phase III trial – INTACT 2. *J Clin Oncol* 2004; 22: 785–794.

22. Gatzemeier U, Pluzanska A, Szczesna A, *et al.* Results of a phase III trial of erlotinib (OSI-774) combined with cisplatin and gemcitabine chemotherapy in advanced non-small-cell lung cancer. *Proc ASCO* 2004; 23: 617.

23. Herbst RS, Prager D, Hermann R, *et al.* TRIBUTE: a phase III trial of erlotinib hydrochloride (OSI-774) combined with carboplatin and paclitaxel chemotherapy in advanced non-small-cell lung cancer. *J Clin Oncol* 2005; 23: 5892–5899.

24. Cappuzzo F, Varella-Garcia M, Shigematsu H, *et al.* Increased HER2 gene copy number is

associated with response to gefitinib therapy in epidermal growth factor receptor-positive non-small-cell lung cancer patients. *J Clin Oncol* 2005; 23: 5007–5018.

25. Bell DW, Lynch TJ, Haserlat SM, *et al.* Epidermal growth factor receptor mutations and gene amplification in non-small-cell lung cancer: molecular analysis of the IDEAL/INTACT gefitinib trials. *J Clin Oncol* 2005; 23: 8081–8092.

26. Eberhard DA, Johnson BE, Amler LC, *et al.* Mutations in the epidermal growth factor receptor and in KRAS are predictive and prognostic indicators in patients with non-small-cell lung cancer treated with chemotherapy alone and in combination with erlotinib. *J Clin Oncol* 2005; 23: 5900–5909.

27. Kelly K, Gaspar LE, Chanksy K, *et al.* SWOG 0023: a randomized phase III trial of cisplatin/etoposide plus radiation therapy followed by consolidation docetaxel then maintenance therapy with gefitinib or placebo in patients with locally advanced unresectable stage III non-small cell lung cancer. *Lung Cancer* 2005; 49: Suppl. 2, S64.

28. Rosell R, Daniel C, Ramlua R, *et al.* Randomized phase II study of cetuximab in combination with cisplatin (C) and vinorelbine (V) *vs.* CV alone in the first-line treatment of patients with epidermal growth factor receptor (EGFR) expressing advanced NSCLC. *J Clin Oncol* 2004; 22: Suppl. 14, 620s.

29. Thienelt CD, Bunn PA Jr, Hanna N, *et al.* Multicenter phase I/II study of cetuximab with paclitaxel and carboplatin in untreated patients with stage IV non-small-cell lung cancer. *J Clin Oncol* 2005; 23: 8786–8793.

30. Robert F, Blumenschein G, Herbst RS, *et al.* Phase I/IIa study of cetuximab with gemcitabine plus carboplatin in patients with chemotherapy-naive advanced non-small-cell lung cancer. *J Clin Oncol* 2005; 23: 9089–9096.

31. Crawford J, Swanson P, Prager D, *et al.* Panitumumab, a fully human antibody, combined with paclitaxel and carboplatin *versus* paclitaxel and carboplatin alone for first line advanced non-small cell lung cancer. *Eur J Cancer* 2005; 3: Suppl. 2, 324.

32. Gatzemeier U, Groth G, Butts C, *et al.* Randomized phase II trial of gemcitabine–cisplatin with or without trastuzumab in HER2-positive non-small-cell lung cancer. *Ann Oncol* 2004; 15: 19–27.

33. Zinner RG, Glisson BS, Fossella FV, *et al.* Trastuzumab in combination with cisplatin and gemcitabine in patients with Her2-overexpressing, untreated, advanced non-small cell lung cancer: report of a phase II trial and findings regarding optimal identification of patients with Her2-overexpressing disease. *Lung Cancer* 2004; 44: 99–110.

34. Langer CJ, Stephenson P, Thor A, Vangel M, Johnson DH. Trastuzumab in the treatment of advanced non-small-cell lung cancer: is there a role? Focus on Eastern Cooperative Oncology Group study 2598. *J Clin Oncol* 2004; 22: 1180–1187.

35. Herbst RS, Onn A, Sandler A. Angiogenesis and lung cancer: prognostic and therapeutic implications. *J Clin Oncol* 2005; 23: 3243–3256.

36. Johnson DH, Fehrenbacher L, Novotny WF, *et al.* Randomized phase II trial comparing bevacizumab plus carboplatin and paclitaxel with carboplatin and paclitaxel alone in previously untreated locally advanced or metastatic non-small-cell lung cancer. *J Clin Oncol* 2004; 22: 2184–2191.

37. Sandler AB, Gray R, Perry M, *et al.* Paclitaxel-carboplatin alone or with bevacizumab for non-small-cell lung cancer. *N Engl J Med* 2006; 355: 2542–2550.

38. Herbst RS, Johnson DH, Mininberg E, *et al.* Phase I/II trial evaluating the anti-vascular endothelial growth factor monoclonal antibody bevacizumab in combination with the HER-1/epidermal growth factor receptor tyrosine kinase inhibitor erlotinib for patients with recurrent non-small-cell lung cancer. *J Clin Oncol* 2005; 23: 2544–2555.

39. Natale R, Bodkin D, Govindan R, *et al.* A comparison of the antitumour efficacy of ZD6474 and gefitinib in patients with NSCLC: results of a randomized, double-blind phase II study. *Lung Cancer* 2005; 49: Suppl. 2, S37.

40. Herbst R, Johnson B, Rowbottom J, *et al.* ZD6474 plus Docetaxel in patients with previously treated NSCLC: results of a randomized, placebo-controlled phase II trial. *Lung Cancer* 2005; 49: Suppl. 2, S35.

41. Shepherd FA, Giaccone G, Seymour L, et al. Prospective, randomized, double-blind, placebo-controlled trial of marimastat after response to first-line chemotherapy in patients with small-cell lung cancer: a trial of the National Cancer Institute of Canada – Clinical Trials Group and the European Organization for Research and Treatment of Cancer. *J Clin Oncol* 2002; 20: 4434–4439.

42. Bissett D, O'Byrne KJ, von Pawel J, et al. Phase III study of matrix metalloproteinase inhibitor prinomastat in non-small-cell lung cancer. *J Clin Oncol* 2005; 23: 842–849.

43. Leighl NB, Paz-Ares L, Douillard J-Y, et al. Randomized phase III study of matrix metalloproteinase inhibitor BMS-275291 in combination with paclitaxel and carboplatin in advanced non-small-cell lung cancer: National Cancer Institute of Canada–Clinical Trials Group Study BR.18. *J Clin Oncol* 2005; 23: 2831–2839.

44. Mascaux C, Iannino N, Martin B, et al. The role of RAS oncogene in survival of patients with lung cancer: a systematic review of the literature with meta-analysis. *Br J Cancer* 2005; 92: 131–139.

45. Adjei AA. An overview of farnesyltransferase inhibitors and their role in lung cancer therapy. *Lung Cancer* 2003; 41: Suppl. 1, S55–S62.

46. Blumenschein G, Ludwig C, Thomas G, et al. A randomized phase III trial comparing lonafarnib/carboplatin/paclitaxel *versus* carboplatin/paclitaxel in chemotherapy-naïve patients with advanced or metastatic non-small cell lung cancer. *Lung Cancer* 2005; 49: Suppl. 2, S30.

47. Paz-Ares L, Douillard JY, Koralewski P, et al. Phase III study of gemcitabine and cisplatin with or without aprinocarsen, a protein kinase C-α antisense oligonucleotide, in patients with advanced-stage non-small-cell lung cancer. *J Clin Oncol* 2006; 24: 1428–1434.

48. Tyagi P. Bexarotene in combination with chemotherapy fails to prolong survival in patients with advanced non-small-cell lung cancer: results from the SPIRIT I and II trials. *Clin Lung Cancer* 2005; 7: 17–19.

49. Giaccone G, Debruyne C, Felip E, et al. Phase III study of adjuvant vaccination with Bec2/bacille Calmette–Guerin in responding patients with limited-disease small-cell lung cancer (European Organisation for Research and Treatment of Cancer 08971-08971B; Silva Study). *J Clin Oncol* 2005; 23: 6854–6864.

50. Butts C, Murray N, Maksymiuk A, et al. Randomized phase IIB trial of BLP25 liposome vaccine in stage IIIB and IV non-small-cell lung cancer. *J Clin Oncol* 2005; 23: 6674–6681.

51. O'Brien ME, Anderson H, Kaukel E, et al. SRL172 (killed *Mycobacterium vaccae*) in addition to standard chemotherapy improves quality of life without affecting survival, in patients with advanced non-small-cell lung cancer: phase III results. *Ann Oncol* 2004; 15: 906–914.

52. Raez LE, Cassileth PA, Schlesselman JJ, et al. Allogeneic vaccination with a B7.1 HLA-A gene-modified adenocarcinoma cell line in patients with advanced non-small-cell lung cancer. *J Clin Oncol* 2004; 22: 2800–2807.

53. Hirschowitz EA, Foody T, Kryscio R, Dickson L, Sturgill J, Yannelli J. Autologous dendritic cell vaccines for non-small-cell lung cancer. *J Clin Oncol* 2004; 22: 2808–2815.

54. Schuler M, Herrmann R, De Greve JLP, et al. Adenovirus-mediated wild-type p53 gene transfer in patients receiving chemotherapy for advanced non-small-cell lung cancer: results of a multicenter phase II study. *J Clin Oncol* 2001; 19: 1750–1758.

55. Kosaka T, Yatabe Y, Endoh H, Kuwano H, Takahashi T, Mitsudomi T. Mutations of the epidermal growth factor receptor gene in lung cancer: biological and clinical implications. *Cancer Res* 2004; 64: 8919–8923.

56. Shigematsu H, Lin L, Takahashi T, et al. Clinical and biological features associated with epidermal growth factor receptor gene mutations in lung cancers. *J Natl Cancer Inst* 2005; 97: 339–346.

57. Jorissen RN, Walker F, Pouliot N, Garrett TP, Ward CW, Burgess AW. Epidermal growth factor receptor: mechanisms of activation and signalling. *Exp Cell Res* 2003; 284: 31–53.

58. Mukohara T, Kudoh S, Matsuura K, et al. Activated Akt expression has significant correlation with EGFR and TGF-α expressions in stage I NSCLC. *Anticancer Res* 2004; 24: 11–17.

59. Sithanandam G, Smith GT, Fields JR, Fornwald LW, Anderson LM. Alternate paths from epidermal growth factor receptor to Akt in malignant *versus* nontransformed lung epithelial cells: ErbB3 *versus* Gab1. *Am J Respir Cell Mol Biol* 2005; 33: 490–499.

60. Pold M, Krysan K, Pold A, *et al.* Cyclooxygenase-2 modulates the insulin-like growth factor axis in non-small-cell lung cancer. *Cancer Res* 2004; 64: 6549–6555.

61. Warshamana-Greene GS, Litz J, Buchdunger E, Garcia-Echeverria C, Hofmann F, Krystal GW. The insulin-like growth factor-I receptor kinase inhibitor, NVP-ADW742, sensitizes small cell lung cancer cell lines to the effects of chemotherapy. *Clin Cancer Res* 2005; 11: 1563–1571.

62. Grunwald V, Hidalgo M. Developing inhibitors of the epidermal growth factor receptor for cancer treatment. *J Natl Cancer Inst* 2003; 95: 851–867.

63. Hirsch FR, Scagliotti GV, Langer CJ, Varella-Garcia M, Franklin WA. Epidermal growth factor family of receptors in preneoplasia and lung cancer: perspectives for targeted therapies. *Lung Cancer* 2003; 41: Suppl. 1, S29–S42.

64. Mendelsohn J, Baselga J. The EGF receptor family as targets for cancer therapy. *Oncogene* 2000; 19: 6550–6565.

65. Maulik G, Kijima T, Ma PC, *et al.* Modulation of the c-Met/hepatocyte growth factor pathway in small cell lung cancer. *Clin Cancer Res* 2002; 8: 620–627.

66. Qiao H, Hung W, Tremblay E, *et al.* Constitutive activation of Met kinase in non-small-cell lung carcinomas correlates with anchorage-independent cell survival. *J Cell Biochem* 2002; 86: 665–677.

67. Song L, Turkson J, Karras JG, Jove R, Haura EB. Activation of Stat3 by receptor tyrosine kinases and cytokines regulates survival in human non-small cell carcinoma cells. *Oncogene* 2003; 22: 4150–4165.

68. Calo V, Migliavacca M, Bazan V, *et al.* STAT proteins: from normal control of cellular events to tumorigenesis. *J Cell Physiol* 2003; 197: 157–168.

69. Qing Y, Stark GR. Alternative activation of STAT1 and STAT3 in response to interferon-γ. *J Biol Chem* 2004; 279: 41679–41685.

70. Cheng CH, Yu KC, Chen HL, *et al.* Blockade of v-Src-stimulated tumour formation by the Src homology 3 domain of Crk-associated substrate (Cas). *FEBS Lett* 2004; 557: 221–227.

71. Lo RK, Cheung H, Wong YH. Constitutively active Gα16 stimulates STAT3 *via* a c-Src/JAK- and ERK-dependent mechanism. *J Biol Chem* 2003; 278: 52154–52165.

72. Su JL, Shih JY, Yen ML, *et al.* Cyclooxygenase-2 induces EP$_1$- and HER-2/Neu-dependent vascular endothelial growth factor-C up-regulation: a novel mechanism of lymphangiogenesis in lung adenocarcinoma. *Cancer Res* 2004; 64: 554–564.

73. Brabek J, Constancio SS, Shin NY, Pozzi A, Weaver AM, Hanks SK. CAS promotes invasiveness of Src-transformed cells. *Oncogene* 2004; 23: 7406–7415.

74. Noda S, Kishi K, Yuasa T, *et al.* Overexpression of wild-type Akt1 promoted insulin-stimulated p70S6 kinase (p70S6K) activity and affected GSK3β regulation, but did not promote insulin-stimulated GLUT4 translocation or glucose transport in L6 myotubes. *J Med Invest* 2000; 47: 47–55.

75. Li YJ, Wei ZM, Meng YX, Ji XR. β-Catenin up-regulates the expression of cyclinD1, c-myc and MMP-7 in human pancreatic cancer: relationships with carcinogenesis and metastasis. *World J Gastroenterol* 2005; 11: 2117–2123.

76. Shin HS, Lee HJ, Nishida M, *et al.* Betacellulin and amphiregulin induce upregulation of cyclin D1 and DNA synthesis activity through differential signaling pathways in vascular smooth muscle cells. *Circ Res* 2003; 93: 302–310.

77. Popper HH, Markert E, Stacher E, *et al.* Differences in growth signaling pathway activation in small cell and non-small cell carcinomas of the lung. *Eur Respir J* 2006; 28: Suppl. 50, 326s.

78. Antoniades HN, Galanopoulos T, Neville-Golden J, O'Hara CJ. Malignant epithelial cells in primary human lung carcinomas coexpress *in vivo* platelet-derived growth factor (PDGF) and PDGF receptor mRNAs and their protein products. *Proc Natl Acad Sci USA* 1992; 89: 3942–3946.

79. Klotz LO, Schieke SM, Sies H, Holbrook NJ. Peroxynitrite activates the phosphoinositide 3-kinase/Akt pathway in human skin primary fibroblasts. *Biochem J* 2000; 352: 219–225.

80. Nakagami H, Morishita R, Yamamoto K, *et al.* Mitogenic and antiapoptotic actions of hepatocyte growth factor through ERK, STAT3, and Akt in endothelial cells. *Hypertension* 2001; 37: 581–586.

81. Sowter HM, Ratcliffe PJ, Watson P, Greenberg AH, Harris AL. HIF-1-dependent regulation of

hypoxic induction of the cell death factors BNIP3 and NIX in human tumours. *Cancer Res* 2001; 61: 6669–6673.

82. Sandau KB, Faus HG, Brune B. Induction of hypoxia-inducible-factor 1 by nitric oxide is mediated *via* the PI 3K pathway. *Biochem Biophys Res Commun* 2000; 278: 263–267.

83. Phillips RJ, Mestas J, Gharaee-Kermani M, *et al.* Epidermal growth factor and hypoxia-induced expression of CXC chemokine receptor 4 on non-small cell lung cancer cells is regulated by the phosphatidylinositol 3-kinase/PTEN/AKT/mammalian target of rapamycin signaling pathway and activation of hypoxia inducible factor-1α. *J Biol Chem* 2005; 280: 22473–22481.

84. Kumar CC, Diao R, Yin Z, *et al.* Expression, purification, characterization and homology modeling of active Akt/PKB, a key enzyme involved in cell survival signalling. *Biochim Biophys Acta* 2001; 1526: 257–268.

85. Lee HY, Srinivas H, Xia D, *et al.* Evidence that phosphatidylinositol 3-kinase- and mitogen-activated protein kinase kinase-4/c-Jun NH$_2$-terminal kinase-dependent pathways cooperate to maintain lung cancer cell survival. *J Biol Chem* 2003; 278: 23630–23638.

86. Burow ME, Weldon CB, Melnik LI, *et al.* PI3-K/AKT regulation of NF-κB signaling events in suppression of TNF-induced apoptosis. *Biochem Biophys Res Commun* 2000; 271: 342–345.

87. Franke TF, Hornik CP, Segev L, Shostak GA, Sugimoto C. PI3K/Akt and apoptosis: size matters. *Oncogene* 2003; 22: 8983–8998.

88. Kennedy SG, Kandel ES, Cross TK, Hay N. Akt/protein kinase B inhibits cell death by preventing the release of cytochrome c from mitochondria. *Mol Cell Biol* 1999; 19: 5800–5810.

89. Kandel ES, Skeen J, Majewski N, *et al.* Activation of Akt/protein kinase B overcomes a G$_2$/M cell cycle checkpoint induced by DNA damage. *Mol Cell Biol* 2002; 22: 7831–7841.

90. Hirsch FR, Varella-Garcia M, Bunn PA Jr., *et al.* Epidermal growth factor receptor in non-small-cell lung carcinomas: correlation between gene copy number and protein expression and impact on prognosis. *J Clin Oncol* 2003; 21: 3798–3807.

91. Popper HH, Ullmann R, Halbwedl I, Kothmaier H, Petzmann S. Complex chromosomal aberrations in pulmonary adenocarcinomas detected by array-CGH. *Mod Path* 2005; 85: Suppl. 1, S1469.

CHAPTER 5

What is a rare tumour and how should it be dealt with clinically?

N. Girard*, M. Barbareschi#, J-F. Cordier*, B. Murer#

*Dept of Respiratory Medicine, Reference Center for Orphan Pulmonary Diseases, Louis Pradel Hospital, Hospices Civils de Lyon, Lyon, France. #Dept of Pathology, Ospeadalde Umberto I, Mestre, Venice, Italy.

Correspondence: J-F. Cordier, Louis Pradel Hospital, Université Claude Bernard, 28 avenue Doyen Lépine, 69677 Lyon Cedex, France. Fax: 33 472357653; E-mail: germop@univ-lyon1.fr

The most common lung tumour is lung carcinoma, with adenocarcinoma, squamous cell carcinoma, large cell carcinoma and small cell carcinoma representing almost 99% of cases [1]. Excluding metastatic lesions in the lung, other histopathological categories account for a total of <1% of lung tumours, but these represent a wide range of diverse tumoral processes, with possible specific clinical and radiological imaging features permitting the clinician to suspect a rare tumour [2]. The role of the pathologist is obviously first to establish the diagnosis, and secondly to allow the clinician to determine and orientate the treatment and prognosis. Although diagnosis may be made on the basis of routinely stained sections, immunohistochemistry is often necessary to define the precise nature of the neoplasm and to evaluate its biological aggressiveness. More sophisticated techniques (flow cytometry and molecular and cytogenetic analysis) have a limited role in diagnosis, but may play a role in predicting clinical behaviour. Since rare pulmonary tumours are usually limited to the lung at the time of diagnosis, and frequently consist of benign or low-grade malignant lesions, the therapeutic strategy often consists of upfront surgical resection when the tumour is limited to the lung, ensuring both diagnosis and the first step of the treatment [3–7]. Thus curability and prognosis may often be better than for nonsmall cell lung cancer (NSCLC) [2, 4].

As rare pulmonary tumours have been mostly described as single case reports and small series [3, 4], an exhaustive review of the literature was undertaken in order to obtain a rigorous overview of rare pulmonary tumours (table 1). As an exhaustive review of all types of rare lung tumour is outside the scope of the present chapter, five rare pulmonary tumours of particular interest to both the pathologist and the clinician, further illustrating the close cooperation between both specialists, were selected: myofibroblastic tumour, sarcomas, epithelioid haemangioendothelioma (EHE), mucoepidermoid carcinoma, and pulmonary lymphoma, especially mucosa-associated lymphoid tissue (MALT) lymphoma.

Methods

A systematic review of the literature was carried out using the PubMed database, initially using the following keywords: "rare" OR "orphan" AND "lung" OR "pulmonary" AND "tumour" OR "cancer". The list of rare lung tumours was then established from the retrieved articles, and was further completed using the World Health

Eur Respir Mon, 2007, 39, 85–133. Printed in UK - all rights reserved. Copyright ERS Journals Ltd 2007; European Respiratory Monograph; ISSN 1025-448x.

Table 1. – Cumulative reported rare pulmonary tumours

Tumour	Features			Spontaneous evolution	Treatment	Curability	Reference
	Clinical	Radiological	PET				
Acinic cell carcinoma	Usu asym	Periph mass		Malignant	Simple R; no adj	Exc after R	[8, 9]
Adenoid cystic carcinoma	Cough, chest pain, haemoptysis, shortness of breath	Hilar or proximal mass, atelectasis	↑uptake#	Malignant	Ext R; adj RT	Good	[10-12]
Adenoma Alveolar/papillary	F predom, 5th–8th D, chest pain, dyspnoea	Well-circ small subpleural nodule, lower lobe predom, het ENH on MRI/CT	No uptake [10]	Benign	Simple R; no adj	Exc	[13-16]
Pleiomorphic	6th–7th D	Well-circ proximal small nodule	No uptake [10]	Malignant	Ext R	Unpred	[17]
Angiomyolipoma Angiosarcoma¶	Usu asym, dyspnoea Haemoptysis	Volum het mass Mult bil nodules surrounded by a halo of GG, reticulonod infiltrates, cauliflower-like appearance on MRI T2	↑uptake#	Benign Malignant	Simple R; no adj Ext R; preop/adj CHT, adj RT	Exc Poor (1-yr surv <10%)	[18-23]
Carcinoid tumour	M predom, 5th–7th D, cor with CS, usu asym	Hilar or periph mass, consolidation, PE	↑uptake [24]	Malignant	Ext R; CHT (neoad/adj)?, adj RT?	Dep on type, (typ/atyp 5-yr surv 90/55%)	[24-29]
Carcinosarcoma	M predom, 6th–9th D, fever, WL, cough, chest pain	Periph nodule, upper lobe predom	↑uptake#	Malignant	Ext R; adj CHT, adj RT	Poor (2-yr surv <10%)	[3, 4, 30-33]
Chemodectoma⁺ Chondroma	F predom, assn to Carney's triad	Well-circ nodule, calcifications, cystic features	↑uptake#	Benign	Simple R; no adj	Exc	[34]
Chondrosarcoma	M predom	Calcifications, cystic changes	↑uptake#	Malignant	Ext R; adj CHT?	Good	[35, 36]
Choriocarcinoma	M predom, feminisation (HCG test)	Mult varying size nodules, reticulonod infiltrates	↑uptake#	Malignant	Ext R; adj CHT, adj RT	Poor (2-yr surv <10%)	[4, 37, 38]

Table 1. – (Continued)

Tumour	Features Clinical	Features Radiological	PET	Spontaneous evolution	Treatment	Curability	Reference
Choristoma Pancreatic	Neonate, assn with other malformation (enteric dup), RD	Het solid and cystic lesion		Benign	Simple R	Poor	[39]
Glial	Neonate, RD, assn with anencephalia	Mult cystic lesions		Benign	No Tx	Poor	[40]
Thyroid	F predom, 6th–9th D, assn with multinod thyroid goitre			Benign	Simple R	Exc	[41]
Desmoplastic small round cell tumour	Dyspnoea, cough, WL	Bil reticulonod infiltrates		Malignant	Ext R; adj CHT	Unpred	[42]
Embryonal carcinoma	Asym	Well-circ coin lesion	↑uptake#	Malignant	Ext R; adj CHT?	Unpred	[43]
Endometriosis	F, 3rd–6th D, menstrual rhythm haemoptysis	Mult nod/alveolar shadows, var in size/vasc ENH during menstrual cycle (CT/MRI)	↑uptake#	Benign	Simple R; HT	Exc	[44, 45]
Ependymoma	Asym		No uptake, uptake on ^{11}C-Met PET#	Benign	Simple R; no adj	Good	[46]
Epithelioid haemangioendothelioma§	F predom, 4th–6th D, haemoptysis, chest pain	Mult bil nodules, perivasc GG	↑uptake [45, 47]	Malignant	Simple R; no adj	Poor (5-yr surv 60%)	[4, 18, 19, 48–54]
Foetal adenocarcinoma^f	7th–8th D, cor with CS	Solitary nodule	↑uptake#	Malignant	Ext R; CHT (neoadj/adj)?, adj RT	Poor (3-yr surv 50%)	[55, 56]
Fibrosarcoma	Usu asym, cough, chest pain	Periph well-circ mass (adult), hilar mass with atelectasis (infant), calcifications	↑uptake#	Malignant	Ext R; adj RT	Dep on grade, usu poor (2-yr surv 30%)	[57–61]
Follicular bronchitis	Immunosuppression, AIDS context, RA, Sjögren's syndrome				Steroids		[62]
Giant cell carcinoma	6th D	Volum periph mass		Malignant	Ext R; adj RT, adj CHT	Poor (5-yr surv 10%)	[63, 64]
Glomus tumor	Asym	Small nodules	↑uptake [63], interest of ^{18}F-dopa-PET	Malignant	Ext R	Exc	[65]

Table 1. – (Continued)

Tumour	Features			Spontaneous evolution	Treatment	Curability	Reference
	Clinical	Radiological	PET				
Hamartoma	M predom, 6th D, usu asym	Solitary subpleural polypoid nodule, coin lesion with popcorn pattern of calcification	↑uptake [66, 67]	Benign	Simple R; no adj	Exc, assn with lung carcinoma in the same lobe (10%)	[66, 68, 69]
Haemangiomatosis	Young adults, dyspnoea, haemoptysis, PH	Bil reticulonod lesions, micronodules, centrilobular GG			HLT	Poor (3-yr surv 50%)	[70]
Haemangiopericytoma	M predom, 6th–7th D, chest pain, dyspnoea, cough, haemoptysis	Well-circ hom large mass	↑ uptake#	Malignant	Ext R; adj RT, adj CHT	Poor	[3, 4, 71,72]
Inflammatory pseudotumour	Young adults (<30 yrs), history of infection, usu asym, cough, haemoptysis	Well-circ solitary hom coin lesion	↑uptake [73]	Benign, local invasion	Simple R; no adj	Good (5-yr surv 80–100%)	[3, 73–84]
Intravascular lymphoma	Dyspnoea, fever	Diffuse interstitial opacities		High grade	IT, CHT	Good	[85]
Kaposi's sarcoma	AIDS infection context, haemoptysis	Diffuse mult periph nodules, peribronchovasc thickening, PE		Malignant	CHT?	Poor	[86]
Leiomyoma	F, usu asym	Well-circ hom proximal mass	No uptake#	Benign	Simple R; no adj	Exc	[3, 87]
Leiomyosarcoma	M predom, 6th D	Het mass, cystic and/or necrotic features	↑uptake#	Malignant	Ext R; adj CHT?, adj RT	Dep on grade, better in infants (5-yr surv 50%)	[3, 4, 57, 58, 88–92]
Lipoma	M predom, 5th–6th D, usu asym	Round well-circ hom hypodense nodule	No uptake [87]	Benign	Simple R; no adj	Exc	[93, 94]
Liposarcoma		Inhom irregular mass, fat signal depending on differentiation	↑uptake#	Malignant	Ext R; preop/adj CHT, adj RT	Good	[95]
Lymphangioleiomyoma	Assn with lymphangioleiomyomatosis or mult endocrine neoplasia	Volum mass, diurnal var in size		Benign	R?	Exc	[96]

Table 1. – (Continued)

Tumour	Features		PET	Spontaneous evolution	Treatment	Curability	Reference
	Clinical	Radiological					
Lymphoepithelioma-like carcinoma	3rd-4th D, exposure to EBV (Asian origin predom), dyspnoea, chest pain, WL	Well-defined hilar mass, peribronchovasc spread, vasc encasement		Malignant	Ext R; adj RT, adj CHT	Poor (2-yr surv 50%)	[97]
Lymphoma Hodgkin's	F predom, cough, dyspnoea, fever, WL, swelling	Mult bil opacities, inhom and cystic features	↑uptake [118]	Malignant	CHT	Poor (5-yr surv 50%)	[62, 85, 98–122] [114]
Non-Hodgkin's Low grade MALT	Usually asym, 4th-6th D	Well-circ localised bil opacities, alveolar pattern with air bronchogram	↑uptake [118]	Low grade	Watchful waiting, simple R; IT, CHT	Good (5-yr surv 75–90%)	[62, 100, 106]
Follicular	Usu asym		↑uptake [118]	Low grade	Watchful waiting; IT, CHT	Good (5-yr surv 75–90%)	
Mantle cell Small lymphocytic	Usu asym		↑uptake [118]	Low grade	Watchful waiting; IT	Good (5-yr surv 75–90%)	[106]
High grade Diffuse large B-cell	Immunosuppression, AIDS context, cough, dyspnoea, fever, WL, swelling	Atelectasis, single pulmonary mass, rapidly progressive	↑uptake [118]	High grade	CHT, IT	Good (5-yr surv 65–75%), poorer in AIDS (2-yr surv 50%)	[62]
Burkitt's	Cough, dyspnoea, fever, WL, swelling Immunosuppression	Mult nod opacities	↑uptake [118]	High grade	CHT	Poor	[62]
T-cell Lymphomatoid granulomatosis	Immunosuppression, AIDS context, M predom, cough, dyspnoea, fever	Bil nodules predom in lower lobes, peribronchovasc dist, poss spont migration or disappearance	↑uptake [118]	High grade	Simple R; CHT, steroids, RT	Poor (5-yr surv 40%)	[108–112]

Table 1. – (Continued)

Tumour	Clinical	Radiological	PET	Spontaneous evolution	Treatment	Curability	Reference
Malignant fibrous histiocytoma##							
Malignant mesenchymoma	F predom, 7th D			Malignant	Ext R; adj CHT?; adj RT?	Poor	[123]
Melanoma	↑ risk in albino types, cough with haemoptysis	Hilar nodules	↑uptake#	Malignant	Ext R; adj CHT, adj IT (IFN)	Poor (5-yr surv 30%)	[3, 4, 124, 125]
Meningioma	F predom, usu asym, assn to neurofibromatosis	Coin lesion usually visible on CXR	↑uptake [126]	Benign	Simple R; no adj	Exc	[127]
Mucoepidermoid carcinoma	Infant, M predom, persistent pneumonia, cough, dyspnoea	Well-circ proximal mass, upper lobe predom	↑uptake [128]	Malignant	Ext R; adj RT	Dep on grade, low/high 5-yr surv 80/30%, better in infant than in adult	[3, 4, 129–134]
Multifocal micronodular pneumocyte hyperplasia	Assn with TS/lymphangioleiomyomatosis, F predom, usu asym, poss RD, cough	Bil mult well-defined micronodules, GG		Benign	R?; no adj	Exc	[135]
Myoepithelial carcinoma	M predom, 5th–6th D		↑ uptake [134]	Malignant	Ext R; no adj	Unpred	[136]
Myoepithelioma	Chest pain, dyspnoea Usu asym	Mult small nodules	↑uptake#	Benign	Simple R; no adj	Exc	[137]
Myofibrosarcoma			↑ uptake [138]	Malignant	Ext R; adj CHT	Unpred	[138]
Neurinoma¶¶			↑uptake#	Malignant	Simple R		[139]
Neurogenic sarcoma	Can be assd with neurofibromatosis	Well-circ het mass, haemorrhagic and/or necrotic features	↑ uptake [139]	Malignant	Ext R; adj CHT, adj RT	Poor, poor (5-yr surv <50%)	[89, 139]
Nodular amyloidosis	7th D, poss assn with Sjögren's syndrome, usu asym	Solitary or mult periph nodules, sharp margins	↑ uptake [140]	Malignant	Simple R; CHT	Unpred	[140–142]
Osteosarcoma	Cough, dyspnoea, chest pain	Volum calcified masses	↑uptake#, uptake on 99mTc scint	Malignant	Ext R; adj CHT	Poor (5-yr surv <10%)	[143]
Paraganglioma	Infant, 5th–6th D, poss HTN, flush (catecholamine secretion), assn with MEN 2, von Hippel–Lindau	Well-circ hilar lobulated tumour	↑uptake#, uptake on MIBG scint	Malignant	Simple R; adj RT?	Poor (5-yr surv 40%)	[144]

Table 1. – (Continued)

Tumour	Features		PET	Spontaneous evolution	Treatment	Curability	Reference
	Clinical	Radiological					
Plasmacytoma	M predom, 7th–8th D, assn with monoclonal gammopathy/multiple myeloma, usu asym	Solitary volum mass, periph nodule	↑uptake[#]	Malignant	Ext R; adj RT, adj CHT	Poor (5-yr surv 50%)	[145, 146]
Pleiomorphic giant/spindle cell carcinoma	M predom, cor with CS, 5th–7th D	Volum periph mass		Malignant	Ext R, mediastinal node R; adj RT, adj CHT	Poor (5-yr surv 5%)	[147]
Pleiomorphic sarcoma	M predom, cough, dyspnoea	Well-circ mass	↑uptake [148]	Malignant	Ext R; adj CHT?, adj RT?	Unpred, dep on grade	[3, 58, 88, 89, 148–150]
Pneumocytoma[++] Pulmonary blastoma[§§] Pleuropulmonary blastoma	Cough, dyspnoea, chest pain, fever, infant <5 yrs, other tumour familial history/lung congenital cysts history	Well-defined multilobulated volum mass, cystic (type I) and/or solid (type II, III) features, PE or pneumothorax, assn to lung cysts	↑uptake [147]	Malignant	Ext R; CHT (neoadj/adj), adj RT	Type I good (5-yr surv 80%), type II/III poor (5-yr surv 40%)	[151–155]
Pneumoblastoma	F predom, adults, 4th–5th D, chest pains, WL, cough, PE	Well-defined periph volum mass	↑uptake [147]	Malignant	Ext R; CHT (neoadj/adj), adj RT	Poor (5-yr surv 15%)	[156, 157]
Pulmonary artery leiomyosarcoma	5th–6th D, F predom, chest pain, dyspnoea, PH	Distension and soft mass in the pulmonary artery, necrotic and/or haemorrhagic features, ENH after injection of Gd on MRI	↑uptake [158]	Malignant	Ext R, vasc reconstruction; adj CHT	Poor (1-yr surv 50%)	[158–166]
Rhabdomyosarcoma	Infant, pneumothorax, assd with congenital pulmonary cysts	Volum het mass, cystic and/or necrotic features	↑uptake[#]	Malignant	Ext R; adj CHT, adj RT	Dep on grade, usu poor (2-yr surv 50%)	[167, 168]

Table 1. – (Continued)

Tumour	Clinical	Features Radiological	PET	Spontaneous evolution	Treatment	Curability	Reference
Schwannoma	F predom, cough, dyspnoea	Well-circ mass	↑uptake#	Malignant	Ext R; no adj	Good	[169]
Sclerosing haemangioma	F predom, usu asym, haemoptysis	Solitary well-circ hom mass, air meniscus sign on CT	↑uptake [171]	Benign	Ext R; no adj	Exc	[170–173]
Sebaceous carcinoma	Asym			Malignant	Ext R; no adj	Good	[174]
Sugar (clear) cell tumour	Asym, usu adults, may occur in infant	Intense post-contrast ENH on CT, well-circ periph nodules, periph coin lesion	↑uptake [174]	Benign	Simple R; no adj	Exc	[175, 176]
Spindle cell carcinoma	M predom, 5th–7th D			Malignant	Ext R; adj RT, adj CHT	Poor (5-yr surv 20%)	[177]
Synovial sarcoma	F predom, usu asym, chest pain, shortness of breath, haemoptysis	Inhom volum mass, necrotic, haemorrhagic and cystic changes	↑uptake#	Malignant	Ext R; adj CHT	Dep on grade, poor (5-yr surv 50%)	[88, 178, 179]
Teratoma	F predom, 1st–4th D, dry cough, chest pain, dyspnoea, haemoptysis, fever, trichoptysis	Upper lobe predom, calcifications, lobulated het mass, periph radiolucent areas, high-signal component on MRI	↑uptake#	Usu benign, 30% malignant	Simple R	Unpred	[180]
Thymoma	No paraneoplastic associated syndrome	Well-circ periph mass, PE	↑uptake#	Malignant	Ext R; adj RT	Good	[181]
Yolk sac tumour	M, 3rd–5th D, cough, dyspnoea	Volum hom mass	↑uptake#	Malignant	Ext R (debulking); adj CHT	Good	[182, 183]

PET: positron emission tomography; MALT: mucosa-associated lymphoid tissue; usu: usually; asym: asymptomatic; periph: peripheral; R: resection; adj: adjuvant treatment; exc: excellent; ext: extensive; RT: radiotherapy; F: female; predom: predominance; D: decade; circ: circumscribed; het: heterogeneous; ENH: enhancement; MRI: magnetic resonance imaging; CT: computed tomography; unpred: unpredictable; volum: voluminous; mult: multiple; bil: bilateral; nod: nodular; GG: ground-glass (attenuation); preop: pre-operative; CHT: chemotherapy; surv: survival; M: male; cor: correlation; CS: cigarette smoking; PE: pleural effusion; neoadj: neoadjuvant; dep: dependent; typ: typical; atyp: atypical; WL: weight loss; assn: association; HCG: human chronic gonadotropin; dup: duplication; RD: respiratory distress; Tx: treatment; var: variation; vasc: vascular; perivasc: perivascular; HT: hormone therapy; Met: methionine; RA: rheumatoid arthritis; dopa: dihydroxyphenylalanine; PH: pulmonary hypertension; HLT: heart and/or lung transplantation; hom: homogeneous; IT: immunotherapy; peribronchovasc: peribronchovascular; EBV: Epstein–Barr virus; dist: distribution; poss: possible; spont: spontaneous; IFN: interferon; CXR: chest radiography; TS: tuberous sclerosis; assd: associated; HTN: hypertension; scint: scintigraphy; MEN: multiple endocrine neoplasia; MIBG: metaiodobenzylguanidine; Gd: gadolinium. #: no specific data available regarding pulmonary localisation, PET feature determined by analogy to other localisation of tumour; *: see epithelioid haemangioendothelioma (low-grade lesion); +: see paraganglioma; §: see angiosarcoma (high-grade lesion); ¶: see pleiomorphic sarcoma; ##: see schwannoma; ++: see sclerosing haemangioma; §§: see foetal adenocarcinoma.

Organization tumour classification atlas [1, 184]. For each tumour identified, a second search on PubMed was then performed using the following keywords: tumour name AND "lung" OR "pulmonary", and tumour name AND "lung" OR "pulmonary" AND "PET scan". Only articles relating to primary tumours were selected, excluding cases reporting any other previous, synchronous or metachronal tumour of any type. Tumours of the chest wall, pleura, mediastinum and trachea were not included in the analysis. A bibliography was eventually completed with the references of the articles. The review was censored on March 1, 2006.

The PubMed search using the above methodology retrieved 1,119 articles, the complete list of which may be obtained from the present authors. All abstracts were read and 502 articles were analysed in depth (67 of the 135 retrieved for inflammatory pseudotumour, 89 of the 146 for sarcoma, 26 of the 51 for EHE, 19 of the 32 for mucoepidermoid carcinoma, 46 of the 63 for lymphoma, and 255 of the 692 for other tumour types).

Rarity as a characteristic feature

From an epidemiological point of view, the overall prevalence of rare pulmonary tumours is <1% of all lung tumours [3, 4]. Carcinoid tumours, accounting for ~0.5% of lung tumours, are included in this definition [2–7]. Since the annual incidence of lung cancer is estimated to exceed 1,000,000 worldwide, rare pulmonary tumours consequently occur in 10,000 patients annually. As a consequence of their rarity, knowledge regarding rare tumours is mainly based upon case reports or small series [3, 4], most of which are dated. Even if sometimes difficult to interpret, they nevertheless provide a good overview of the results of surgical resection. Moreover, publication bias regarding not only the proportion of cases reported but also the recruitment of patients (medical, surgical or pathological studies) may lead to overestimation of the incidence of exceptionally rare tumours, as well as to underestimation of the prevalence of the less rare entities (table 1) [2, 5–7]. Nonetheless, the present chapter identified the more frequent among the rare pulmonary tumours as carcinoid tumours, hamartoma, sclerosing haemangioma, inflammatory pseudotumour, pneumoblastoma and MALT lymphoma (table 1).

From a clinical point of view, rare pulmonary tumours may also correspond to common tumours arising in an unexpected population. Thus, for example, carcinoma represent 99% of pulmonary tumours in adults, but are regarded as rare tumours in childhood, even if representing 20% of pulmonary tumours in infants; conversely, EHE and blastoma are frequent tumours in childhood, but are quite rare in the whole population (table 2) [185, 186].

Table 2. – Pathology of rare lung tumours in infants

Benign	Malignant
Inflammatory pseudotumour	Carcinoid tumour
Adenoma	Carcinoma (bronchogenic, mucoepidermoid, neuroendocrine, adenoid cystic)
Mucosal cystadenoma	Sarcoma (fibrosarcoma, leiomyosarcoma, rhabdomyosarcoma, chondrosarcoma)
Hamartoma	Pneumoblastoma
Leiomyoma	Epithelioid haemangioendothelioma
Haemangioma	Haemangiopericytoma
Lymphangioma	Paraganglioma
Schwannoma	Plasmacytoma
Granular cell tumour	

Data adapted from [185, 186].

From a pathological point of view, since 99% of lung cancers are adenocarcinoma, squamous cell carcinoma, large cell carcinoma or small-cell carcinoma, and any tumoral lung lesion presenting with other histological features may be defined as a rare pulmonary tumour [1, 2, 184], pathologists are familiar with the most common pulmonary carcinomas; however, a large array of other benign and malignant tumours can present as primary lung tumours. These include epithelial, mesenchymal or mixed rare entities that may give rise to problems in diagnosis, particularly on small biopsy. Although, in most instances, the diagnosis may be made on the basis of routinely stained sections, immunohistochemistry can be useful in defining the nature of the neoplasm and evaluating its biological aggressiveness. More sophisticated studies (flow cytometry and molecular and cytogenetic analysis) may have a limited role in the diagnosis, but probably play a role in predicting clinical behaviour in some tumours, such as sarcoma (table 3). Since most of the neoplasms discussed in this chapter may also arise from extrapulmonary sites, the determining point in defining a rare pulmonary tumour is ensuring that it is primary in nature, with a detailed clinical history and accurate imaging evaluation. This requires clinical input since histological findings do not reveal the site of origin. Excluding secondary tumours, three pathological groups can be actualised depending upon the tissue of origin of the rare pulmonary neoplasm [184]: 1) rare tumours derived from (minority) orthotopic tissues (table 4) [2, 5, 7]; 2) rare lung tumours derived from ectopic tissues (mostly derived from embryonic residues; table 5) [6, 7]; and 3) rare lung tumours derived from haematopoietic tissues (table 6) [62]. Finally, the determination of differentiation and malignant potential and the definition of low- and high-grade neoplasm rely on the pathologist.

Inflammatory myofibroblastic pseudotumour

Inflammatory myofibroblastic pseudotumours (IPTs) comprise a fairly wide spectrum of lesions previously variously termed inflammatory pseudotumour, fibroma, fibroxanthoma, fibrous histiocytoma, solitary granuloma and pseudosarcomatous tumour [1]. They are composed of a mixture of inflammatory cells, myofibroblastic cells and collagen, and destroy the underlying lung architecture [187]. Attempts at subclassifying these tumours meet with the fact that nearly all myofibroblastic tumours show both benign and malignant features [1].

Older case reports emphasised that, in as many as 30% of cases, chronic or repeated infections could be a potential cause, but this concept was reconsidered, with more recent reports containing computed tomography (CT) studies suggesting that recurrent pulmonary infections were rather a consequence of bronchial obstruction by the tumour [73–75]. However, more recently, the identification of pro-viral sequences of human herpes virus (HHV) 8, a virus responsible for Kaposi's sarcoma in immunodeficient patients, in tumoural tissues from nonimmunodeficient patients has led to suspicion of a viral origin of IPT [73].

Clinical features

IPTs mostly occur before the fourth decade of life, and, especially, account for >50% of pulmonary tumours in children [187]. The sex distribution is equal [74, 75, 187]. Patients are asymptomatic in ~60% of cases, or may present with nonspecific manifestations, including chronic cough, dyspnoea or, rarely, haemoptysis [76, 77, 187].

Table 3. – Pathological features of primary pulmonary sarcomas

	Morphology	IHC expression	Molecular/chromosomal abnormalities
Leiomyosarcoma, low grade (fig. 3)	Fascicles of spindle cells at right angles and/or epithelioid growth pattern; fibrillary cytoplasm and cigar-shape nuclei; >3 mitosis·10 HPF^{-1}	Strong expression: SMA, h-caldesmon and vimentin; desmin +/-; CKs: may be + (focal)	R-cyclin D pathway (90%); p53 mutation (20%); loss 13q14–21; loss 10q; gains 17p, 8q and 1p; monosomy 1p12-pter
Leiomyosarcoma, high grade (fig. 4)	Marked hypercellularity and pleomorphism; irregular nuclear chromatin; prominent nucleoli; necrosis, haemorrhage; >10 mitosis·10 HPF^{-1}	Like low-grade variant; only vimentin is positive	R-cyclin D pathway (90%); p53 mutation (20%); loss 13q14–21; l 10q; gains 17p, 8q and 1p; monosomy 1p12-pter
Synovial sarcoma, monophasic (fig. 5)	Interweaving fascicles of densely packed spindle cells, rarely round cells; haemangiopericytoma-like pattern; nuclei: dark, round to oval; scant cytoplasm; stroma: scant and focally myxoid; 2–20 mitosis·10 HPF^{-1}	Useful positive diagnostic markers: EMA, pan-CK, E-cadherin and CD34; other positive markers: CK 14 and CK-KL1, CD99 and Bcl-2, which is of little relevance	Translocation: t(X;18)(p11.2;q11.2) syt-ssx1 fusion type#
Synovial sarcoma, biphasic (fig. 6)	Epithelial and spindle cell proliferation; epithelial component with cleft-like glandular spaces lined with cuboidal cells with round nuclei	Like monophasic variant	Translocation: t(X;18)(p11.2;q11.2) syt-ssx2 fusion type#
Pleomorphic sarcoma (fig. 7)	Intraparenchymal well-circumscribed lesion; storiform growth pattern; atypical spindle cells; marked pleomorphism; giant cells with multiple and bizarre nuclei and prominent nucleoli; >10 mitosis·HPF^{-1}	Nonspecific; vimentin: +; positive reaction in giant cells: desmin, SMA, CD68 and CD34	Mutation of ink4a, rbl and p53 genes on Chrs 7, 2 and 13
Chondrosarcoma	Lobulated nodular mass; atypical chondrocytes; slightly bizarre nuclei	Nonspecific	Not known in lung

Table 3. – (Continued)

	Morphology	IHC expression	Molecular/chromosomal abnormalities
Osteosarcoma	Bizarre spindle cells; osteoid formation; haemorrhage and necrosis; high mitotic index	Nonspecific	Not known in lung
Rhabdomyosarcoma	Alveolar/embryonal type	Muscle markers	Not known in lung
Pulmonary artery sarcoma (fig. 9)	Pleomorphic spindle cell proliferation; areas of leiomyosarcoma, fibrosarcoma, rhabdomyosarcoma, chondrosarcoma and angiosarcoma; tumours tend to spread along the intima	Vimentin: +; variable reactivity: SMA, CD31 and CD34	Amplification of 12q13–q15, containing *sas/cdk4*, *mdm2* and *gli*
Epithelioid haemangioendothelioma (fig. 11)	Polypoid lesion spreading into the alveolar spaces; invasion of arteries, veins and lymphatics 1–2 mitosis·HPF^{-1}(low-grade tumours)	+: vimentin, CD31, CD34, FVIII, CK (25% of cases); Weibel–Palade bodies on electron microscopy	Translocation: Chrs 7 and 22 [50], Chrs 1 and 3: t(1;3)(p36.3;q25) and *pax7* on 1p36; Robertsonian translocation: Chr 14
Angiosarcoma	Solid areas of large cells with central hyperchromatic nuclei, prominent nucleoli and abundant cytoplasm showing small vacuoles; anastomosing vascular channels lined with atypical endothelium; necrosis and haemorrhage; frequent mitosis	+: vimentin and, among endothelial markers, FVIII	Similar genetics as in EHE

IHC: immunohistochemistry; HPF: high-power field; h-caldesmon: high-molecular-weight caldesmon; SMA: smooth muscle actin; +: positive; -: negative; +/-: slightly positive; CK: cytokeratin; EMA: epithelial membrane antigen; KL-1: pan-keratin 1; Bcl-2: B-cell leukaemia/lymphoma 2 gene product; *syt*: synaptotagmin I gene; *ssx1*: synovial sarcoma, X breakpoint 1 gene; *ink4a*: cyclin-dependent kinase inhibitor 2A gene; *rb1*: retinoblastoma gene; *p53*: tumour protein p53 gene; Chr: chromosome; *sas*: sialic acid synthase gene; *cdk4*: cyclin-dependent kinase 4 gene; *mdm2*: mouse double minute 2 homologue gene; *gli*: glioma-associated oncogene homologue 1 gene; FVIII: factor VIII; *pax7*: paired box gene 7; EHE: epithelioid haemangioendothelioma. #: of synovial sarcoma.

Table 4. – Pathological classification of rare lung tumours from orthotopic tissues

Miscellaneous benign epithelial tumour
  Adenoma
  Micronodular pneumocyte hyperplasia
  Myoepithelioma
Hamartoma
Salivary gland type
  Adenoid cystic carcinoma
  Mucoepidermoid carcinoma
  Acinic cell carcinoma
Large cell carcinoma variants
  Lymphoepithelioma-like carcinoma
Adenocarcinoma, variants
  Foetal adenocarcinoma
Fibrous tumour (benign)
  Inflammatory pseudotumour
  Fibroma: solitary fibrous tumour
Smooth muscle tumour
  Leiomyoma
  Lymphangioleiomyoma
  Angiomyolipoma
Vascular tumour
  Haemangiomatosis
  Lymphangioma
  Haemangiopericytoma
Cartilage/bone-forming sarcoma
  Chondroma
Fatty tumour
  Lipoma
Neurogenic tumour (benign)
  Neurinoma
Sarcoma
Fibrous tumour
  Fibrosarcoma
  Lymphangioma
Smooth muscle tumour
  Leiomyosarcoma
Skeletal muscle tumour
  Rhabdomyosarcoma
Vascular tumour
  Epithelioid haemangioendothelioma
  Angiosarcoma
  Kaposi's sarcoma
  Pulmonary artery leiomyosarcoma
Cartilage/bone-forming sarcoma
  Chondrosarcoma
  Osteosarcoma
Neurogenic tumour
  Neurogenic sarcoma
Fatty tumour
  Liposarcoma
Others
  Synovialosarcoma
  Desmoplastic tumour
  Malignant mesenchymoma
Sarcomatoid carcinoma
  Carcinosarcoma
  Pulmonary blastoma
  Spindle cell carcinoma
  Giant cell carcinoma
  Pleomorphic carcinoma

Table 4. – (Continued)

Neuroendocrine tumour
  Carcinoid
  Paraganglioma/chemodectoma
Miscellaneous tumours of uncertain histogenesis
  Pneumocytoma/sclerosing haemangioma
  Clear cell tumour (sugar tumour)
  Granular cell tumour

Data adapted from [1, 2, 5, 7, 184].

Imaging features

IPTs appear as solitary well-circumscribed masses, ranging 2–15 cm in diameter. They are usually peripheral, but have been reported to occur as tracheobronchial lesions in 10–40% of cases [75, 77]. They are associated with obstructive atelectasis in 30% of cases [73, 75–77]. The usual stability in size is the more important imaging diagnostic criterion. Multifocal and bilateral forms are exceptional, and are considered as overlap forms of low-grade fibrosarcoma or malignant fibrous histiocytoma [74]. Myofibroblastic tumours are a well-known source of positron emission tomography (PET) false positives [78]. Pre-operative diagnosis using endoscopic or percutaneous biopsy remains difficult due to the heterogeneous structure of these tumours [75].

Pathological features

IPTs may appear macroscopically as an intraparenchymatous well-circumscribed mass or an endobronchial polypoid lesion of variable size. They are characterised histologically as an irregular proliferation of fibroblasts and myofibroblasts intermixed with an infiltrate of inflammatory cells, mainly lymphocytes and plasma cells (fig. 1). Eosinophils, histiocytes and multinucleate giant cells are the other inflammatory cells present in this lesion. Three distinct histological patterns are described [188]: 1) inflammatory myxoid proliferation with fascicles of spindled fibroblasts or myofibroblasts, collagen, and abundant lymphocytes and plasma cells; 2) a compact spindle cell pattern simulating a fibrous histiocytoma characterised by a myxoid proliferation of fibroblasts and myofibroblasts arrayed in a pattern associated with

Table 5. – Pathological classification of rare lung tumours from ectopic tissues

Thymoma
Neurectodermal tumour
  Glomus tumour
  Meningioma
  Ependymoma
  Melanoma
  Sebaceous carcinoma
Germ cell tumour
  Teratoma
  Seminoma
  Nonseminomatous tumour
    Embryonal carcinoma
    Yolk sac tumour
    Choriocarcinoma
Choristoma (thyroid, pancreas, adrenal)
Endometriosis

Table 6. – Pathological classification of rare lung tumours from haematopoietic tissues

Non-Hodgkin's lymphoma
  Mature B-cell lymphoma
    Extranodal marginal zone lymphoma: MALT/BALT
    Lymphomatoid granulomatosis
    Diffuse large B-cell lymphoma
    Angiotropic/intravascular lymphoma
    Plasmacytoma
    Nodular amyloidosis
    Mantle cell lymphoma
    Burkitt's lymphoma
    Small lymphocytic lymphoma
    Lymphoplasmacytoid lymphoma (Waldenström's disease)
  Mature T-cell lymphoma
    T-cell/NK-cell lymphoma
Hodgkin's lymphoma

MALT: mucosa-associated lymphoid tissue; BALT: bronchus-associated lymphoid tissue; NK: natural killer. Data adapted from [62].

plasma cells, xanthoma cells and rare giant cells; and 3) hypocellular, characterised by dense collagen with sparse spindle cells and inflammatory cells. Vascular invasion and obliterative phlebitis may also be present, particularly in the inflammatory myofibro-blastic variant. Foci of necrosis, mitotic figures and calcification are infrequently seen. The proliferating spindle cells usually stain for vimentin and smooth muscle actin. Focal immunoreaction has been described for desmin, cytokeratin, CD30 and histiocytic marker (KP-1). The plasma cells are polyclonal, and, in adults, may exhibit a strong cytoplasmic immunoglobulin (Ig) G4 reaction, associated with retroperitoneal and mediastinal fibrosis and high serum IgG4 levels [189]. A similar pattern has been observed in sclerosing pancreatitis, suggesting that an IgG4-related immunopathological process might be involved in the pathogenesis of IPT. Epstein–Barr virus (EBV) RNA and HHV8 DNA have recently been detected in IPTs, and it is postulated that they may play a role in their histogenesis *via* expression of cytokines such as interleukin (IL)-6 and IL-8 and cyclin D1, expressed in a few cases of IPT [74].

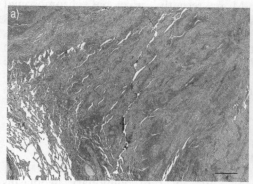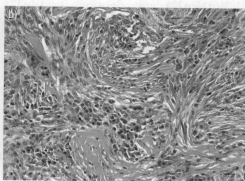

Fig. 1. – Pathology of primary pulmonary inflammatory pseudotumour. a) Inflammatory pseudotumour/myo-fibroblastic tumour of the lung showing fascicles of spindled fibroblasts or myofibroblasts, collagen and an abundant infiltrate of inflammatory cells. b) At higher magnification, an irregular proliferation of fibroblasts and myofibroblasts intermixed with inflammatory cells, mainly lymphocytes and plasma cells, is present. Scale bars= a) 500 µm, b) 40µm.

Tumours composed of fibroblasts and myofibroblasts are considered in the differential diagnosis, and many of these overlap with IPTs. These lesions include benign and malignant fibrous histiocytoma, myofibroblastoma, low grade myxofibrosarcoma, inflammatory fibrosarcoma and follicular dendritic tumours.

Treatment

Even if myofibroblastic tumours are considered to be benign lesions, with possible spontaneous regression [79], surgical resection is recommended due to their tendency to progress and relapse, with local pleural, parietal or mediastinal invasiveness in 3–5% of cases [76, 190]. Since the tumour occurs with a fibrous envelope, usually allowing easy surgical delineation, the need for adjuvant treatment in case of incomplete resection/ uncommon pathological features has not been evaluated. Pre-operative treatment with radiotherapy has occasionally been reported in patients with mediastinal involvement [191]. In inoperable patients, focal conformal radiotherapy is now preferred to treatment with corticosteroids, although they induced an objective response of as high as 50% in an older series [79]. In recurrent or multifocal lesions, chemotherapy may consist of the same protocols as in soft-tissue sarcoma [74].

Prognosis

Patients who undergo surgical resection of an inflammatory myofibroblastic tumour exhibit a 5-yr overall survival ranging 75–100% [73–79, 188–190]. Transformation into low- and/or high-grade fibrosarcoma has exceptionally been reported (<10 cases in the literature), and may correspond to initially misdiagnosed high-grade tumours [1]. There are no clear histological features which might be predictive of aggressive behaviour. However, some morphological findings associated with poor prognosis include necrosis involving >15% of the total microscopic area, bizarre ganglion-like cells, mitosis of >3 mitosis·50 high-power fields $(HPF)^{-1}$, high cellularity with fascicular pattern, and nuclear atypia and poor circumscription. Other factors are metastasis and local recurrence. Some genetic and molecular alterations seem to be potentially predictive of clinical behaviour, particularly in younger patients. Cytogenetic analysis has shown abnormal karyotype 47,XX+r (ring) and the clonal abnormalities translocation t(1.2)(q21;p23) and deletion del(4)(q27). More recently, a clonal chromosomal aberration involving the 2p23 and anaplastic lymphoma kinase (ALK) gene regions has been reported in young patients with IPT. This specific chromosomal aberration is associated with overexpression of ALK in the nuclei and cytoplasm of spindle cells in IPTs. Strong expression of p53 and aneuploid DNA has also been observed in more aggressive cases. Together, these molecular and genetic studies suggest that some IPTs are low-grade sarcomas and may be important in predicting clinical behaviour and in surgical management.

Pulmonary parenchymal sarcomas

Primary pulmonary sarcomas account for ~40% of rare pulmonary neoplasms [4]. They comprise parenchymal sarcomas (leiomyosarcoma, rhabdomyosarcoma, fibrosarcoma, malignant fibrous histiocytoma, osteosarcoma, chondrosarcoma and liposarcoma), and great- and small-vessel sarcomas (leiomyosarcoma, fibrosarcoma, angiosarcoma and haemangiopericytoma). The pathological findings are identical to those of their soft-tissue counterparts, with a spectrum of differentiation from low-to-high grade.

Primary pulmonary sarcomas mainly occur between the sixth and eighth decades of life [57, 58, 88, 89, 192]. Clinical symptoms are nonspecific, and usually consist of cough, dyspnoea and haemoptysis, depending on the size and location of the lesions; performance status is generally conserved at the time of diagnosis [88]. Radiological imaging shows a voluminous solitary heterogeneous well-defined round lesion, ranging 4–25 cm in diameter and frequently presenting with cystic, necrotic or haemorrhagic features (fig. 2). PET shows increased uptake. The sarcomas progress mainly by local extension. The systemic metastases occurring in advanced disease are rare at the time of diagnosis (<2%) [57, 192]. Pathological confirmation of the diagnosis has been reported to be obtained *via* transparietal or endobronchial biopsy, but the sensitivity of such techniques remains uncertain [192]. As mediastinal involvement is rare, mediastinoscopy is not recommended [57, 192]. A definite diagnosis is often obtained by examination of the resected tumour.

The pathological diagnosis of a primary sarcoma in the lung must first consider and rule out the possibility of a pulmonary metastasis from a soft-tissue sarcoma, and secondly distinguish it from primary epithelial carcinomas of the lung that may assume a sarcomatoid or biphasic appearance and exhibit a different behaviour: pleomorphic carcinoma, spindle cell carcinoma, giant cell carcinoma, carcinosarcoma, and pulmonary blastoma. In addition, the possibility of "benign" metastases from the uterus (metastasising leiomyoma) or bone (giant cell tumour) must be considered. Moreover, most mesenchymal tumours of the lung have both benign and malignant counterparts. Finally, since grading is useful in the treatment decision for some adult sarcomas, it should be provided in order to plan therapy. In this setting, a well-reproducible scheme is the three-grade system of the French Federation of Cancer Centers Sarcoma Group (Paris, France), in which three distinct parameters are considered: tumour differentiation, mitotic rate and amount of necrosis. In some sarcomas, the presence of specific genetic alterations plays an important role in defining the outcome of the disease.

Surgery is the most efficient treatment for primary pulmonary sarcoma. As most of them are limited, resection rates are as high as 80% [88]. Similar to other soft-tissue sarcomas, post-operative radiotherapy is debated in the case of incomplete resection and/or high-grade lesions [58, 88]. More studies are required to better evaluate radiotherapy in a modern setting. Conversely, the indication for adjuvant chemotherapy mostly depends upon the grade of the lesion [89, 90]. Contrary to other soft-tissue sarcomas, neoadjuvant strategies have been disappointing, and, thus, are not recommended [58, 88]. In the case of unresectable lesions, chemoradiation may be the best therapeutic strategy [88, 90].

Prognosis mainly depends upon the possibility of complete resection (50–80% of cases in published surgical studies), which, combined with the grade of the lesion, is the best predictive factor of local and systemic recurrence and survival. The influence of size as a prognostic factor remains the subject of debate, and seems to be less important than in other soft-tissue sarcomas [57, 58, 88, 89, 192]. The 5-yr overall survival of primary pulmonary sarcoma ranges 40–50% [57, 58, 88–90, 192].

Leiomyosarcoma

Primary pulmonary leiomyosarcoma, accounting for 0.03% of pulmonary tumours [3, 4], is one of the most common pulmonary sarcomas [57, 58, 88, 89, 192]. It occurs in both middle-aged adults and infants [91, 92, 193]. Macroscopically, primary leiomyosarcomas show the microscopic findings of their uterine or soft-tissue counterparts, revealing a spectrum of differentiation that ranges from low- to high-grade leiomyosarcoma (figs 3 and 4). Their histological patterns are summarised in table 3.

The differential diagnosis includes other primary spindle cell tumours, such as fibrosarcoma, synovial sarcoma and metastasis from uterine, soft tissue or gastrointestinal tract stromal tumours. Immunohistochemical characteristics and clinical evaluation are generally useful in defining the correct diagnosis.

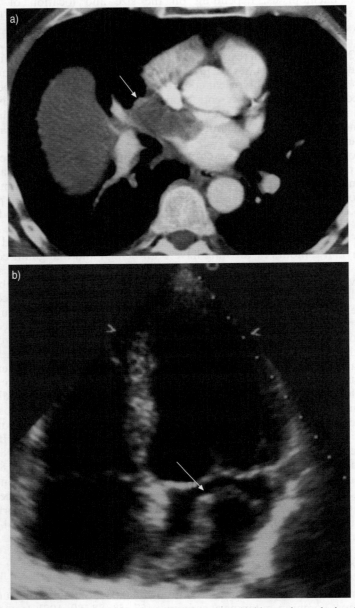

Fig. 2. – Primary pulmonary fibrosarcoma. A 54-yr-old male presented with transient aphasia related to a vascular ischaemic accident. Imaging disclosed a voluminous tumour (arrow) of the right lung invading the homo- and contralateral mediastinum and the left atrium (a), with a floating atrial neoplastic thrombus (arrow) partially obstructing the mitral valve inflow (b). The patient underwent complete tumoural resection, with extensive right pneumonectomy, atriotomy and excision of the thrombus, which was neoplastic. Pathological analysis revealed a round-cell high-grade fibrosarcoma.

Prognosis. Overall 5-yr survival tends to be better than in other types of pulmonary sarcoma, especially in infants, and ranges 50–60% [91, 92, 193, 194]. Predictors of prognosis include the presence or absence of metastasis, the histological grade of differentiation (low- and intermediate-grade *versus* high-grade lesions), based on the arrangement of tumour cells, mitotic activity, nuclear pleomorphism and atypia, and the presence or absence of necrosis and haemorrhage. In primary pulmonary leiomyosarcomas, tumour size is a less important prognostic factor [195]. The prognostic significance of the chromosomal and molecular abnormalities is not well established.

Synovial sarcoma

Pulmonary synovial sarcomas occur in young-to-middle-aged adults, with a slight female predominance [178, 179, 196, 197]. Histologically, pulmonary synovial sarcomas

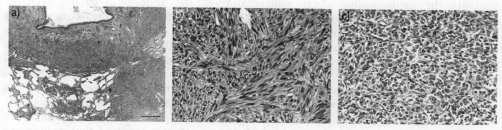

Fig. 3. – Pathology of primary pulmonary low-grade leiomyosarcoma. a) Low-grade leiomyosarcoma with spindle cell proliferation around the bronchus infiltrating the bronchial wall. The neoplasm extends to the surrounding lung parenchyma. b) At higher magnification, the tumour shows fascicles of plump elongated cells intersecting at right angles. The spindle cells have a scant fibrillary cytoplasm and typically elongated cigar-shaped nuclei. The nuclear chromatin tends to be coarse and nucleoli are slightly enlarged. A few mitotic figures are seen. c) Some cases have a prominent epithelioid growth pattern, showing large round-to-oval cells with abundant eosinophilic cytoplasm, round nuclei and prominent nucleoli. Scale bars=a) 500µm, b and c) 20 µm.

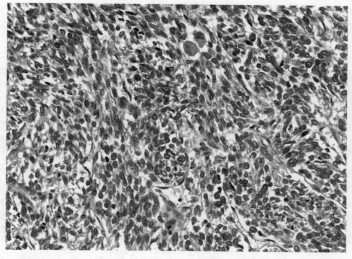

Fig. 4. – Pathology of primary pulmonary high-grade leiomyosarcoma showing marked hypercellularity with nuclear irregularity and pleomorphism. The nuclear chromatin is coarse and irregular and nucleoli are prominent. Mitotic figures are frequent. Scale bar=40 µm.

are identical to their soft-tissue counterparts even though they present a prevalent monophasic growth pattern (figs 5 and 6; table 3). Currently, detecting the translocation t(X;18)(p11.2;q11.2) in a spindle or round cell sarcoma is virtually synonymous with synovial sarcoma diagnosis [198]. This translocation, found in >90% of synovial sarcomas regardless of histological type, results in the fusion of two genes, synaptotagmin I (*syt*) and synovial sarcoma, X breakpoint (*ssx*) 1 or 2, to give *syt-ssx1* and *syt-ssx2*.

The most important differential diagnosis is with spindle cell carcinoma, which shows more prominent nuclear pleomorphism, an infiltrative growth pattern and greater mitotic activity. In addition, areas of adenocarcinoma or squamous cell carcinoma differentiation are frequently seen in spindle cell carcinomas.

Prognosis. Primary pulmonary synovial sarcomas tend to exhibit locoregional spread involving the mediastinum, chest wall, diaphragm or abdominal cavity; systemic metastases are frequent (25% of cases), and mainly occur in the liver, bone, brain and lung itself [178, 196, 197]. Overall prognosis is poor regardless of therapy, and mainly depends upon the pathological grade (5-yr survival ranges 30–40%). The characteristic gene expression of soft tissue synovial sarcoma is of interest not only in diagnosing synovial sarcoma but also in predicting prognosis. Patients with synovial sarcomas that express the *syt-ssx1* fusion type seem to show significantly shorter metastasis-free survival than *syt-ssx2* patients, with a 5-yr progression-free survival rate of 42 *versus* 89%, respectively. Whether this genetic pattern has the same prognostic significance in the pulmonary synovial sarcomas remains to be established. It was recently reported that pulmonary synovial sarcoma with the *syt-ssx2* phenotype was associated with a rapidly progressive downhill course [199]. Other genetic or biological alterations can correlate with clinical outcome. In particular, increased expression of p53, cyclin A, cyclin E and cyclin D1, together with a high Ki67 proliferative index, are associated with poor outcome and/or increased risk of tumour relapse. Low expression of p27 (knotted1-interacting protein) also seems to be associated with dismal outcome, whereas overexpression of β-catenin, with or without mutations, seems to contribute to the development and progression of synovial sarcoma.

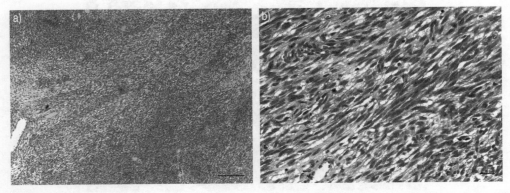

Fig. 5. – Pathology of primary pulmonary monophasic synovial sarcoma. a) The predominant spindle cell proliferation grows in interweaving fascicles. b) The spindle cells are densely packed with dark round-to-oval nuclei and scant amphophilic cytoplasm. The stroma is scant and focally myxoid. Numerous mitoses are present. Scale bars=a) 500µm, b) 40µm.

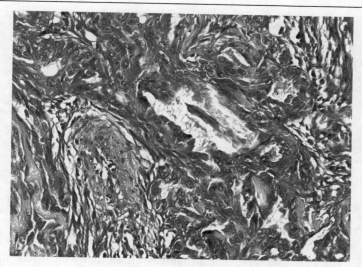

Fig. 6. – Pathology of primary pulmonary biphasic synovial sarcoma. The epithelial component is characterised by the presence of cleft-like glandular spaces. These glandular spaces are lined with cuboidal cells with scant cytoplasm and round nuclei and contain mucoid secretions. Scale bar=40µm.

Pleiomorphic sarcoma

Pleiomorphic sarcoma, previously named malignant fibrous histiocytoma, has been reported as the most frequent soft-part sarcoma in middle-aged adults, and also shows rare occurrence as a primary lung tumour (~0.04% of lung tumours [4]) [148–150, 200]. In the differential diagnosis, pleomorphic carcinoma, fibrosarcoma, malignant solitary fibrous tumour, inflammatory pseudotumour and metastatic disease should be considered. Correct use of immunohistochemical stains and careful evaluation of the morphology drive the correct diagnosis (fig. 7; table 3). Metastatic epithelioid and pleomorphic sarcomas might be very difficult to distinguish, but there are additional markers which assist in this respect. Finally, inflammatory pseudotumour may be confused with storiform/inflammatory pleiomorphic sarcoma. The presence of necrosis, atypical cells and a marked number of mitoses favour the diagnosis of pleiomorphic sarcoma.

Prognosis. The prognosis in pleiomorphic sarcoma is usually dismal and largely depends upon the stage of the disease at the time of diagnosis [148–150]. Tumour size and reduced expression of p21 are considered poor prognostic factors. However, surgery is as efficient at treating recurrences as the initial tumour, and then outcome can be better than expected, with a third of patients dying from the disease [150].

Other primary pulmonary parenchymal sarcomas

Osteo- and chondrosarcomas occur in patients older than those with bone osteosarcomas, and are very rare (0.01% of lung tumours [4]). They have been reported in adults in their fifth decade of life with a male predominance, and present with nodular parenchymal or peribronchial heterogeneous voluminous masses with calcified and cystic changes [35, 36]. Increased uptake on technetium-99m scintigraphy is usual in osteosarcoma [143]. Peripheral lesions must be differentiated from primary chest wall tumours. The pathological features of these tumours are described in table 3. Surgery

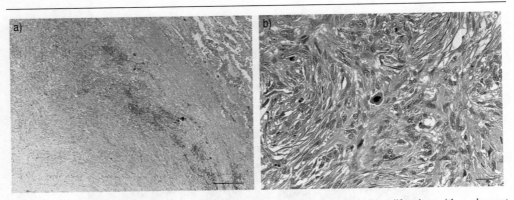

Fig. 7. – Pathology of primary pulmonary pleiomorphic sarcoma. a) Spindle cell proliferation with a clear-cut storiform pattern. b) The spindle-shaped cells resemble fibroblasts and contain irregular hyperchromatic nuclei with mitotic activity. Scale bars=a) 500µm, b) 40 µm.

seems to offer the best outcome. The prognosis differs between osteo- and chondro-sarcoma; since most osteosarcomas are unresectable, treatment is mainly based on chemotherapy, and the 5-yr overall survival is <10%, whereas extensive resection of chondrosarcoma leads to a good prognosis, with 5-yr survival of >80% [167, 168].

Pure primary pulmonary rhabdomyosarcomas are extremely rare, and mostly occur in infants [167]. Of the reported cases, >50% occur in close association with a history of congenital cystic malformation of the lung, thus regarded as a risk factor for rhabdomyosarcoma [167, 168]. Areas of rhabdomyosarcoma differentiation may also be present in lesions in children, such as pleuropulmonary blastoma, and in other tumours observed in adults, such as carcinosarcomas, pulmonary blastomas and pulmonary artery sarcoma. Pure rhabdomyosarcomas are extremely rare and present as an intraparenchymal or endobronchial mass (table 3).

Only a few cases of primary liposarcomas of the lung have been described. The histological features are identical to those described in their soft-tissue counterparts. Multimodal therapy relies on extensive resection, followed by adjuvant chemotherapy and radiotherapy. The prognosis is usually poor, with a 2-yr survival of ~50% [95].

Pulmonary vascular tumours

Pulmonary artery leiomyosarcoma

Clinical features. Pulmonary artery sarcomas mainly occur in patients in their fifth to sixth decade of life [158, 160–166]. There is no sex predominance, although a female predominance has been reported [158, 160, 161, 164]. The usual manifestations combine dyspnoea, chest pain, cough and haemoptysis, often initially leading to a diagnosis of pulmonary embolism [158]. However, failure of anticoagulant therapy in this setting, as well as weight loss and fever (arising in 40% of cases), may rectify this misdiagnosis [158, 161, 164]. Clinical examination may show systolic ejection murmur on cardiac auscultation and cyanosis [160, 161, 163].

Imaging features. Radiographic findings include hilar enlargement (50% of cases), pulmonary nodules (40% of cases), pericarditis (30% of cases) and possibly ground-glass opacities or pleural effusion (fig. 8) [158, 160, 164]. CT typically reveals a large polypoid filling defect in the central pulmonary circulation (cloverleaf appearance) [160]. In contrast to the abrupt narrowing and cut-off observed in cruoric thromboembolic disease, sarcoma forms a contiguously soft smooth tapering tissue filled into the pulmonary artery, with vascular distension and possible extravascular nodular spread in the parenchyma [160, 163, 164]. Cases of sarcoma present with a heterogeneous appearance, including areas of necrosis, haemorrhages and peripheral ossification, dependent on the histological type [159, 166]. Magnetic resonance imaging features differ from those of emboli, with T1 heterogeneous enhancement, T2 peripheral enhancement and increased uptake of gadolinium, which are not found in emboli [160, 163, 164]. PET shows increased uptake [165]. Classical arteriographic findings are a characteristic motion of the pediculate or lobulated lesions stalk (to and fro motion), and a pressure gradient between the artery trunk and the artery [160, 163, 164]. However, ventilation/perfusion scintigraphic and echocardiographic findings are similar to those in pulmonary embolism [158, 161].

Pathological features. Macroscopically, the tumour appears as a polypoid intraluminal mass or nodular sessile mass that spreads along the intima of the vessel, resembling an organised thrombus. It may be multifocal, and tends to grow down into the pulmonary valve or distally into the small branches of the pulmonary artery. Histologically, this tumour is usually characterised by undifferentiated spindle cell proliferation with marked cellular pleomorphism and a variable mitotic count (fig. 9, table 3). The most frequent histological feature consists of leiomyosarcoma, but other sarcoma subtypes, such as fibrosarcoma and synovial sarcoma, have also been reported in the pulmonary artery location. Differential diagnosis essentially includes metastatic sarcomas and thrombus.

Treatment. Surgery is the recommended treatment for pulmonary artery sarcoma, with resectability rates ranging 60–75%. It consists of complete excision from the vascular bed of the tumour, with or without graft reconstruction of the pulmonary arteries [158, 160–166]. In the case of voluminous and/or invading lesions, extensive resection with pneumonectomy, and even heart and lung transplantation, has been reported [160, 163, 164]. A slight improvement in overall survival has been reported to occur with adjuvant chemotherapy and/or radiotherapy.

Prognosis. Patients mostly die of right heart failure due to progressive outflow peripheral vascular obstruction and emboli. The grading system for soft-tissue sarcomas may be used for defining differentiation and prognosis, even though, with the dismal prognosis, definition of the grade of the tumour is prognostically irrelevant. Outcome is poor, and mainly depends upon the opportunity to perform complete resection. In recent series, life expectancy is ~6–12 months, and 1-yr survival is ~50% [161, 164].

Epithelioid haemangioendothelioma

Two types of peripheral intravascular sarcomatous tumours are described, namely EHE and high-grade angiosarcoma. EHE is a low-to-intermediate-grade mixed epithelioid, endothelial and vascular tumour, mostly arising in the skin and deep soft tissues [1]. The lung is unusual as a primary location, and it was initially considered an intravascular and intra-alveolar extension of bronchioloalveolar carcinoma, and thus called intravascular bronchoalveolar tumour [1, 48]. EHE accounts for 0.03% of lung primary tumours [3].

Clinical features. EHE mostly occurs in Caucasian females (80% of reported cases), in the age range 12–65 yrs [48, 49]. The tumour is frequently discovered on routine chest radiography; nonspecific symptoms reported in ~50% of patients include pleuritic chest

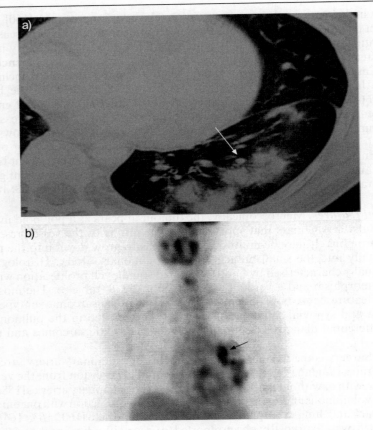

Fig. 8. – Primary pulmonary artery sarcoma. A 38-yr-old female presented with acute chest pain, haemoptysis and dyspnoea. Computed tomography (CT) revealed complete obstruction of the left inferior lobar artery and parenchymal opacities (arrow) of the left inferior lobe, leading to a diagnosis of pulmonary embolism with infarction. However, the opacities were atypical, irregular and plurifocal, and without pleural contact (a). Despite effective heparin treatment, the symptoms recurred 3 months later. CT showed an increase in peripheral nodule diameter, associated with enlargement of the pulmonary artery and increased uptake on positron emission tomography (arrow), suggesting a diagnosis of pulmonary artery sarcoma (b). The patient underwent pulmonary endarteriectomy, complete resection of the tumour and extensive left pneumonectomy. Pathological examination showed spindle-cell sarcoma, and confirmed parenchymal pulmonary metastases. Despite adjuvant chemotherapy, the patient died 4 months after surgery.

pain, nonproductive cough, dyspnoea and haemoptysis [48, 49]. Physical examination may reveal inspiratory crackles (30% of cases) [48–50].

Imaging features. The most characteristic imaging features of EHE are multiple bilateral slow-growing perivascular nodules, usually located in relation with small vessels or bronchi. Nodule sizes range 3–50 mm (mean diameter 20 mm), and their lesion number ranges 10–20 lesions (fig. 10) [18, 48–50]. Despite evidence of microscopic calcifications on pathological examination, nodules are not calcified on imaging. Another radiological feature is mainly infiltrative ground-glass opacities, simulating carcinomatous lymphangitis [18, 48–51]. Pleural effusion and mediastinal involvement arise in <10% of cases [49]. EHE shows increased uptake on PET [50].

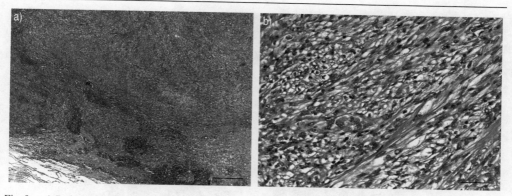

Fig. 9. – a) Pathology of primary pulmonary artery leiomyosarcoma. b) Undifferentiated spindle cell proliferation resembling a leiomyosarcoma, with marked cellular pleomorphism and a variable mitotic count resembling a leiomyosarcoma or fibrosarcoma. Scale bars=a) 500µm, b) 40 µm.

Pathological features. Diagnosis is performed by means of lung biopsy; transbronchial biopsy has recently been reported to yield sufficient tissues to permit a pathological diagnosis [48, 50]. EHE can diffusely involve the pleura, simulating diffuse malignant mesothelioma. Microscopically, low-grade EHE is characterised by polypoid nodules growing into the alveolar spaces with an angiocentric growth pattern, hence the old term of intravascular sclerosing bronchiolar alveolar tumour (fig. 11; table 3).

The differential diagnosis includes sclerosing haemangioma (an epithelial neoplasm with cells positive for epithelial membrane antigen and surfactant apoprotein A), metastasis from epithelioid sarcomas and malignant mesothelioma. Other benign lesions, such as amyloid nodules, old granulomas or infarction, should be considered in the differential diagnosis.

Little is known about the genetics of EHE. A recent study revealed an identical translocation involving chromosomes 1 and 3, and paired box gene (PAX) 7, localised to 1p36, is considered a potential gene which may be rearranged in EHE 1;3 translocation [52]. Similar to other sarcomas, this translocation may prove central to the diagnosis of this tumour.

Treatment. The only effective treatment for EHE is complete extensive surgical resection of the pulmonary nodules. Partial lung resection, such as segmentectomy or wedge resection, is associated with a short disease-free interval and poor outcome [48–50]. Surgery remains the most effective therapeutic option even in the case of localised recurrence, implying the need for a short follow-up period after the initial treatment [53]. Chemotherapy and radiotherapy are ineffective in EHE [48–50]. However, some spontaneous regressions have been reported, arising 5–15 yrs after the diagnosis, thus supporting a watch-and-wait approach in asymptomatic patients with low-grade EHE [48–50].

Prognosis. Even if the overall prognosis in EHE is characterised by a median survival of 5–6 yrs, this rare tumour is slow-growing, rarely causes metastases and thus might be considered a chronic disease, as in a female patient who underwent 13 operations for localised recurrent pulmonary EHE over a 24-yr period [53]. Endobronchial spread, pleural effusion and extended endovascular disease have been identified as unfavourable prognostic factors [48–50, 54].

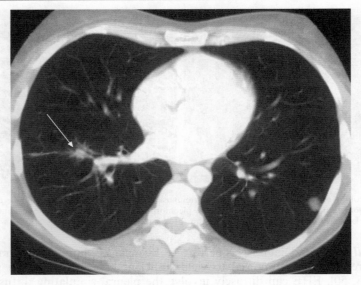

Fig. 10. – Primary pulmonary epithelioid haemangioendothelioma. A 45-yr-old female presented with cough leading to the discovery of multiple bilateral small nodules, one of which had a juxtahilar location and fusiform pattern on computed tomography (arrow). Positron emission tomography revealed increased uptake by this nodule. Surgical biopsy specimens showed epithelioid haemangioendothelioma. The patient received two lines of chemotherapy with liposomal anthracycline and imatinib, leading to transient stabilisation of the lesions. The patient then developed right chronic pleural effusion associated with hypertrophic osteoarthropathy.

Angiosarcoma

High-grade primary pulmonary vascular tumours correspond to epithelioid angio-sarcoma, very rarely reported in the literature, and Kaposi's sarcoma, arising in patients with AIDS [49]. No direct filiation from EHE to angiosarcoma has been reported to date.

The clinical features of angiosarcoma are similar to those of EHE, but high-grade angiosarcomas are frequently revealed by massive haemoptysis [18]. Radiologically, angiosarcoma cases present with multiple bilateral nodules surrounded by a halo of ground-glass attenuation, with a typical specific cauliflower-like appearance on T2

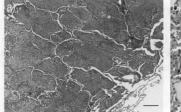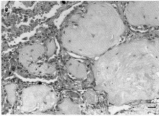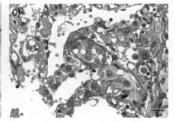

Fig. 11. – Pathology of primary pulmonary epithelioid haemangioendothelioma. a) Polypoid nodules growing into the alveolar spaces. b) The cellular proliferation in the periphery of the nodules is embedded in a myxoid stroma assuming a chondroid appearance. At the centre of the masses, the intercellular matrix tends to undergo to sclerosis and hyalinisation, and, in long-standing lesions, the entire tumour may appear extensively sclerotic and sometimes calcified. c) They are composed of large polygonal cells with round-to-oval nuclei with intranuclear inclusions and inconspicuous nucleoli. The cytoplasm is large and eosinophilic with vacuoles, some containing erythrocytes, which are one of the diagnostic hallmarks of the lesion. Scale bars=a) 500µm, b and c) 40 µm.

magnetic resonance imaging [19]. The differential diagnosis includes metastatic cardiac angiosarcoma.

Pathological features. Epithelioid angiosarcoma cases tend to present with large solitary masses with necrotic and haemorrhagic areas on the cut surface. The histological patterns are described in figure 12 and table 3.

Treatment. The management of angiosarcoma is not established; surgical resection is rarely possible due to local and regional invasion; radiotherapy and chemotherapy are less efficient than in other localisations [18]. A minor antitumoural effect of intratumoural and/or systemic high doses of IL-2 has recently been reported [19].

The prognosis in epithelioid angiosarcoma is especially poor, with most patients dying within 1 yr after diagnosis, whatever therapy is engaged.

Mucoepidermoid carcinoma

Mucoepidermoid carcinoma represents the most frequent variant of salivary gland-like tumours of the bronchus. It is a mixed malignant tumour characterised by the presence of squamous cells, mucin-secreting cells and cells of intermediate type [1]. The tumours are classified as low-, intermediate- and high-grade lesions [128–130]. Mucoepidermoid carcinoma accounts for 0.06–0.12% of lung tumours [3, 4].

Clinical features

Mucoepidermoid carcinoma shows an equal sex distribution, with a slight male predominance [130, 131]. The age range is 3–78 yrs, with 50% of tumours occurring between the third and fourth decades of life [128, 130, 131]. High-grade tumours are usually diagnosed in older patients [128, 130]. The symptoms are related to bronchial obstruction, including dyspnoea, cough and haemoptysis. Most mucoepidermoid carcinomas in childhood are diagnosed following a history of recurrent pneumonia [131–133].

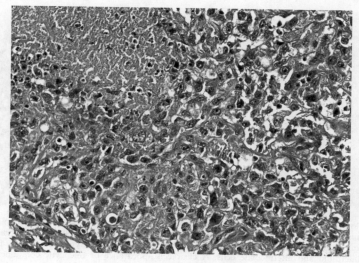

Fig. 12. – Pathology of primary pulmonary high-grade angiosarcoma. The cells are large, with central hyperchromatic, pleomorphic and atypical nuclei and prominent nucleoli. The cytoplasm is abundant and eosinophilic, with small vacuoles. Mitoses and necrosis are easily identified. In solid areas, the stroma is less prominent and lacks the sclerotic appearance that characterises the low-grade lesions.

Imaging features

Imaging studies reveal a well-circumscribed smoothly oval or lobulated homogeneous mass, often presenting with cystic and/or calcification features [130]. The lesion is solitary in 40–70% of cases [128–131], and shows mild central enhancement on CT [131]. Hilar involvement is infrequent, and is the hallmark of high-grade lesions [133]. PET reveals increased uptake [132]. Proximal mucoepidermoid tumours exhibit an iceberg-like appearance, with partial exophytic endobronchial growth that makes diagnostic endobronchial biopsy possible [130, 133].

Pathological features

Pulmonary mucoepidermoid carcinoma exhibits identical pathological features to the salivary gland of the same name. Cases may present with a polypoid endobronchial mass covered with bronchial mucosa that can be focally ulcerated or can present with a peripheral mass. The cut surface of the tumour has a cystic or solid appearance with abundant mucus. High-grade tumours appear larger with necrotic and haemorrhagic areas and tend to infiltrate the lung parenchyma.

Mucoepidermoid tumours are classified as either low or high grade based on morphological and cytological features. An example of a low-grade mucoepidermoid tumour can be seen in figure 13, in which mucus-filled cystic as well as solid areas are evident. The stroma may be myxoid or fibrotic, sometimes with a dense hyalinised material and calcification. A prominent lymphoplasmacytic infiltrate may be associated with the tumour. The high-grade mucoepidermoid carcinoma shows a predominance of solid areas composed of epidermoid and intermediate cells. It is characterised by marked nuclear pleomorphism, high mitotic counts (>4 mitosis·10 HPF^{-1}), and areas of necrosis and haemorrhage. Immunohistochemically, these tumours stain with pancytokeratins and cytokeratin (CK) 7 and are negative with CK20 and thyroid transcription factor 1. The epidermoid component shows a positive reaction to CK5/6. Low-grade

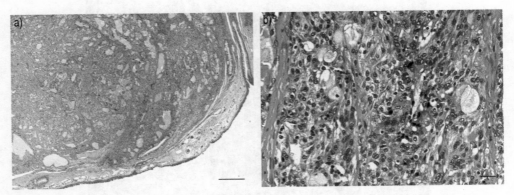

Fig. 13. – Pathology of primary pulmonary mucoepidermoid carcinoma. a) Low-grade mucoepidermoid tumour with a predominantly endobronchial location, showing mucus-filled cystic as well as solid areas. The cysts are lined with columnar goblet-type cells and low cuboidal cells with bland atypia. The solid areas are mainly composed of epidermoid and intermediate cells. A clear cell appearance or oncocytic component may be seen. b) At higher magnification, three cell types, mucinous, nonkeratinising squamoid and intermediate, can be seen. The mucin-producing cells are round or columnar with a large vacuolated cytoplasm. The nuclei are uniform, small and eccentrically placed. The intermediate epidermoid cells have centrally placed round nuclei, denser cytoplasm and distinct cell borders. Scale bars=a) 500µm, b) 40 µm.

mucoepidermoid tumours are sometimes difficult to differentiate from mucous gland adenomas. The presence of intermediate cells and squamous differentiation are characteristic of the mucoepidermoid tumours. High-grade mucoepidermoid tumours should be differentiated from squamous cell carcinomas, which lack the glandular differentiation, and from adenosquamous carcinomas, which is much more difficult and controversial. Compared with adenosquamous carcinoma, mucoepidermoid tumours are centrally located with an endobronchial growth pattern and areas of low-grade mucoepidermoid tumour with intermediate/squamous cells and isolated pearl formation. In addition, they lack the *in situ* carcinoma of the surface bronchial epithelium. In contrast with other rare tumours for which there are no criteria for cytological diagnosis, mucoepidermoid carcinoma may be diagnosed on cytological smears. The presence of three cell types, mucinous, nonkeratinising squamoid and intermediate, at times with extracellular mucin or cellular debris, supports the diagnosis of mucoepidermoid carcinoma. High-grade tumours contain numerous markedly atypical cells with pleiomorphic nuclei and prominent nucleoli.

Treatment

Extensive surgical resection including mediastinal lymph node dissection is the only effective treatment for mucoepidermoid carcinoma [128–133]. Endobronchial resection had been proposed to remove bronchial obstruction, but cannot be recommended due to the need for complete resection [127]. High-grade lesions have often been reported to receive post-operative radiotherapy and chemotherapy, without a clearly evaluated benefit [128, 130].

Prognosis

The prognosis for mucoepidermoid carcinoma is strongly related to the grade of the lesion: low-grade lesions mostly occur in children and young adults, usually do not present with hilar involvement and show a 5-yr survival ranging 70–80 % [129, 130]. The prognosis is even better in children than in adults, as no tumour-related death has ever been reported in children, who underwent follow-up until 21 yrs after the initial exclusively surgical resection [133]. High-grade tumours have a substantially worse prognosis, with a 5-yr survival of only 30–45% [130]. Patients with N2 involvement show the worst outcome, with a median survival of 6–10 months, due to rapid metastatic spread [130].

Primary pulmonary lymphoma

Primary pulmonary lymphoma is defined as a lymphoma affecting one or both lungs (parenchyma, bronchus or both), without evidence of extrapulmonary involvement or bone-marrow disease on diagnosis or during the subsequent 3 months [62]. Exceptions to these criteria have been occasionally considered when the lung is the main site of involvement, associated with satellite mediastinal and/or systemic nodes [61, 98–100]. Primary pulmonary lymphoma represent 0.4% of all lymphoma [100, 103], and 15–30% of rare pulmonary tumours [3, 4]. The main types are marginal zone B-cell lymphoma of the MALT type and lymphomatoid granulomatosis (LG); primary pulmonary high-grade B-cell lymphoma, intravascular large B-cell lymphoma and Hodgkin's lymphoma occur infrequently.

Marginal zone B-cell lymphoma of the MALT type

Pulmonary MALT lymphoma represents a low-grade malignant extranodal marginal zone B-cell lymphoma sharing the same pathological features as MALT lymphomas seen in other sites, especially gastric lymphoma. It accounts for 0.5% of all lymphoma, and 70–90% of primary pulmonary lymphomas, thus being one of the more frequent rare pulmonary tumours [3, 4]. A strong relationship has been established between MALT gastric lymphoma and chronic inflammation due to *Helicobacter pylori* infection [102]. Other infectious associations with MALT lymphoma have been reported with a less significant level of evidence, for example infection with *Chlamydia psittaci* and MALT lymphoma of the ocular adnexae. However, to date no chronic infectious condition has been identified in association with pulmonary MALT lymphoma, although concurrent progression with chronic hepatitis C has been described [102]. However, it is thought that MALT is absent in normal bronchial tree tissue, and only develops after inflammation due to long-term antigen stimulation (smoking, infections and autoimmune conditions, such as Sjögren's syndrome) [102].

Clinical features. Two populations are especially concerned with MALT lymphoma: patients aged >45 yrs, and younger patients with underlying immunosuppression, especially HIV infection, with a slight male predominance [99–101, 103]. MALT lymphoma is discovered on routine chest radiography in ~40% of cases; when present, respiratory signs usually include cough, dyspnoea and chest pain [99–101, 103, 104]. B signs (fever, swelling and weight loss) are uncommon. Blood tests show a monoclonal gammopathy in 30% of cases [99, 100].

Imaging features. Three imaging patterns of MALT lymphoma have been reported; the most suggestive is the pneumonia-like alveolar consolidation of variable density found on air bronchography, frequently localised in the middle lobe (fig. 14); other patterns are the tumour-like aspect with a solitary alveolar nodular opacity with sharper margins ranging 2–25 cm in diameter (30% of cases) and air bronchogram, by which medium air bronchioles are air-filled within a parenchymal consolidation and the infiltrative aspect with poorly-defined ground-glass opacities, observed at early stages before the invasion within the alveolar spaces of the lymphoproliferative tissue [99–102]. Some patients present with combined opacities, such as a focal nodular opacity with a peripheral peribronchovascular ground-glass attenuation halo. Other imaging features include frequently positive angiographic signs, bronchial dilatation included in an alveolar pattern and localised ground-glass opacities [99–102]. There is usually no hilar, mediastinal or extrapulmonary involvement [99–102]. Staging according to Ann Arbor Classification is either I extranodal (E; unilateral or bilateral involvement) or IIE (hilar/mediastinal lymph nodes) [105].

Pathological features. Diagnosis often requires surgical lung biopsy; although bronchoalveolar lavage and fine-needle biopsy may show the B-cell infiltration, they fail to exclude differential diagnoses, such as reactional lymphoid proliferation [99, 103, 104]. The histological diagnostic criteria are distinctive, and most cases can be diagnosed on the basis of routinely stained sections (fig. 15). At low magnification, the lymphoid infiltrate shows a typical lymphangitic growth pattern, spreading along bronchovascular bundles and interlobular septa, and producing a nodular interstitial pattern. The lymphoid infiltrate tends to expand into the lung parenchyma, forming solid nodules that obliterate the lung architecture with destruction of alveolar walls and filling of the alveolar spaces. The involvement of the visceral pleura is common, whereas less frequent is the

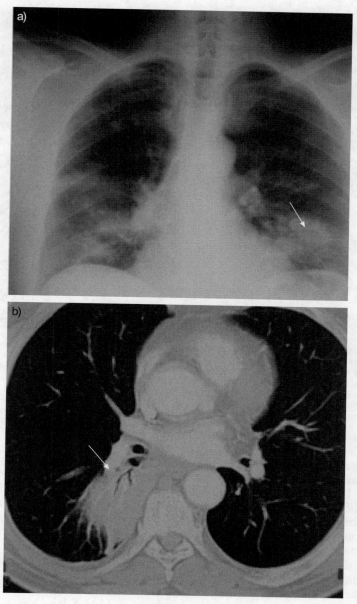

Fig. 14. – Primary pulmonary mucosa-associated lymphoid tissue lymphoma. A 67-yr-old asymptomatic patient without smoking history was referred after a persistent alveolar consolidation in the inferior lobes (arrows) had been discovered at a) routine work examination chest roentgenogram and b) computed tomography. Lung biopsy showed a monomorphic lymphoid infiltrate, with, at immunophenotypic studies, expression of pan-B marker CD20. Marginal B-cells expressed CD43, and were negative for CD5, CD10 and CD23. Gastroscopy disclosed *Helicobacter pylori* gastritis, and the patient received treatment with amoxicillin and omeprazole, without any changes in the pulmonary lesion. The patient has remained asymptomatic for 4 yrs, without specific cytotoxic treatment.

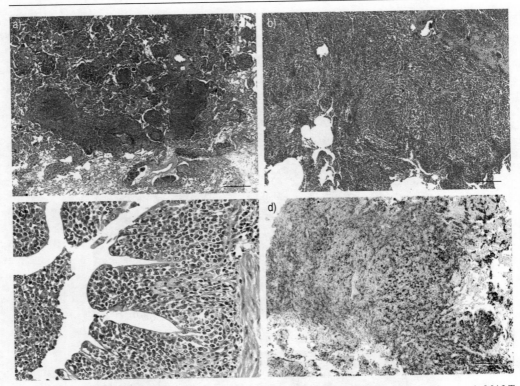

Fig. 15. – Pathology of primary pulmonary mucosa-associate lymphoid tissue (MALT) lymphoma. a) MALT lymphoma shows a typical lymphangitic growth producing a nodular interstitial pattern. b) The lymphoid infiltrate tend to expand into the lung parenchyma forming solid nodules that obliterate the lung architecture with destruction of alveolar wall and filling of the alveolar spaces. c) The involvement of bronchovascular bundles is associated with the presence of lymphoepithelial lesions in which the neoplastic cells invade the bronchial epithelium. The lymphoid infiltrate is relatively monomorphic and have a centrocyte-like appearance, with slightly irregular nuclear contours and scant or abundant clear cytoplasm. d) The neoplastic cells of MALT lymphoma of the lung have the immunophenotypic features of marginal zone B-lymphocytes, with expression of the pan-B-markers (CD 20 positive reaction in MALT lymphoma). Scale bars=a and d) 500μm, b) 100 μm.

involvement of the parietal pleura, a finding that is diagnostic of lymphoma. Pleural effusion is absent. Scattered plasmacytoid lymphocytes or mature plasma cells with intranuclear Dutcher bodies may be present, as well as small regular lymphocytes and a variable number of large transformed cells, a finding of uncertain prognostic significance. Randomly distributed lymphoid follicles with germinal centres infiltrated by lymphomatous cells (mantle zone colonisation) are relatively frequent. Additional histological features include the presence of giant cells with occasional non-necrotising granulomas that can mimic sarcoidosis, hypersensitivity pneumonia or infections. The prominent monomorphic lymphoid infiltrate and the typical distribution of lymphoma can define the lesions. Giant lamellar bodies, sclerosis towards the centre of the nodular masses or amyloid deposits are additional findings in MALT lymphomas.

The neoplastic cells exhibit the immunophenotypic features of marginal zone B-lymphocytes, with expression of the pan-B markers CD20, PAX5 and CD79. These cells are negative for CD5, CD10, CD23, B-cell chronic lymphocytic leukaemia (CLL)/lymphoma 6 (BCL6) and cyclin D1 (BCL1). The marginal zone B-cells express BCL2 and CD43, in >50% of cases; nuclear expression of BCL10 is found in lymphomas with a t(11;18) or a t(1;14) translocation. They typically express IgM but not IgD, and a light chain restriction is observed in the plasmacytic component. These immunohisto-chemical features may also define the monotypy of the proliferation. Follicular dendritic cells, stained with CD21, CD23 and CD35, can be useful for demonstrating residual germinative centres that have been colonised by lymphomatous cells. The tumour cells may show homing receptors such as $\alpha_4\beta_7$ integrin, favouring dissemination through other mucosal sites. MALT lymphomas are associated with different chromosomal changes that are represented by translocations and aneuploidy. The translocations that appear essentially specific for MALT lymphoma of the lung are t(1;14)(p22;q32) involving the *bcl10* and *igh* genes and t(11;18)(q21,q21) with involvement of *api2* and *malt1* genes [106]. Other translocations documented in MALT lymphomas include t(14;18)(q32,q21), t(1;2)(p22;p12). The precise mechanisms involved in the development of these translocations remain unknown. Translocations may be associated with aneuploidy, particularly trisomy of chromosome 3. Interestingly, the MALT lymphomas with the translocation t(11;18)(*api2/malt1*) do not present with aneuploidy. MALT lymphomas with a large cell component may present additional mutations involving such as *c-myc*, *p53* and *p16*. These molecular alterations have become a useful diagnostic tool and can be detected by interphase fluorescence *in situ* hybridisation and/or by an RT-PCR in paraffin embedded material. In cases with the t(1;14)(*bcl10/igh*), involving the *bcl10* gene, a strong nuclear overexpression of BCL10 can be detected by immunohistochemistry. A weak nuclear expression of BCL10 is also observed in cases of advanced MALT lymphomas with translocation t(11;18)(*api2/malt1*). In addition, cases with t(14;18)(*igh/malt1*) show a strong cytoplasmic overexpression of MALT1 and BCL10. However the overexpression of these molecules has no clinical utility, as they are neither specific for specific translocations nor to MALT lymphoma.

The differential diagnosis of MALT-type pulmonary lymphomas typically involves the benign lymphoproliferative disorders, which include follicular bronchitis/bronchiolitis, lymphocytic interstitial pneumonia and localised nodular lymphoid hyperplasia [106]. Difficulties in making the diagnosis occur more frequently with small biopsy specimens in which the typical distribution of lymphoma is lacking. In these cases, in addition to the clinical and imaging data, the presence of a marked infiltration destroying the alveolar architecture and showing a lymphangitic distribution, and the presence of monomorphic centrocytic/monocytic cells with more pronounced lymphoepithelial lesions, with a CD20+/CD43+/bcl2+/CD5-/CD10- immunoprofile, are suggestive of lymphoma. In benign lymphoproliferative lesions, the infiltrate is more localised and polymorphic, with rare lymphoepithelial complexes that have the immunoprofile CD20+/CD43-. Molecular analysis (evaluation of monoclonality) may assist in the diagnosis. Lung involvement in CLL may be confused with a MALT lymphoma. Histologically, the lymphoid infiltrate is limited to the bronchovascular bundles with relative sparing of the lung parenchyma. The cells of CLL are B-lymphocytes, expressing the pan-B markers CD20, PAX5 and CD79a. They also express CD5, CD43, CD23 and Bcl2. They are negative for CD10, BCL6 and BCL1/cyclin D1. Approximately 10–20% of tumoural cells are positive for Ki67. Mantle cell lymphoma may involve the lung and be confused with a MALT lymphoma with diffuse infiltration of monomorphic small lymphocytes. These cells have a characteristic immunophenotype. They express the B-cell markers (CD20, PAX5 and CD79a), as well as CD5, CD43, BCL2 and BCL1/cyclin D1. They are negative for CD10, CD23 and BCL6. Ki67 is expressed by many more cells than in other small lymphocytic proliferations, ranging 20–50%. In follicular lymphoma, the infiltration assumes a nodular pattern containing small and large cleaved cells (centrocytes) and large noncleaved cells (centroblasts). These cells express the B-cell markers, BCL2, BCL6 and CD10; they are negative for CD5, CD43 and CD23. Ki67 is variable, ranging 10–40%.

Treatment. At the time of pathological surgical diagnosis, extensive resection is frequently performed in the case of a limited resectable lesion [99–102]. However, in asymptomatic patients, a watch-and-wait approach may be preferred to aggressive treatment (fig. 15) [62, 99–102]. In symptomatic patients, resection or exclusive radiotherapy had been proposed in older studies, as well as, in more advanced stages, principles of treatment of low-grade nodal lymphoma based in first intention on single-agent chemotherapy (chlorambucil, fludarabine or rituximab) [99–102]. Rituximab, an anti-CD20 antibody, is particularly effective and well-tolerated in MALT lymphoma [62, 98–104]. Comparison between rituximab and surgery has not been carried out. However, considering that MALT lymphoma is now regarded as a multifocal disease of mucosal immunity, the role of systemic treatment has increased, and adjuvant/exclusive chemotherapy with rituximab is recommended [100].

Prognosis. MALT lymphomas have an indolent course, and they remain localised until late in their history, carrying a better prognosis than other lymphoma [99–104, 107]. The overall prognosis of MALT lymphoma is excellent, with 5-yr survival ranging 84–94% [99–104, 107]. Recurrences occur in ~50% of cases, but are controllable. Progression to high-grade B-cell lymphoma occurs in <5% of cases [62, 102–104, 106, 107]. Apart from age, no clinical predictive or prognostic factors have been identified; in particular, the extent of the surgical resection does not influence the outcome, which is an argument against extensive pneumonectomy [103]. There are no clear histological parameters useful in predicting the prognosis of MALT lymphomas of the lung. However, the presence of intratumoural amyloid seems to be associated with adverse outcome, whereas predominance of lymphoepithelial lesions appears to be associated with a better outcome [100]. Involvement of the pleura and/or regional lymph nodes does not appear to modify the outcome of the lesion. Despite the strong evidence for an important role of t(11;18)(q21;q21) in MALT lymphoma progression and the overexpression of $\alpha_4\beta_7$ integrin, the prognostic significance of these molecular alterations and other translocations observed in MALT lymphoma of the lung are unknown and remain to be studied. However, the molecular alterations in this specific type of lymphomas are attractive targets for the development of new treatment strategies.

Lymphomatoid granulomatosis

LG, currently called angiocentric lymphoma or angiocentric immunoproliferative lesion, was initially thought not to be a lymphoid malignancy, but rather an inflammatory granulomatous disease, since its radioclinical presentation is somewhat similar to other granulomatoses, such as Wegener's disease [62, 108, 109]. Involving many organs, such as brain, skin and liver, lung is the most frequent site [62, 108, 109].

Clinical features. LG occurs in middle-aged adults, with a marked male predominance [62, 108, 109]. Nearly all patients present with respiratory and systemic symptoms, consisting of cough, dyspnoea, chest pain, fever and weight loss. Peripheral and thoracic lymphadenopathy are absent.

Imaging features. LG cases present with multiple smooth bilateral nodules, with a peribronchovascular pattern, ranging 2–10 cm and mainly localised in the lower lobes [62, 108, 109]. Excavation of convergent nodules tends to occur and leads to cavitated pseudotumoural masses [62, 108, 109].

Pathological features. The diagnosis of LG is based upon histological examination of surgical pulmonary biopsy specimens (endoscopic samples are rarely diagnostic).

Macroscopically, LG forms multiple and confluent nodules, which are poorly circumscribed, of variable size, often large and involve the entire lobe. The cut surface is tan/grey or yellowish, with areas of necrosis. LG is characterised histologically by pulmonary nodules composed of an angiocentric, polymorphous and usually atypical lymphoreticular infiltrate with a variable, but often extensive, coagulative necrosis involving arterioles and veins. Vessels display mural infiltrates of small lymphocytes and atypical large cells with vesicular nuclei and large basophilic nucleoli or crumpled and darkly stained nuclei. The lymphoid cells infiltrate the subendothelial and adventitial zones and erode and obliterate the vessel wall and lumen. Granulomatous formations are occasionally seen. Central necrosis, often prominent in the nodules of LG, may be due to the angiocentric character of the infiltrate or the interferon (IFN)-γ-induced elaboration of cytokines, such as IFN-γ-inducible protein (IP) 10 and the monokine induced by IFN-γ, which results in tissue necrosis and vascular damage. The production of IFN-γ is induced by IL-12, secreted by EBV-infected B-cells. Increased serum levels of IP-10 in patients with LG is often associated with the skin lesions of LG. Immunohistochemistry shows a rich T-cell infiltrate (predominantly CD4+ T-lymphocytes), with scattered atypical cells of the B-phenotype. Various studies have identified colocalisation of EBV RNA and expression of a pan-B-cell marker in atypical cells, suggesting that LG represents a T-cell-rich EBV-associated B-cell lymphoproliferative disorder. This interpretation is supported by the demonstration of Ig heavy chain rearrangement in many cases. In addition, large B-cells proliferate at a greater rate than the numerous T-cells, and the rate of B-cell proliferation correlates with the grade of the lesion and overlaps with that of B-cell lymphomas in grade III lesions.

Differentiation from other disorders with a vasculitic component, including Wegener's granulomatosis and other malignant lymphomas, may be difficult. Wegener's granulomatosis differs from LG in that the cellular granuloma is composed of acute and chronic inflammatory cells, and vasculitis consists of focal wall necrosis rather than transmural infiltration by lymphoid cells. The identification of diagnostic Reed–Sternberg cells is required to distinguish Hodgkin's lymphoma from LG. More problematic is the differentiation from angiotropic non-Hodgkin's lymphomas with vascular involvement. The diagnosis of LG should be reserved for lesions characterised by a polymorphic lymphoid infiltrate, vascular infiltration and necrosis. The presence of a polymorphic infiltrate is useful in distinguishing LG from non-Hodgkin's lymphomas. Vascular infiltration alone is not diagnostic for LG. There are rare cases with a histological appearance similar to that of LG in which the atypical cells have a T-cell phenotype or express a positive reaction for CD56. These are now considered peripheral T-cell lymphomas that are similar to LG, and immunophenotypic evaluation is important in distinguishing between the two entities.

Treatment. Chemotherapy based on high-dose steroids associated with cyclophosphamide is the most-reported treatment. The use of more recent cytotoxic or targeted agents has not been evaluated to date. For the rare localised tumours, radiotherapy and/or surgery have been successfully used [62, 108, 109].

Prognosis. Although some series have reported possible spontaneous resolution and complete remissions, the overall prognosis remains grim, with a 5-yr survival of 30–40%. Progression to nodal diffuse aggressive lymphoma has been reported in 12–47% of patients. The main prognostic factors are age, extension of the lesions and complete remission after first-line chemotherapy [62, 108, 109]. Grading of LG may provide prognostic data. It has been subdivided into three grades according to the quantity and degree of cellular atypia and presence or absence of necrosis. Grade I LG is characterised by a predominance of reactive T-lymphocytes and histiocytes. Large atypical cells are rare, with absent or sporadic mitotic figures. Necrosis is absent or focal. In grade II LG, the atypical B-cells represent ~1% of the total population and show scattered mitosis. Necrosis is focal, when present. In grade III LG, the large cells are numerous, comprising ~20% of the total population. Mitotic figures are easily detected and necrosis may be extensive. A more recent study has shown that the proliferation index within the B-cell population, evaluated using DNA topoisomerase IIα, correlates with the histological grade [110]. In particular, a high proliferation index (mean 36%) has been observed in grade III LG, suggesting that chemotherapy is more likely to be effective in these cases than in LG grades I and II, in which the proliferative index is lower (0% in grade I and 17% in grade II). In addition, histological grade has been related to the number of EBV-positive cells identified on *in situ* hybridisation. In grade I lesions, EBV-positive cells are absent or scarce; in grade II, EBV-positive cells represent <100 cells·HPF^{-1}; and, in grade III, EBV-positive cells occur at >100 cells·HPF^{-1}. The quantification of the number of EBV-positive B-cells and proliferative index are particularly useful in distinguishing grade III from grade II LG [111, 112]. In addition, all these data seem to suggest that only grade III LG might be regarded as a high-grade lymphoma.

Other lymphoma

The prevalence of primary pulmonary high-grade B-cell lymphoma may be under-estimated since its rapid spread to mediastinal nodes and other extrathoracic sites may obscure its pulmonary origin [99]. It typically occurs in patients in their sixth or seventh decade of life, often presenting with marked B signs (fever, weight loss and sweats). Radiologically, primary pulmonary high-grade B-cell lymphoma cases usually present as multiple well-defined rounded solid masses of various size, more frequently localised in the subpleural areas of the lower lobes [98–101, 104]. Histologically, they show the characteristics of the large B-cell lymphomas at other sites, with large cleaved and noncleaved cells showing centroblastic or immunoblastic morphology, with large round nuclei, dispersed chromatin, and variable prominent nucleoli. The cytoplasm is relatively abundant and mitoses are numerous. The neoplastic cells exhibit a B-cell phenotype (CD20, CD19, CD22 and CD79a expression) with Ig light chain restriction. Occasionally, they may be positive for BCL2 and a small group express a nuclear protein staining for forkhead box protein P1 [113]. A background composed of reactive CD3-positive T-lymphocytes is usually present, and, occasionally, it may be prominent (T-cell-rich variant). Chemotherapy is based on the same multi-agent regimens as used in high-grade nodal lymphomas, prednisone and rituximab [99–101, 104, 106, 107]. Overall prognosis is much worse than for MALT lymphoma, with 5-yr survival ranging 50–70% [99–101, 104, 106, 107].

In patients with HIV infection, pulmonary MALT lymphomas are less frequent than high-grade lymphomas, mostly with a B-cell phenotype [62, 98, 106, 107]. Survival is poor, with a median survival of 4 months following diagnosis, due not only to lymphoma progression but also to infectious consequences of the underlying immunological status, precluding the delivery of optimal chemotherapy [99, 107].

Intravascular large cell lymphoma is an exceptional variant of non-Hodgkin's lymphoma presenting with puzzling clinical manifestations, dependent on the proximal or peripheral location of the tumour, which is characterised by proliferation of neoplastic lymphoid cells within the lumen of small and intermediately sized blood vessels, resulting in thrombotic and ischaemic complications [62, 85]. Lymphadenopathy is usually absent, and pulmonary imaging features include bilateral ground-glass opacities and/or, sometimes, migratory atelectasis shadows [85]. Pathologically, the vessels are filled with noncohesive large atypical mononuclear cells with round vesicular nuclei, prominent nucleoli and a moderately amphophilic cytoplasm. The cells may fill the vessels and proliferate in the subendothelial layer. The neoplastic cells stain for CD45RB and B-cell markers; however, they lack the leukocyte adhesion molecule CD11a/CD18. Disseminated carcinomas or melanoma may mimic intravascular large cell lymphoma. Clinical history and immunostaining are helpful in making a distinction. Transbronchial biopsy may provide diagnostic tissue and can assist with the diagnosis. Treatment with conventional combination chemotherapy with or without rituximab leads to remission with prolonged survival [62, 85, 102].

Primary pulmonary Hodgkin's lymphoma is very rare [114], affecting females more frequently than males. Radiologically, it appears as either a solitary mass with cystic and heterogeneous features, typically involving the superior lobes, or a multinodular disease [114]. Its pathological features include multiple macronodules, associated with satellite micronodules and patchy interstitial infiltrates distributed along lymphatic routes. Necrosis is common, sometimes simulating granulomatous lesions. Diagnosis is based on recognition of characteristic Reed–Sternberg cells. The immunophenotypic features are as those described in primary nodal Hodgkin's lymphoma. Treatment consists of intensive polychemotherapy associated with radiotherapy, and, exceptionally, surgical resection in the case of localised disease. Factors correlated with a poorer prognosis include B symptoms, bilateral disease, multilobar involvement, invasion of the pleura and cavitation [114]. Overall outcome is worse than in nodal Hodgkin's lymphoma [114].

How should rare tumours be dealt with clinically?

Diagnosis

Although rare pulmonary tumours are often asymptomatic, the first step in the diagnosis of a rare pulmonary tumour would be to recognise specific clinical and radiological features, which, even if infrequent, are pathognomonic or strongly suggestive of the diagnosis, e.g. trichoptysis in teratoma, catecholamine secretion syndrome in paraganglioma, popcorn calcifications in hamartoma, air bronchoalveolo-gram in parenchymal consolidation at chest radiography in MALT lymphoma or the air meniscus sign in sclerosing haemangioma (table 1). Moreover, the clinical history may be helpful in suspecting a rare pulmonary tumour, e.g. B signs and lymphoma, or feminisation and choriocarcinoma in males (table 1). The absence of a smoking history, especially in males, can also invoke the possibility of a rare tumour.

Once a pathological diagnosis has been obtained, the next and crucial step in the clinical diagnostic strategy for rare pulmonary tumours is to ensure their primary nature. Indeed, metastasis in the lung from another occult tumour constitutes the majority of cases of pulmonary tumours of uncommon histological type (e.g. melanoma in the skin, adenoid cystic carcinoma in the salivary gland, lymphoma in lymphatic nodes and choriocarcinoma in the male genitalia) [7]. Contrary to metastatic tumour cases, which usually present as multiple bilateral pulmonary nodules, most primary pulmonary rare tumour cases present as a unique solitary lesion. However, some of them may present with multinodular and/or bilateral reticulonodular infiltrative imaging features (e.g. EHE/angiosarcoma, LG and choriocarcinoma; table 1). Therefore, accurate screening for any previous history of extrathoracic tumour, as well as complete investigations and follow-up for other synchronous and metachronous cancers, is required to establish a diagnosis of primary pulmonary tumour.

The strategy for confidently establishing the lack of an extrapulmonary primary tumour mainly relies on CT imaging centred particularly on areas determined by the pathological diagnosis (*i.e.* where a primary tumour with the same pathology is more likely to be found). Furthermore, other specific investigations may be necessary in order to ensure the primary nature of the tumour (*e.g.* bone marrow biopsy for lymphoma). PET currently represents a determining tool in searching for a primary tumour. However, false negative results occur depending on the tumour type and size (especially if <10 mm in diameter). Even if experience is limited in the field of rare tumours, many recent case reports include the PET features of these tumours. The present review of the literature indicates that most benign tumours do not exhibit uptake of fluorine-18-fluoro-2-deoxyglucose, and, conversely, most malignant lesions are PET-positive (table 1) [132, 200]. Thus, in addition to being a diagnostic tool for establishing the primary nature of rare pulmonary tumours, PET could also be useful in evaluating post-therapy changes, determining prognosis and, eventually, performing accurate follow-up.

Therapeutic strategies

The first step in the therapeutic strategy for rare pulmonary tumours is to define the requirement for and extent of surgical resection; in all cases, the degree of malignancy must be established, especially in high-risk patients (table 7). Even when faced with a well-circumscribed homogeneous nodule thought to be a benign tumour, surgical resection is required [201]. Indeed, in many older case reports of rare pulmonary tumours, the pulmonary lesion was primarily thought to be an early-stage NSCLC, and upfront resection ensured both the diagnosis and the first-step of the therapeutic strategy (table 1).

However, regarding the potential morbidity of thoracic surgery, extensive pulmonary resection has to be well balanced. As well as benign tumours, some rare pulmonary tumours, pathologically considered to be malignant (such as haemangioendothelioma, acinic cell carcinoma, paraganglioma and neurinoma) should definitely be treated with simple excision, and do not require extensive lung resection. Conversely, benign tumours (such as myofibroblastic tumours or teratoma) may exhibit a locally invasive, recurrent and even metastatic behaviour; hence the old prefix pseudo (pseudolymphoma and

Table 7. – Reported malignant rare pulmonary tumours by curability and prognosis[#]

Excellent/good (>80%)	Intermediate/unpredictable	Poor (<20%)
Acinic cell carcinoma	Carcinoid tumour	Fibrosarcoma
Adenoid cystic carcinoma	Mucoepidermoid carcinoma	Angiosarcoma
Chondrosarcoma	Pleuropulmonary blastoma	Carcinosarcoma
Liposarcoma	Desmoplastic tumour	Choriocarcinoma
Schwannoma	Neurinoma	Osteosarcoma
Glomus tumour	Neurogenic sarcoma	Rhabdomyosarcoma
Sebaceous carcinoma	Paraganglioma	Synovial sarcoma
Thymoma	Embryonal carcinoma	Malignant mesenchymoma
Yolk sac tumour	Myoepithelial carcinoma	Giant/spindle cell carcinoma
MALT lymphoma	Myofibrosarcoma	Foetal adenocarcinoma
Low-grade lymphoma	Leiomyosarcoma	Pneumoblastoma
Intravascular lymphoma	Malignant fibrous histiocytoma	Pulmonary artery leiomyosarcoma
	Diffuse large B-cell lymphoma	Haemangiopericytoma
	Epithelioid haemangioendothelioma	Kaposi's sarcoma
	Plasmacytoma	Melanoma
		Lymphomatoid granulomatosis
		Lymphoepithelioma-like carcinoma
		Haemangiomatosis

MALT: mucosa-associated lymphoid tissue. [#]: 5-yr survival shown in parenthesis.

pseudotumour), thus requiring the same surgical procedure as malignant tumours (table 1).

As surgery represents the upfront treatment for rare pulmonary tumours, the only means of completing the therapeutic programme in cases of malignant tumour remains to administer adjuvant radiotherapy and/or chemotherapy. From a similar rationale to that for NSCLC [201], post-operative radiotherapy is mostly performed in the case of incomplete resection or positive resection margins. Conversely, chemotherapy has been mainly reported to be administered in aggressive tumours with a high risk of locoregional and/or systemic recurrence, such as sarcoma, germ cell tumours, high-grade lymphoma and carcinomas (table 1). Chemotherapy regimens consist of cytotoxic agent combinations effective in tumours of a similar histological type arising at other sites [57, 88, 192]. More recently, regarding evolving concepts in thoracic oncology [202], the usefulness of neoadjuvant chemotherapy has been highlighted for sarcomas [57, 88, 192], pulmonary blastoma [151] and carcinoid tumours [25]. These strategies ensure that all patients receive all of the components of multimodal treatment, permitting surgical resection under better local conditions, and could possibly increase systemic control rates [203]. This approach may also help the clinician to evaluate the efficacy of chemotherapy in rare pulmonary tumours, by making the evaluation of the pathological tumoural response available before surgery. Neoadjuvant treatments require a definite pathological diagnosis, especially in the case of local and/or mediastinal invasiveness precluding complete resection; since pathological studies on small specimens may be less accurate in the case of mixed or poorly differentiated tumours, surgical biopsy may be necessary.

Finally, there is an urgent need for collaborative pathological studies of the molecular features of rare pulmonary tumours, especially regarding molecular pathways implicated in their carcinogenesis, which may be specifically targeted by available agents, such as gefitinib, directed against epidermal growth factor receptor, and imatinib, directed against c-kit (CD119) [204]. Haematological malignancies constitute a separate group of rare pulmonary tumours, in which surgery may be helpful in the case of a localised lesion, but for which the principles of treatment of more advanced systemic malignancies apply above all, including multiagent intensive chemotherapy and haematopoietic stem cell transplantation in aggressive diseases [62]. These malignancies constitute a model of the therapeutic impact of precise pathological characterisation, since their immunological phenotype directly leads to the use of targeted therapies, such as rituximab in the CD20+ primary pulmonary lymphomas.

As for most rare pulmonary diseases, a consequence of their rarity is the lack of evidence-based recommendations for treatment in the absence of randomised therapeutic trials. This emphasises the need for cooperative collaboration in constituting cohorts and launching clinical trials.

Prognosis

The prognosis of rare pulmonary tumours depends upon both their aggressiveness and their curability (tables 1 and 6). As well as benign tumours, a large proportion of malignant tumours, such as adenoid cystic carcinoma, chondrosarcoma, liposarcoma, yolk sac tumours and low-grade lymphoma, are associated with prolonged survival with accurate treatment. As most rare pulmonary tumours are benign or low-grade malignant lesions, and, moreover, are frequently localised in the lung without lymph node involvement at the time of diagnosis, their overall prognosis remains better than that for NSCLC; in the series of rare pulmonary tumours reported by MILLER et al. [4], overall 5-yr survival was 39%, higher than the 20% reported for NSCLC [1].

Conclusion

The management of rare pulmonary tumours is a model of cooperation between clinicians and pathologists from establishing the diagnosis to treatment and evaluation of prognosis. On this basis, collaborative studies, *via* specialised centres for rare diseases, involving pulmonologists, specialised pathologists, surgical and medical oncologists, and radiotherapists, are warranted in order to collect more actualised and multidisciplinary, and especially therapeutic, data about these tumours.

Summary

The management of rare primary pulmonary tumours is a paradigm of the cooperation between clinicians and pathologists from establishment of the diagnosis to treatment. From a pathological point of view, rare primary pulmonary tumours are defined as tumours of unusual histological type in the lung. From an epidemiological point of view, they may be defined by an overall prevalence of <1% of all lung tumours. Rare pulmonary tumours represent a wide range of diverse tumoral processes, which may be classified into three main pathological groups: 1) rare tumours derived from orthotopic tissues; 2) rare lung tumours derived from ectopic tissues; and 3) rare lung tumours derived from haematopoietic tissues.

The first step in the diagnosis of rare primary pulmonary tumours is to recognise possible specific clinical and radiological features that, even if infrequent, may suggest the diagnosis. The second is to establish the definite pathological diagnosis, and the third to ensure that it is primary in nature. In order to illustrate the close cooperation between the pathologist and the clinician, five rare primary pulmonary tumours of special interest are described in this chapter: myofibroblastic tumour; sarcomas; epithelioid haemangioendothelioma; mucoepidermoid carcinoma; and pulmonary lymphoma, especially mucosa-associated lymphoid tissue lymphoma.

Therapeutic strategy consists of upfront surgical resection when possible, ensuring both the diagnosis and the first step of treatment. The role of radiotherapy and/or chemotherapy mainly depends upon the aggressiveness and curability of the tumour. The overall prognosis of rare pulmonary neoplasms remains better than that of nonsmall cell lung cancer. Large multicentric observational studies to establish pathological databases, to generate basic research and therapeutic trials, and eventually to assess actualised state-of-the-art recommendations for management and treatment are warranted to improve knowledge of rare primary pulmonary tumours.

Keywords: Epithelioid haemangioendothelioma, lymphoma, mucoepidermoid carcinoma, myofibroblastic tumour, rare tumour, sarcoma.

References

1. Travis WB, Brambilla A, Muller-Hermelinck HK, Harris CC. World Health Organization Classification of Tumours. Pathology and Genetics of Tumours of the Lung, Pleura, Thymus and Heart. Lyon, IARC Press, 2004.
2. Miller DL. Rare pulmonary neoplasms. *Semin Respir Crit Care Med* 1997; 18: 405–415.

3. Sekine I, Kodama T, Yokose T, *et al.* Rare pulmonary tumors – a review of 32 cases. *Oncology* 1998; 55: 431–434.

4. Miller DL, Allen MS. Rare pulmonary neoplasms. *Mayo Clin Proc* 1993; 68: 492–498.

5. Allan JS. Rare solitary benign tumors of the lung. *Semin Thorac Cardiovasc Surg* 2003; 15: 315–322.

6. Marchevsky AM. Lung tumors derived from ectopic tissues. *Semin Diagn Pathol* 1995; 12: 172–184.

7. Pierce WC, Figlin RA. Primary tumors of the lung other than lung cancer. *Curr Opin Oncol* 1993; 5: 343–352.

8. Lee HY, Mancer K, Koong HN. Primary acinic cell carcinoma of the lung with lymph node metastasis. *Arch Pathol Lab Med* 2003; 127: e216–e219.

9. Ukoha OO, Quartararo P, Carter D, Kashgarian M, Ponn RB. Acinic cell carcinoma of the lung with metastasis to lymph nodes. *Chest* 1999; 115: 591–595.

10. Kanematsu T, Yohena T, Uehara T, *et al.* Treatment outcome of resected and nonresected primary adenoid cystic carcinoma of the lung. *Ann Thorac Cardiovasc Surg* 2002; 8: 74–77.

11. Maziak DE, Todd TR, Keshavjee SH, Winton TL, Van Nostrand P, Pearson FG. Adenoid cystic carcinoma of the airway: thirty-two-year experience. *J Thorac Cardiovasc Surg* 1996; 112: 1522–1531.

12. Dalton ML, Gatling RR. Peripheral adenoid cystic carcinoma of the lung. *South Med J* 1990; 83: 577–579.

13. Noda M, Tabata T, Yamane Y. [Pleomorphic adenoma of the lung; report of a case.] *Kyobu Geka* 2002; 55: 1073–1076.

14. Burke LM, Rush WI, Khoor A, *et al.* Alveolar adenoma: a histochemical, immunohistochemical, and ultrastructural analysis of 17 cases. *Hum Pathol* 1999; 30: 158–167.

15. Hara M, Sato Y, Kitase M, *et al.* CT and MR findings of a pleomorphic adenoma in the peripheral lung. *Radiat Med* 2001; 19: 111–114.

16. Halldorsson A, Dissanaike S, Kaye KS. Alveolar adenoma of the lung: a clinicopathological description of a case of this very unusual tumour. *J Clin Pathol* 2005; 58: 1211–1214.

17. Gloeckner-Hofmann K, Krismann M, Feller AC. Angiomyolipom der Lunge. [Angiomyolipoma of the lung.] *Pathologe* 2000; 21: 260–263.

18. Lopez L, Iriberri M, Cancelo L, Gomez A, Uresandi F, Atxotegui V. Persistent hemoptysis secondary to extensive epithelioid angiosarcoma. *Arch Bronconeumol* 2004; 40: 188–190.

19. Atasoy C, Fitoz S, Yigit H, Atasoy P, Erden I, Akyar S. Radiographic CT and MRI findings in primary pulmonary angiosarcoma. *Clin Imaging* 2001; 25: 337–340.

20. Kojima K, Okamoto I, Ushijima S, *et al.* Successful treatment of primary pulmonary angiosarcoma. *Chest* 2003; 124: 2397–2400.

21. Savona G, Frau G, D'Alia G. Angiosarcoma del polmone. [Angiosarcoma of the lung. Clinical case.] *Minerva Chir* 1990; 45: 429–432.

22. Pandit SA, Fiedler PN, Westcott JL. Primary angiosarcoma of the lung. *Ann Diagn Pathol* 2005; 9: 302–304.

23. Attanoos RL, Appleton MA, Gibbs AR. Primary sarcomas of the lung: a clinicopathological and immunohistochemical study of 14 cases. *Histopathology* 1996; 29: 29–36.

24. Travis WD, Rush W, Flieder DB, *et al.* Survival analysis of 200 pulmonary neuroendocrine tumors with clarification of criteria for atypical carcinoid and its separation from typical carcinoid. *Am J Surg Pathol* 1998; 22: 934–944.

25. Hasleton PS, Gomm S, Blair V, Thatcher N. Pulmonary carcinoid tumours: a clinico-pathological study of 35 cases. *Br J Cancer* 1986; 54: 963–967.

26. Schrevens L, Vansteenkiste J, Deneffe G, *et al.* Clinical-radiological presentation and outcome of surgically treated pulmonary carcinoid tumours: a long-term single institution experience. *Lung Cancer* 2004; 43: 39–45.

27. Fink G, Krelbaum T, Yellin A, *et al.* Pulmonary carcinoid: presentation, diagnosis, and outcome in 142 cases in Israel and review of 640 cases from the literature. *Chest* 2001; 119: 1647–1651.

28. Beasley MB, Thunnissen FB, Brambilla E, *et al.* Pulmonary atypical carcinoid: predictors of survival in 106 cases. *Hum Pathol* 2000; 31: 1255–1265.

29.	Jain M, Yung E, Trow T, Katz DS. F-18 FDG positron emission tomography demonstration of pulmonary carcinoid. *Clin Nucl Med* 2004; 29: 370–371.

30.	Reynolds S, Jenkins G, Akosa A, Roberts CM. Carcinosarcoma of the lung: an unusual cause of empyema. *Respir Med* 1995; 89: 73–75.

31.	Huwer H, Kalweit G, Straub U, Feindt P, Volkmer I, Gams E. Pulmonary carcinosarcoma: diagnostic problems and determinants of the prognosis. *Eur J Cardiothorac Surg* 1996; 10: 403–407.

32.	Matsukawa M, Terashima H, Shimada T, Aida H, Meguro A, Kondoh K. [Primary carcinosarcoma of TE lung – a report of two cases.] *Nippon Kyobu Geka Gakkai Zasshi* 1996; 44: 970–977.

33.	Heremans A, Verbeken E, Deneffe G, Demedts M. Carcinosarcoma of the lung. Report of two cases and review of the literature. *Acta Clin Belg* 1989; 44: 110–115.

34.	Kiryu T, Kawaguchi S, Matsui E, Hoshi H, Kokubo M, Shimokawa K. Multiple chondromatous hamartomas of the lung: a case report and review of the literature with special reference to Carney syndrome. *Cancer* 1999; 85: 2557–2561.

35.	Parker LA, Molina PL, Bignault AG, Fidler ME. Primary pulmonary chondrosarcoma mimicking bronchogenic cyst on CT and MRI. *Clin Imaging* 1996; 20: 181–183.

36.	Hayashi T, Tsuda N, Iseki M, Kishikawa M, Shinozaki T, Hasumoto M. Primary chondrosarcoma of the lung. A clinicopathologic study. *Cancer* 1993; 72: 69–74.

37.	Arslanian A, Pischedda F, Filosso PL, *et al.* Primary choriocarcinoma of the lung. *J Thorac Cardiovasc Surg* 2003; 125: 193–196.

38.	Chen F, Tatsumi A, Numoto S. Combined choriocarcinoma and adenocarcinoma of the lung occurring in a man: case report and review of the literature. *Cancer* 2001; 91: 123–129.

39.	de Krijger RR, Albers MJ, Bogers AJ, Mooi WJ. Heterotopic pancreatic tissue presenting as a solid and cystic lung lesion: a very unusual bronchopulmonary foregut malformation. *Pediatr Dev Pathol* 2004; 7: 204–209.

40.	Morgan T, Anderson J, Jorden M, Keller K, Robinson T, Hintz S. Pulmonary glial heterotopia in a monoamniotic twin. *Pediatr Pulmonol* 2003; 36: 162–166.

41.	Bando T, Genka K, Ishikawa K, Kuniyoshi M, Kuda T. Ectopic intrapulmonary thyroid. *Chest* 1993; 103: 1278–1279.

42.	Syed S, Haque AK, Hawkins HK, Sorensen PH, Cowan DF. Desmoplastic small round cell tumor of the lung. *Arch Pathol Lab Med* 2002; 126: 1226–1228.

43.	Eggerath A, Klose KC. Embryonal Krebsgeschwür des Lugenflügels–ein Beitrag zur differentialen Diagnose der Lungenmünze Verletzungen. [Embryonal carcinoma of the lung–a contribution to the differential diagnosis of pulmonary coin lesions.] *Z Erkr Atmungsorgane* 1986; 166: 290–293.

44.	Shimizu I, Nakanishi R, Yoshino I, Yasumoto K. An endometrial nodule in the lung without pelvic endometriosis. *J Cardiovasc Surg* 1998; 39: 867–868.

45.	Cassina PC, Hauser M, Kacl G, Imthurn B, Schroder S, Weder W. Catamenial hemoptysis. Diagnosis with MRI. *Chest* 1997; 111: 1447–1450.

46.	Crotty TB, Hooker RP, Swensen SJ, Scheithauer BW, Myers JL. Primary malignant ependymoma of the lung. *Mayo Clin Proc* 1992; 67: 373–378.

47.	Fagen K, Silverman ED, Cole RL. Detection of a pulmonary epithelioid hemangioendothelioma by FDG PET scan. *Clin Nucl Med* 2004; 29: 758–759.

48.	Dail DH, Liebow AA, Gmelich JT, *et al.* Intravascular, bronchiolar, and alveolar tumor of the lung (IVBAT). An analysis of twenty cases of a peculiar sclerosing endothelial tumor. *Cancer* 1983; 51: 452–464.

49.	Kitaichi M, Nagai S, Nishimura K, *et al.* Pulmonary epithelioid haemangioendothelioma in 21 patients, including three with partial spontaneous regression. *Eur Respir J* 1998; 12: 89–96.

50.	Cronin P, Arenberg D. Pulmonary epithelioid hemangioendothelioma: an unusual case and a review of the literature. *Chest* 2004; 125: 789–793.

51.	Ross GJ, Violi L, Friedman AC, Edmonds PR, Unger E. Intravascular bronchioloalveolar tumor: CT and pathologic correlation. *J Comput Assist Tomogr* 1989; 13: 240–243.

52.	Boudousquie AC, Lawce HJ, Sherman R, Olson S, Magenis RE, Corless CL. Complex translocation [7;22] identified in an epithelioid hemangioendothelioma. *Cancer Genet Cytogenet* 1996; 92: 116–121.

53. Miettinen M, Collan Y, Halttunen P, Maamies T, Vilkko P. Intravascular bronchioloalveolar tumor. *Cancer* 1987; 60: 2471–2475.

54. De-Luca S, Sanguinetti CM, Bearzi I, Murer B. Intravascular bronchioloalveolar tumour. *Eur Respir J* 1990; 3: 346–348.

55. Nakatani Y, Kitamura H, Inayama Y, *et al.* Pulmonary adenocarcinomas of the fetal lung type: a clinicopathologic study indicating differences in histology, epidemiology, and natural history of low-grade and high-grade forms. *Am J Surg Pathol* 1998; 22: 399–411.

56. Sheehan KM, Curran J, Kay EW, Broe P, Grace A. Well differentiated fetal adenocarcinoma of the lung in a 29 year old woman. *J Clin Pathol* 2003; 56: 478–479.

57. Janssen JP, Mulder JJ, Wagenaar SS, Elbers HR, van den Bosch JM. Primary sarcoma of the lung: a clinical study with long-term follow-up. *Ann Thorac Surg* 1994; 58: 1151–1155.

58. Porte HL, Metois DG, Leroy X, Conti M, Gosselin B, Wurtz A. Surgical treatment of primary sarcoma of the lung. *Eur J Cardiothorac Surg* 2000; 18: 136–142.

59. Kunst PW, Sutedja G, Golding RP, Risse E, Kardos G, Postmus PE. Unusual pulmonary lesions: case 1. A juvenile bronchopulmonary fibrosarcoma. *J Clin Oncol* 2002; 20: 2745–2751.

60. Logrono R, Filipowicz EA, Eyzaguirre EJ, Sawh RN. Diagnosis of primary fibrosarcoma of the lung by fine-needle aspiration and core biopsy. *Arch Pathol Lab Med* 1999; 123: 731–735.

61. Picard E, Udassin R, Ramu N, *et al.* Pulmonary fibrosarcoma in childhood: fiber-optic bronchoscopic diagnosis and review of the literature. *Pediatr Pulmonol* 1999; 27: 347–350.

62. Cadranel J, Wislez M, Antoine M. Primary pulmonary lymphoma. *Eur Respir J* 2002; 20: 750–762.

63. Ginsberg SS, Buzaid AC, Stern H, Carter D. Giant cell carcinoma of the lung. *Cancer* 1992; 70: 606–610.

64. Rossi G, Cavazza A, Sturm N, *et al.* Pulmonary carcinomas with pleomorphic, sarcomatoid, or sarcomatous elements: a clinicopathologic and immunohistochemical study of 75 cases. *Am J Surg Pathol* 2003; 27: 311–324.

65. Hishida T, Hasegawa T, Asamura H, *et al.* Malignant glomus tumor of the lung. *Pathol Int* 2003; 53: 632–636.

66. Xu R, Murray M, Jagirdar J, Delgado Y, Melamed J. Placental transmogrification of the lung is a histologic pattern frequently associated with pulmonary fibrochondromatous hamartoma. *Arch Pathol Lab Med* 2002; 126: 562–566.

67. Ruiz-Hernandez G, Gonzalez A, de Juan R, *et al.* Tomografia por emission de positrons mediante PET-18FDG en lesions pulmonares radiologicamente indeterminadas. [Diagnostic accuracy of semiquantitative analysis of positron emission tomography in radiologically indeterminate lung lesions.] *Rev Esp Med Nucl* 2002; 21: 403–409.

68. Cottin V, Thomas L, Loire R, Chalabreysse L, Gindre D, Cordier JF. Mesenchymal cystic hamartoma of the lung in Cowden's disease. *Respir Med* 2003; 97: 188–191.

69. Wang SC. [Lung hamartoma: a report of 30 cases and review of 477 cases.] *Zhonghua Wai Ke Za Zhi* 1992; 30: 540–542.

70. Almagro P, Julia J, Sanjaume M, *et al.* Pulmonary capillary hemangiomatosis associated with primary pulmonary hypertension: report of 2 new cases and review of 35 cases from the literature. *Medicine (Baltimore)* 2002; 81: 417–424.

71. Kiefer T, Wertzel H, Freudenberg N, Hasse J. Long-term survival after repetitive surgery for malignant hemangiopericytoma of the lung with subsequent systemic metastases: case report and review of the literature. *Thorac Cardiovasc Surg* 1997; 45: 307–309.

72. Hercot O, Giron J, Joffre P, Senac JP, Mary H, Baldet P. [Pulmonary hemangiopericytoma. Apropos of a case and review of the literature.] *J Radiol* 1988; 69: 443–448.

73. Cerfolio RJ, Allen MS, Nascimento AG, *et al.* Inflammatory pseudotumors of the lung. *Ann Thorac Surg* 1999; 67: 933–936.

74. Boman F, Champigneulle J, Boccon-Gibod L, *et al.* Tumeur myofibroblastique inflammatoire pulmonaire à forme endobronchique, infiltrante, multifocale et récidivante. [Inflammatory

myofibroblastic tumor of the lung with endobronchial, infiltrating, multifocal and recurrent form.] *Ann Pathol* 1995; 15: 207–210.

75. Sakurai H, Hasegawa T, Watanabe S, Suzuki K, Asamura H, Tsuchiya R. Inflammatory myofibroblastic tumor of the lung. *Eur J Cardiothorac Surg* 2004; 25: 155–159.

76. Gomez-Roman JJ, Sanchez-Velasco P, Ocejo-Vinyals G, Hernandez-Nieto E, Leyva-Cobian F, Val-Bernal JF. Human herpesvirus-8 genes are expressed in pulmonary inflammatory myofibroblastic tumor (inflammatory pseudotumor). *Am J Surg Pathol* 2001; 25: 624–629.

77. Kim TS, Han J, Kim GY, Lee KS, Kim H, Kim J. Pulmonary inflammatory pseudotumor (inflammatory myofibroblastic tumor): CT features with pathologic correlation. *J Comput Assist Tomogr* 2005; 29: 633–639.

78. Slosman DO, Spiliopoulos A, Keller A, *et al.* Quantitative metabolic PET imaging of a plasma cell granuloma. *J Thorac Imaging* 1994; 9: 116–119.

79. Ishioka S, Maeda A, Yamasaki M, Yamakido M. Inflammatory pseudotumor of the lung with pleural thickening treated with corticosteroids. *Chest* 2000; 117: 923.

80. Tokumoto H, Nomura S, Yamaguchi K, Yoshizumi M, Kamoshida S. [Primary pulmonary hemangiopericytoma detected on routine chest X-ray examination.] *Nihon Kyobu Shikkan Gakkai Zasshi* 1996; 34: 1125–1129.

81. Melloni G, Carretta A, Ciriaco P, *et al.* Inflammatory pseudotumor of the lung in adults. *Ann Thorac Surg* 2005; 79: 426–432.

82. Tuncozgur B, Ustunsoy H, Bakir K, Ucak R, Elbeyli L. Inflammatory pseudotumor of the lung. *Thorac Cardiovasc Surg* 2000; 48: 112–113.

83. Crimm PD, Kiechle FL. Fibroma of the lung; case report. *J Thorac Surg* 1952; 23: 205–209.

84. Deavers M, Guinee D, Koss MN, Travis WD. Granular cell tumors of the lung. Clinicopathologic study of 20 cases. *Am J Surg Pathol* 1995; 19: 627–635.

85. Goh SG, Chuah KL, Tan PH. Intravascular lymphomatosis of the lung and liver following eyelid lymphoma in a Chinese man and review of primary pulmonary intravascular lymphomatosis. *Pathology* 2002; 34: 82–85.

86. Gruden JF, Huang L, Webb WR, Gamsu G, Hopewell PC, Sides DM. AIDS-related Kaposi sarcoma of the lung: radiographic findings and staging system with bronchoscopic correlation. *Radiology* 1995; 195: 545–552.

87. Gal AA, Brooks JS, Pietra GG. Leiomyomatous neoplasms of the lung: a clinical, histologic, and immunohistochemical study. *Mod Pathol* 1989; 2: 209–216.

88. Penel N, Lartigau E, Fournier C, *et al.* Sarcomes des tissues mous thoraciques de l'adulte: etude retrospective de 40 cas. [Primary soft tissue sarcoma of the chest in adults: a retrospective study of 40 cases.] *Ann Chir* 2003; 128: 237–245.

89. Etienne-Mastroianni B, Falchero L, Chalabreysse L, *et al.* Primary sarcomas of the lung: a clinicopathologic study of 12 cases. *Lung Cancer* 2002; 38: 283–289.

90. Keel SB, Bacha E, Mark EJ, Nielsen GP, Rosenberg AE. Primary pulmonary sarcoma: a clinicopathologic study of 26 cases. *Mod Pathol* 1999; 12: 1124–1131.

91. Takeda F, Yamagiwa I, Ohizumi H, Shiono S. Leiomyosarcoma of the main bronchus in a girl: a long-time survivor with multiple lung metastases. *Pediatr Pulmonol* 2004; 37: 368–374.

92. Conte B, Leitner J. Leiomyosarcoma of the lung. *J Thorac Cardiovasc Surg* 1993; 105: 1119–1120.

93. Hirata T, Reshad K, Itoi K, Muro K, Akiyama J. Lipomas of the peripheral lung – a case report and review of the literature. *Thorac Cardiovasc Surg* 1989; 37: 385–387.

94. Muraoka M, Oka T, Akamine S, *et al.* Endobronchial lipoma: review of 64 cases reported in Japan. *Chest* 2003; 123: 293–296.

95. Loddenkemper C, Perez-Canto A, Leschber G, Stein H. Primary dedifferentiated liposarcoma of the lung. *Histopathology* 2005; 46: 710–712.

96. Avila NA, Bechtle J, Dwyer AJ, Ferrans VJ, Moss J. Lymphangioleiomyomatosis: CT of diurnal variation of lymphangioleiomyomas. *Radiology* 2001; 221: 415–421.

97. Barroso A, Nogueira R, Lencastre H, Seada J, Parente B. Primary lymphoepithelioma-like carcinoma of the lung. *Lung Cancer* 2000; 28: 69–74.

98. Bazot M, Cadranel J, Benayoun S, Tassart M, Bigot JM, Carette MF. Primary pulmonary AIDS-related lymphoma: radiographic and CT findings. *Chest* 1999; 116: 1282–1286.

99. Cordier JF, Chailleux E, Lauque D, *et al.* Primary pulmonary lymphomas. A clinical study of 70 cases in nonimmunocompromised patients. *Chest* 1993; 103: 201–208.

100. Kurtin PJ, Myers JL, Adlakha H, *et al.* Pathologic and clinical features of primary pulmonary extranodal marginal zone B-cell lymphoma of MALT type. *Am J Surg Pathol* 2001; 25: 997–1008.

101. Graham BB, Mathisen DJ, Mark EJ, Takvorian RW. Primary pulmonary lymphoma. *Ann Thorac Surg* 2005; 80: 1248–1253.

102. Bertoni F, Zucca E. State-of-the-art therapeutics: marginal-zone lymphoma. *J Clin Oncol* 2005; 23: 6415–6420.

103. Ferraro P, Trastek VF, Adlakha H, Deschamps C, Allen MS, Pairolero PC. Primary non-Hodgkin's lymphoma of the lung. *Ann Thorac Surg* 2000; 69: 993–997.

104. Begueret H, Vergier B, Parrens M, *et al.* Primary lung small B-cell lymphoma *versus* lymphoid hyperplasia: evaluation of diagnostic criteria in 26 cases. *Am J Surg Pathol* 2002; 26: 76–81.

105. Musshoff K. Prognostic and therapeutic implications of staging in extranodal Hodgkin's disease. *Cancer Res* 1971; 31: 1814–1827.

106. Cortot A, Cottin V, Issartel B, Meyronet D, Coiffier B, Cordier JF. Lymphome pulmonaire du MALT révélant un sida. [Pulmonary MALT lymphoma revealing AIDS.] *Rev Mal Respir* 2006; 23: 353–357.

107. Ray P, Antoine M, Mary-Krause M, *et al.* AIDS-related primary pulmonary lymphoma. *Am J Respir Crit Care Med* 1998; 158: 1221–1229.

108. Taniere P, Thivolet-Bejui F, Vitrey D, *et al.* Lymphomatoid granulomatosis–a report on four cases: evidence for B phenotype of the tumoral cells. *Eur Respir J* 1998; 12: 102–106.

109. Pisani RJ, DeRemee RA. Clinical implications of the histopathologic diagnosis of pulmonary lymphomatoid granulomatosis. *Mayo Clin Proc* 1990; 65: 151–163.

110. Guinee DG Jr, Perkins SL, Travis WD, Holden JA, Tripp SR, Koss MN. Proliferation and cellular phenotype in lymphomatoid granulomatosis: implications of a higher proliferation index in B cells. *Am J Surg Pathol* 1998; 22: 1093–1100.

111. Wilson WH, Kingma DW, Raffeld M, Wittes RE, Jaffe ES. Association of lymphomatoid granulomatosis with Epstein–Barr viral infection of B lymphocytes and response to interferon-α2b. *Blood* 1996; 87: 4531–4537.

112. Jaffe ES, Wilson WH. Lymphomatoid granulomatosis: pathogenesis, pathology and clinical implications. *Cancer Surv* 1997; 30: 233–248.

113. Barrans SL, Fenton JA, Banham A, Owen RG, Jack AS. Strong expression of FOXP1 identifies a distinct subset of diffuse large B-cell lymphoma (DLBCL) patients with poor outcome. *Blood* 2004; 104: 2933–2935.

114. Radin AI. Primary pulmonary Hodgkin's disease. *Cancer* 1990; 65: 550–563.

115. Varona JF, Guerra JM, Grande C, Villena V, Gonzalez-Lois C, Martinez MA. Primary pulmonary lymphoma: diagnosis and follow-up of 6 cases and review of an uncommon entity. *Tumori* 2005; 91: 24–29.

116. Dacic S, Colby TV, Yousem SA. Nodular amyloidoma and primary pulmonary lymphoma with amyloid production: a differential diagnostic problem. *Mod Pathol* 2000; 13: 934–940.

117. Koss MN, Hochholzer L, Nichols PW, Wehunt WD, Lazarus AA. Primary non-Hodgkin's lymphoma and pseudolymphoma of lung: a study of 161 patients. *Hum Pathol* 1983; 14: 1024–1038.

118. Burton C, Ell P, Linch D. The role of PET imaging in lymphoma. *Br J Haematol* 2004; 126: 772–784.

119. Sugai S. Mucosa-associated lymphoid tissue (MALT) lymphoma and primary amyloidosis in the lung in Sjögren's syndrome. *Intern Med* 2002; 41: 251–252.

120. Roggeri A, Agostini L, Vezzani G, Sabattini E, Serra L. Primary malignant non-Hodgkin's lymphoma of the lung arising in mucosa-associated lymphoid tissue (MALT). *Eur Respir J* 1993; 6: 138–140.

121. Goldstraw P. Primary B-cell malignant lymphoma of the lung. *Ann Thorac Surg* 1994; 58: 606.

122. Dobrilovic N, Wright CB, Vester SR, Patel MA, Fannin EA. Unusual chest lesion: giant primary pulmonary lymphoma. *Ann Thorac Surg* 2005; 80: 1134.

123. Watson DC, Hasan A. Mesenchymoma of the lung. *Thorax* 1988; 43: 946–947.

124. Wilson RW, Moran CA. Primary melanoma of the lung: a clinicopathologic and immuno-histochemical study of eight cases. *Am J Surg Pathol* 1997; 21: 1196–1202.

125. Ost D, Joseph C, Sogoloff H, Menezes G. Primary pulmonary melanoma: case report and literature review. *Mayo Clin Proc* 1999; 74: 62–66.

126. Cura M, Smoak W, Dala R. Pulmonary meningioma: false-positive positron emission tomography for malignant pulmonary nodules. *Clin Nucl Med* 2002; 27: 701–704.

127. Prayson RA, Farver CF. Primary pulmonary malignant meningioma. *Am J Surg Pathol* 1999; 23: 722–726.

128. Moran CA. Primary salivary gland-type tumors of the lung. *Semin Diagn Pathol* 1995; 12: 106–122.

129. Yousem SA, Hochholzer L. Mucoepidermoid tumors of the lung. *Cancer* 1987; 60: 1346–1352.

130. Vadasz P, Egervary M. Mucoepidermoid bronchial tumors: a review of 34 operated cases. *Eur J Cardiothorac Surg* 2000; 17: 566–569.

131. Kim TS, Lee KS, Han J, *et al.* Mucoepidermoid carcinoma of the tracheobronchial tree: radiographic and CT findings in 12 patients. *Radiology* 1999; 212: 643–648.

132. Shim SS, Lee KS, Kim BT, Choi JY, Chung MJ, Lee EJ. Focal parenchymal lung lesions showing a potential of false-positive and false-negative interpretation on integrated PET/CT. *AJR Am J Roentgenol* 2006; 186: 639–648.

133. Welsh JH, Maxson T, Jaksic T, Shahab I, Hicks J. Tracheobronchial mucoepidermoid carcinoma in childhood and adolescence: case report and review of the literature. *Int J Pediatr Otorhinolaryngol* 1998; 45: 265–273.

134. Kantar M, Cetingul N, Veral A, Kansoy S, Ozcan C, Alper H. Rare tumors of the lung in children. *Pediatr Hematol Oncol* 2002; 19: 421–428.

135. Kobashi Y, Yoshida K, Miyashita N, Niki Y, Matsushima T, Irei T. Multifocal micronodular pneumocyte hyperplasia in a man with tuberous sclerosis. *Intern Med* 2005; 44: 462–466.

136. Masuya D, Haba R, Huang CL, Yokomise H. Myoepithelial carcinoma of the lung. *Eur J Cardiothorac Surg* 2005; 28: 775–777.

137. Nguyen BD. F-18 FDG PET imaging of metastases from soft tissue myoepithelioma. *Clin Nucl Med* 2005; 30: 201–202.

138. Morawietz L, Kuhnen C, Katenkamp D, Le Coutre P, Ladhoff A, Petersen I. Unusual sarcomatoid neoplasm of the lung suggesting a myofibrosarcoma. *Virchows Arch* 2005; 447: 990–995.

139. Manabe H, Umemoto T, Takagi H, *et al.* Primary neurogenous sarcoma of the lung; report of a case. *Kyobu Geka* 2005; 58: 337–340.

140. Cordier JF. Pulmonary amyloidosis in hematological disorders. *Semin Respir Crit Care Med* 2005; 26: 502–513.

141. Tamura K, Nakajima N, Makino S, Maruyama R, Kohno T, Koga Y. Primary pulmonary amyloidosis with multiple nodules. *Eur J Radiol* 1988; 8: 128–130.

142. Lee SC, Johnson H. Multiple nodular pulmonary amyloidosis. A case report and comparison with diffuse alveolar-septal pulmonary amyloidosis. *Thorax* 1975; 30: 178–185.

143. Kadowaki T, Hamada H, Yokoyama A, *et al.* Two cases of primary pulmonary osteosarcoma. *Intern Med* 2005; 44: 632–637.

144. Aubertine CL, Flieder DB. Primary paraganglioma of the lung. *Ann Diagn Pathol* 2004; 8: 237–241.

145. Etienne G, Grenouillet M, Ghiringhelli C, *et al.* Plasmocytome pulmonaire: à propos de deux nouvelles observations et revue de la littérature. [Pulmonary plasmacytoma: about two new cases and review of the literature.] *Rev Med Interne* 2004; 25: 591–595.

146. Scherwitz P, Kruger I, Eidt S. Extramedullary plasmocytoma of the bronchial system. *Chirurg* 1997; 68: 821–824.

147. Raveglia F, Mezzetti M, Panigalli T, *et al.* Personal experience in surgical management of pulmonary pleomorphic carcinoma. *Ann Thorac Surg* 2004; 78: 1742–1747.

148. Hornick JL, Jaffe ES, Fletcher CD. Extranodal histiocytic sarcoma: clinicopathologic analysis of 14 cases of a rare epithelioid malignancy. *Am J Surg Pathol* 2004; 28: 1133–1144.

149. Kato N, Yamazaki S, Komatu H. Pulmonary fibrous histiocytoma. *Ryoikibetsu Shokogun Shirizu* 1994; 4: 254–257.

150. Kimizuka G, Okuzawa K, Yarita T. Primary giant cell malignant fibrous histocytoma of the lung: a case report. *Pathol Int* 1999; 49: 342–346.

151. Larsen H, Sorensen JB. Pulmonary blastoma: a review with special emphasis on prognosis and treatment. *Cancer Treat Rev* 1996; 22: 145–160.

152. Force S, Patterson GA. Clinical-pathologic conference in general thoracic surgery: pulmonary blastoma. *J Thorac Cardiovasc Surg* 2003; 126: 1247–1250.

153. Parsons SK, Fishman SJ, Hoorntje LE, *et al.* Aggressive multimodal treatment of pleuropulmonary blastoma. *Ann Thorac Surg* 2001; 72: 939–942.

154. Walker RI, Suvarna K, Matthews S. Case report: pulmonary blastoma: presentation of two atypical cases and review of the literature. *Br J Radiol* 2005; 78: 437–440.

155. Wright JR Jr. Pleuropulmonary blastoma: a case report documenting transition from type I (cystic) to type III (solid). *Cancer* 2000; 88: 2853–2858.

156. Robert J, Pache JC, Seium Y, de Perrot M, Spiliopoulos A. Pulmonary blastoma: report of five cases and identification of clinical features suggestive of the disease. *Eur J Cardiothorac Surg* 2002; 22: 708–711.

157. Surmont VF, van Klaveren RJ, Nowak PJ, Zondervan PE, Hoogsteden HC, van Meerbeeck JP. Unexpected response of a pulmonary blastoma on radiotherapy: a case report and review of the literature. *Lung Cancer* 2002; 36: 207–211.

158. Yi CA, Lee KS, Choe YH, Han D, Kwon OJ, Kim S. Computed tomography in pulmonary artery sarcoma: distinguishing features from pulmonary embolic disease. *J Comput Assist Tomogr* 2004; 28: 34–39.

159. Tsunezuka Y, Oda M, Takahashi M, Minato H, Watanabe G. Primary chondromatous osteosarcoma of the pulmonary artery. *Ann Thorac Surg* 2004; 77: 331–334.

160. Cox JE, Chiles C, Aquino SL, Savage P, Oaks T. Pulmonary artery sarcomas: a review of clinical and radiologic features. *J Comput Assist Tomogr* 1997; 21: 750–755.

161. Parish JM, Rosenow EC 3rd, Swensen SJ, Crotty TB. Pulmonary artery sarcoma. Clinical features. *Chest* 1996; 110: 1480–1488.

162. Okano Y, Satoh T, Tatewaki T, *et al.* Pulmonary artery sarcoma diagnosed using intravascular ultrasound images. *Thorax* 1999; 54: 748–749.

163. Gerard A, Durieu I, Cordier JF, Champsaur G, Loire R, Vital Durand D. Sarcome primitive de l'artère pulmonaire. A propos d'une observation. [Primary sarcoma of the pulmonary artery. Case report.] *Rev Med Interne* 1999; 20: 705–708.

164. Devouassoux M, Thivolet Bejui F, Tabone E, *et al.* Saromes de l'artère pulmonaire. [Sarcoma of the pulmonary artery.] *Rev Mal Respir* 1998; 15: 295–299.

165. Thurer RL, Thorsen A, Parker JA, Karp DD. FDG imaging of a pulmonary artery sarcoma. *Ann Thorac Surg* 2000; 70: 1414–1415.

166. Kim JH, Gutierrez FR, Lee EY, Semenkovich J, Bae KT, Ylagan LR. Primary leiomyosarcoma of the pulmonary artery: a diagnostic dilemma. *Clin Imaging* 2003; 27: 206–211.

167. Ozcan C, Celik A, Ural Z, Veral A, Kandiloglu G, Balik E. Primary pulmonary rhabdomyosarcoma arising within cystic adenomatoid malformation: a case report and review of the literature. *J Pediatr Surg* 2001; 36: 1062–1065.

168. Gray JA, Nguyen GK. Primary pulmonary rhabdomyosarcoma diagnosed by fine-needle aspiration cytology. *Diagn Cytopathol* 2003; 29: 181–182.

169. Shao J, Zhu XH, Shi JY, Ma J, Ge XJ, You ZQ. Primary pulmonary schwannoma: clinical analysis of 7 cases and review of the literature. *Zhonghua Jie He He Hu Xi Za Zhi* 2003; 26: 3–6.

170. Iyoda A, Hiroshima K, Shiba M, *et al.* Clinicopathological analysis of pulmonary sclerosing hemangioma. *Ann Thorac Surg* 2004; 78: 1928–1931.

171. Devouassoux-Shisheboran M, Hayashi T, Linnoila RI, Koss MN, Travis WD. A

clinicopathologic study of 100 cases of pulmonary sclerosing hemangioma with immuno-histochemical studies: TTF-1 is expressed in both round and surface cells, suggesting an origin from primitive respiratory epithelium. *Am J Surg Pathol* 2000; 24: 906–916.

172. Gaucher L, Patra P, Despins P, Delumeau J, Ordronneau J, Audouin AF. Une tumeur rare: l'hémangiome sclérosant bénin intra-scissural. [A rare tumor: benign sclerosing pneumocytoma with an intrascissural development.] *Poumon Coeur* 1983; 39: 321–326.

173. Katzenstein AL, Gmelich JT, Carrington CB. Sclerosing hemangioma of the lung: a clinicopathologic study of 51 cases. *Am J Surg Pathol* 1980; 4: 343–356.

174. Borczuk AC, Sha KK, Hisler SE, Mann JM, Hajdu SI. Sebaceous carcinoma of the lung: histologic and immunohistochemical characterization of an unusual pulmonary neoplasm: report of a case and review of the literature. *Am J Surg Pathol* 2002; 26: 795–798.

175. Mishina T, Suzuki I, Fujino M, *et al.* A benign clear cell tumor of the lung that grew gradually over five years. *Nihon Kyobu Shikkan Gakkai Zasshi* 1995; 33: 765–770.

176. Brook OR, Bar-Shalom R, Guralnik L, *et al.* 18F-FDG PET of clear cell (sugar) tumour of the lung. *Nuklearmedizin* 2005; 44: n35.

177. Magro G, Fraggetta F, Manusia M, Mingrino A. Hyalinizing spindle cell tumor with giant rosettes: a previously undescribed lesion of the lung. *Am J Surg Pathol* 1998; 22: 1431–1433.

178. Dennison S, Weppler E, Giacoppe G. Primary pulmonary synovial sarcoma: a case report and review of current diagnostic and therapeutic standards. *Oncologist* 2004; 9: 339–342.

179. Okamoto S, Hisaoka M, Daa T, Hatakeyama K, Iwamasa T, Hashimoto H. Primary pulmonary synovial sarcoma: a clinicopathologic, immunohistochemical, and molecular study of 11 cases. *Hum Pathol* 2004; 35: 850–856.

180. Srivastava A, Padilla O, Alroy J, *et al.* Primary intrapulmonary spindle cell thymoma with marked granulomatous reaction: report of a case with review of literature. *Int J Surg Pathol* 2003; 11: 353–356.

181. Kakkar N, Vasishta RK, Banerjee AK, Garewal G, Deodhar SD, Bambery P. Primary pulmonary malignant teratoma with yolk sac element associated with hematologic neoplasia. *Respiration* 1996; 63: 52–54.

182. Okur E, Halezeroglu S, Somay A, Atasalihi A. Unusual intrathoracic location of a primary germ cell tumour. *Eur J Cardiothorac Surg* 2002; 22: 651–653.

183. Inoue H, Iwasaki M, Ogawa J, *et al.* Pure yolk-sac tumor of the lung. *Thorac Cardiovasc Surg* 1993; 41: 249–251.

184. Beasley MB, Brambilla E, Travis WD. The 2004 World Health Organization classification of lung tumors. *Semin Roentgenol* 2005; 40: 90–97.

185. Kubin K, Hormann M, Riccabona M, Wiesbauer P, Puig S. Benigne und maligne Lungentumoren im Kindesalter. [Benign and malignant pulmonary tumors in childhood.] *Radiologe* 2003; 43: 1095–1102.

186. Hancock BJ, Di Lorenzo M, Youssef S, Yazbeck S, Marcotte JE, Collin PP. Childhood primary pulmonary neoplasms. *J Pediatr Surg* 1993; 28: 1133–1136.

187. Ramirez-Chavez G, Truy E, Felix-Page D, *et al.* Diagnostic des hamartomes pulmonaires. A propos de 50 cas. [Diagnosis of pulmonary hamartoma. Apropos of 50 cases.] *Ann Radiol (Paris)* 1985; 28: 35–42.

188. Coffin CM, Dehner LP, Meis-Kindblom JM. Inflammatory myofibroblastic tumor, inflammatory fibrosarcoma, and related lesions: an historical review with differential diagnostic considerations. *Semin Diagn Pathol* 1998; 15: 102–110.

189. Zen Y, Sawazaki A, Miyayama S, Notsumata K, Tanaka N, Nakanuma Y. A case of retroperitoneal and mediastinal fibrosis exhibiting elevated levels of IgG4 in the absence of sclerosing pancreatitis (autoimmune pancreatitis). *Hum Pathol* 2006; 37: 239–243.

190. Berman M, Georghiou GP, Schonfeld T, *et al.* Pulmonary inflammatory myofibroblastic tumor invading the left atrium. *Ann Thorac Surg* 2003; 76: 601–603.

191. Hoover SV, Granston AS, Koch DF, Hudson TR. Plasma cell granuloma of the lung, response to radiation therapy: report of a single case. *Cancer* 1977; 39: 123–125.

192. Regnard JF, Icard P, Guibert L, de Montpreville VT, Magdeleinat P, Levasseur P. Prognostic

factors and results after surgical treatment of primary sarcomas of the lung. *Ann Thorac Surg* 1999; 68: 227–231.

193. Odashiro AN, Miiji LO, Nguyen GK. Primary lung leiomyosarcoma detected by bronchoscopy cytology. *Diagn Cytopathol* 2005; 33: 220–222.

194. Wick MR, Scheithauer BW, Piehler JM, Pairolero PC. Primary pulmonary leiomyosarcomas. A light and electron microscopic study. *Arch Pathol Lab Med* 1982; 106: 510–514.

195. Moran CA, Suster S, Abbondanzo SL, Koss MN. Primary leiomyosarcomas of the lung: a clinicopathologic and immunohistochemical study of 18 cases. *Mod Pathol* 1997; 10: 121–128.

196. Bode-Lesniewska B, Hodler J, von Hochstetter A, Guillou L, Exner U, Caduff R. Late solitary bone metastasis of a primary pulmonary synovial sarcoma with *SYT-SSX1* translocation type: case report with a long follow-up. *Virchows Arch* 2005; 446: 310–315.

197. Niwa H, Masuda S, Kobayashi C, Oda Y. Pulmonary synovial sarcoma with polypoid endobronchial growth: a case report, immunohistochemical and cytogenetic study. *Pathol Int* 2004; 54: 611–615.

198. Pelmus M, Guillou L, Hostein I, Sierankowski G, Lussan C, Coindre JM. Monophasic fibrous and poorly differentiated synovial sarcoma: immunohistochemical reassessment of 60 t(X;18)(*SYT-SSX*)-positive cases. *Am J Surg Pathol* 2002; 26: 1434–1440.

199. Boroumand N, Raja V, Jones DV, Haque AK. *SYT-SSX2* variant of primary pulmonary synovial sarcoma with focal expression of CD117 (c-Kit) protein and a poor clinical outcome. *Arch Pathol Lab Med* 2003; 127: e201–e204.

200. Jadvar H, Fischman AJ. Evaluation of rare tumors with [F-18]fluorodeoxyglucose positron emission tomography. *Clin Positron Imaging* 1999; 2: 153–158.

201. Marchevsky AM, Changsri C, Gupta I, Fuller C, Houck W, McKenna RJ Jr. Frozen section diagnoses of small pulmonary nodules: accuracy and clinical implications. *Ann Thorac Surg* 2004; 78: 1755–1759.

202. Socinski MA. Adjuvant therapy of resected non-small-cell lung cancer. *Clin Lung Cancer* 2004; 6: 162–169.

203. Betticher DC, Rosell R. Neoadjuvant treatment of early-stage resectable non-small-cell lung cancer. *Lung Cancer* 2004; 46: Suppl. 2, S23–S32.

204. Blay JY, Le Cesne A, Alberti L, Ray-Coquart I. Targeted cancer therapies. *Bull Cancer* 2005; 92: E13–E18.

CHAPTER 6

Smoking-induced lung disease

H.H. Popper*, W. Timens[#]

*Dept of Pathology, Laboratories for Molecular Cytogenetics, Environmental and Respiratory Pathology, Medical University of Graz, Austria. [#]Dept of Pathology, University Medical Center Groningen, University of Groningen, Groningen, the Netherlands.

Correspondence: H.H. Popper, Dept of Pathology, Laboratories for Molecular Cytogenetics, Environmental and Respiratory Pathology, Medical University of Graz, Auenbruggerplatz 25, Graz, A-8036, Austria. Fax: 43 31638583646; E-mail: Helmut.popper@meduni-graz.at

Effects of tobacco smoke on the respiratory tract

Tobacco smoking results in inhalation of various amounts of toxins, which can induce a wide variety of effects on different cell systems in the respiratory tract. The toxins are acidic as well as basic, and, additionally, heat harms the respiratory tract. However, there is also a protective system working, which can reduce the effects of this toxic inhalation. The present chapter discusses the toxic effects of tobacco substances and, briefly, the protective system, and finally focuses on nontumorous tobacco smoke-induced lung diseases.

In most reports, the main focus is the oncogenic effects of tobacco smoke products. Usually, it is not mentioned that prior to an oncogenic effect, there is usually a toxic effect, with cell death, inflammation and repair. Activation of proliferation and angiogenesis also affects normal cells, and, as such, exerts changes in lung structure and cellular constituents, and might have effects on matrix proteins, long before the development of precancerous lesions starts.

Effects of toxins

Among more than 5,000 compounds in tobacco smoke are carcinogens such as nitrosamines, irritants such as phenolic compounds, volatile compounds such as carbon monoxide, various metal oxides, in part depending upon the location and nutrition of the tobacco plants, and, of course, nicotine. Nicotine itself has quite complex actions, mediated in part by nicotinic cholinergic receptors that may show extraneuronal as well as neuronal distribution. Nicotine is a potent angiogenic agent. It hijacks an endogenous nicotinic cholinergic pathway present in endothelial cells, which is involved in physiological as well as pathological angiogenesis [1]. ZHU et al. [2] demonstrated that environmental tobacco smoke results in tumour angiogenesis, and provide evidence that the responsible factor is nicotine. Although a weak carcinogen, nicotine promotes carcinogenesis by a number of different mechanisms [2].

The most toxic substances, which cause respiratory epithelium damage, occur within the vapour phase of tobacco sidestream smoke [3]. Many tobacco smoke constituents are potent inducers of oxygen radicals, thus causing DNA strand breaks, DNA adducts, oxidative DNA damage, chromosomal aberrations and micronuclei formation [4]. In addition, they can also affect the mitotic spindle apparatus and influence the methylation of the promoter region of tumour suppressor genes [5–8]. Multiple different compounds

Eur Respir Mon, 2007, 39, 134–152. Printed in UK - all rights reserved. Copyright ERS Journals Ltd 2007; European Respiratory Monograph; ISSN 1025-448x.

have been identified in tobacco main- and sidestream smoke, including tar (in filterless cigarettes), polycyclic aromatic hydrocarbons (PAHs), N-nitrosamines, many different N-nitroso compounds, such as butanones and nitroso-anatabines, and volatile N-nitrosamines. Within the PAHs alone, 150 different substances have been identified [9]. In addition, many metal oxides, such as chromium, cadmium and arsenic oxides, are generated during tobacco burning. Many of these can either generate oxygen radicals themselves, or act as catalysing agents in concert with nitroso compounds in generating radicals. Depending on environmental contamination, many other unusual metals can occur (e.g. lead contaminates tobacco plants grown close to highways) [10–12]. A comprehensive list of tobacco constituents can be found in articles published by ZARIDZE et al. [13] and STABBERT et al. [14], as well as on the website of the International Agency for Research on Cancer [15]. For some of these components the mechanisms of their toxic and carcinogenic action has been elucidated.

Nitrosamine 4-(methylnitrosamino)-1-(3-pyridyl)-1-butanone (NNK) is formed by nitrosation of nicotine. NNK simultaneously stimulates phosphorylation of B-cell leukaemia/lymphoma 2 gene product (Bcl-2) and myelocytomatosis oncogene (c-Myc) through activation of both extracellular signal-regulated kinase 1/2 and protein kinase Cα, which is required for NNK-induced survival and proliferation. Phosphorylation of Bcl-2 promotes a direct interaction between Bcl-2 and c-Myc in the nucleus and on the outer mitochondrial membrane that significantly enhances the half-life of c-Myc. Thus, NNK induces a functional cooperation between Bcl-2 and c-Myc in promoting cell survival and proliferation [16].

Nicotine and NNK activate the Akt kinase (Akt) pathway and increase cell proliferation and survival. Nicotinic activation of Akt increases phosphorylation of multiple downstream substrates of Akt, including glycogen synthase kinase 3, forkhead homologue in rhabdomyosarcoma, tuberin, mammalian target of rapamycin and ribosomal protein S6 kinase (70 kDa), polypeptide 2 (p70S6K1), in a time-dependent manner. Nicotine or NNK binds to cell-surface nicotinic acetylcholine receptors. Only nicotine decreases apoptosis. The protection conferred by nicotine is nuclear factor (NF)-κB-dependent. Collectively, these results identify tobacco component-induced Akt-dependent proliferation and NF-κB-dependent survival of cancer cells [17].

Carcinogenic effects

In 1950, the first large-scale epidemiological studies demonstrated that lung cancer is causatively associated with cigarette smoking. Although cigarette consumption has gradually decreased in most industrialised countries, death due to lung cancer has reached a high among males and females. In the younger cohorts, the lung cancer death rate is decreasing in both males and females. Conversely, a steeper increase in lung adenocarcinoma incidence has been seen since the 1980s. Contributors to this change in the histological types of lung cancer are a decrease in the mean nicotine and tar delivery of cigarettes from ∼2.7 and ∼38 mg, respectively, in 1955 to ∼1.0 and ∼13.5 mg in 1993. Other major factors relate to changes in the composition of the cigarette tobacco blend and general acceptance of cigarettes with filter tips. However, smokers compensate for the reduced nicotine content by inhaling the smoke more deeply and smoking more intensely. Under these conditions, the peripheral lung is exposed to increased amounts of the smoke carcinogens, which are suspected to lead to lung adenocarcinoma. Importantly, due to the efficacy of the filters, particulate matter with bound carcinogens is withheld in the filters, but vaporised toxins and carcinogens are enriched in the tobacco smoke and delivered to the alveolar periphery. Among the important changes in the composition of the tobacco blend is a significant increase in nitrate content (from 0.5 to 1.2–1.5%), which raises the yields of nitrogen oxides and *N*-nitrosamines in the smoke. Furthermore, the more intense smoking by consumers of low-yield cigarettes increases levels of *N*-nitrosamines in the smoke two- or three-fold. Among the *N*-nitrosamines is NNK (see above), a powerful lung carcinogen in animals that is exclusively formed from nicotine. This organ-specific tobacco-specific nitrosamine (TSNA) induces adenocarcinoma of the lung [18].

The effect of using filters has been evaluated in animal experiments. Mice were exposed to either full tobacco smoke or filtered tobacco smoke devoid of particulate matter. Analysis of the filtered smoke showed reduced concentrations of PAHs and TSNAs of <18%. Concentrations of aldehydes and other volatile organic compounds, such as 1,3-butadiene, benzene or acrolein, were not reduced as much (~50–90%). Some potentially carcinogenic metals reached levels in filtered smoke ranging from <1–77%. However, mice exposed to the filtered smoke atmosphere showed practically identical lung tumour multiplicities and incidence as animals exposed to full smoke. The authors concluded that 1,3-butadiene might be an important contributor to lung tumorigenesis in this mouse model of tobacco smoke carcinogenesis [19].

Temperature

Inhaled tobacco smoke is usually hot, with the temperature at the tip of the cigarette ranging 400–800°C. When tobacco smoke aerosols were generated in the range 250–550°C, there were no mutagenic components below a generator temperature of 400°C, but mutagens were found above this temperature. This underlines the importance of the pyrolysis temperature [20]. The pyrolysis of tobacco depends on various conditions, one of them the temperature and another the pH of the various substances, such as hydrogen cyanide, benzo[a]pyrene, aldehydes, volatile organic compounds, phenolics and aromatic amines. A few compounds are significantly affected by the pH [21]. The temperature of the inhaled smoke condensate reaching the distal airways is still >60°C.

Tobacco smoke, especially sidestream smoke, contains a high concentration of fine dust. Particles smaller than those with a 50% cut-off aerodynamic diameter of 10 μm (PM10; fine dust, respirable size <5 μm) are thought to impact on genotoxicity, as well as on cell proliferation *via* their ability to generate oxidants such as reactive oxygen species (ROS) and reactive nitrogen species. For mechanistic purposes, a discrimination should be made between: 1) the oxidant-generating properties of the particles themselves (*i.e.* acellular), which are mostly determined by the physicochemical characteristics of the particle surface; and 2) the ability of the particles to stimulate cellular oxidant generation. Since particles can induce an inflammatory response, a further subdivision needs to be made into the primary (*i.e.* particle-driven) and secondary (*i.e.* inflammation-driven) formation of oxidants. Particles may also affect genotoxicity by virtue of their ability to carry surface-adsorbed carcinogenic components into the lung. Each of these pathways can impact on genotoxicity and proliferation, as well as on feedback mechanisms involving DNA repair or apoptosis [22]. It should be remembered that toxins and carcinogens, such as NNK, bound to the surface of PM2.5 not only reach the alveolar periphery but also, due to the surface activity and low degradation rate, can act much longer on epithelial cells.

From studies on mutations of the tumour protein p53 gene, which usually precede the development of dysplasia, as well as carcinomas, and can be found in apparently normal epithelial cells, it has become clear that many of the different tobacco carcinogens leave behind a specific fingerprint, interacting specifically with some of the genes within the cell cycle [23].

Other factors relevant to the action of toxic and carcinogenic substances/particles

The architecture of the human bronchial system, as well as the composition of the epithelial lining system, is another factor in the modification of the action of inhaled substances, especially tobacco smoke. In humans, as in primates, the branching of the bronchial tree is asymmetric. A bronchus divides into a main branch with a diameter two-thirds that of the bronchus and a smaller branch with a diameter a third that of the bronchus. This gives rise to air flow turbulence at the bifurcations, causing deposition of particulate matter according to size; the larger the particles, the more they are deposited at larger bronchial bifurcations. The particle phase of tobacco smoke is composed of ash, but also contains incompletely combusted particles from tobacco plants, such as nitrosamines, PAHs and metal oxides. Coal and incompletely combusted plant particles have the tendency to bind PAHs and nitrosylated hydrocarbons, either chemically or physically, and thus prolong the duration of contact of the harmful chemicals with the respiratory epithelium. This has resulted in a toxin- and carcinogen-rich particle fraction acting at larger bifurcations in the era of the filterless cigarette.

The repair programme and its impact on the reaction of the epithelium towards inhaled toxins

After the acute inflammatory reaction, the epithelium is normally restored to full function. However, when the inhalation of toxic substances persists, adaptive changes take place. This is dependent upon the location of the lesion. Although columnar cell hyperplasia followed by goblet cell hyperplasia, and finally transitional and squamous cell metaplasia, are the main steps of repair and protection in the large bronchi [24], proliferation of Clara cells and secretory and goblet cell hyperplasia, as well as type II pneumocyte proliferation, resulting in the so-called cuboidal transformation of the epithelium, can be found in the bronchioloalveolar region. In the large bronchi, this can result in squamous and transitional cell dysplasia [24]. Other types of dysplasia, however, are seen in bronchioles (bronchiolar columnar cell dysplasia [25]) and alveoli (atypical adenomatous hyperplasia [26]). Rarely, squamous cell metaplasia can be encountered in the peripheral lung, most often associated with effects of cytotoxic drugs.

Neuroendocrine cell hyperplasia is another reactive lesion particularly found in patients with obstructive lung disease, such as chronic obstructive pulmonary disease (COPD), bronchiectasis and emphysema [27–29]. Neuroendocrine cells, normally found as scattered single cells along bronchi and bronchioles [30], start to proliferate upon chronic stimulation by disturbed airflow. It is supposed that the aim of this proliferation is to restore normal lung architecture and thus function. However, neuroendocrine hyperplasia itself causes thickening of bronchial/bronchiolar walls and thus stenosis [31, 32].

The defence system

Mucociliary escalator and clearance. One of the oldest defence systems is the mucociliary escalator. The cilia are constantly beating in synchrony towards the larynx, and move the mucus, produced by the bronchial glands and goblet and secretory columnar cells, in that direction. This mucus overlays the epithelium as a thin layer, and protects the epithelium against toxic substances. Since constant movement occurs, the duration of contact and, therefore, the action of toxins is reduced to a few seconds. Coughing and/or ingestion of the mucus together with substances dissolved in it quickly remove most of the harmful inhaled material from the bronchial system.

The phagocytic system. In the alveolar periphery, another old protection system is effective, the phagocytic cell system. Alveolar macrophages constantly enter the alveoli, patrol along the surface, phagocytose all inhaled material and vanish, either into the mucus, if irreversibly damaged by the ingested material, or by entering the lymphatics and reaching the draining lymph nodes, presenting the processed foreign material to dendritic cells and lymphocytes for a probable immune reaction.

The enzymes. The action of enzymes with respect to tobacco toxins and carcinogens is not as simple as it might appear at first glance. Various substances are inhaled within the tobacco smoke; some of them are primarily toxic and carcinogenic, whereas others require activation. Cytochrome P_{450}, family 2, subfamily A, polypeptide 13 (CYP2A13), an enzyme expressed predominantly in the human respiratory tract, exhibits high efficiency in the metabolic activation of tobacco carcinogen NNK. A CT or TT instead of CC genotype in the CYP2A13 gene causes substitution of arginine 257 with cysteine and so results in significantly reduced activity towards NNK and other substrates. By genotyping patients with lung cancer and controls for the variant CYP2A13 genotype, a substantially reduced risk of lung adenocarcinoma was found. This reduced risk of lung adenocarcinoma was associated with the genotype as well as light smokers, but not other types of lung cancer [33].

Phase II enzymes are implicated in the detoxication of many carcinogens and ROS, thereby protecting cells against DNA damage and subsequent malignant transformation. The induction of phase II enzymes is usually considered beneficial. However, in some cases, these enzymes also bioactivate several hazardous chemicals. Furthermore, from the study on the protective action of certain enzymes found in vegetables (*e.g.* isothiocyanate sulphoraphane in broccoli), the fact that these enzymes can also have adverse effects on phase I enzymes, which can subsequently bioactivate a variety of other carcinogens, should not be overlooked. For example, the bioprecursor of sulphoraphane slightly induced phase II detoxifying enzymes, but powerfully induced phase I carcinogen-activating enzymes. It also concomitantly generated ROS [34].

Microsomal epoxide hydrolase 1, a phase I enzyme, plays an important role in both the activation and detoxification of tobacco-derived carcinogens. The low-activity variant genotype of microsomal epoxide hydrolase 1 (polymorphism in exon 3) is associated with a decreased risk of lung cancer. In contrast, the high-activity variant genotype (polymorphism in exon 4) is associated with a modest increase in the risk of lung cancer [35].

The cytochrome P_{450} family of enzymes is responsible for many of the initial metabolic conversions of pro-carcinogenic compounds in tobacco smoke to reactive metabolites. However, other enzyme-based systems, such as myeloperoxidase, may also be involved. Myeloperoxidase is a phase I metabolic enzyme that has a polymorphic region upstream of the gene that appears to reduce transcriptional activity. The polymorphic guanine to adenine shift is associated with a reduction in lung cancer risk in males, younger individuals and current smokers, but not in former smokers and those who have never smoked [36].

In a lung cancer risk assessment study, the effect of different phase I and II enzymes were studied. By analysing the activities of aryl hydrocarbon hydroxylase, ethoxycoumarin *O*-deethylase, epoxide hydrolase, uridine diphosphate glucuronosyltransferase and glutathione-*S*-transferase (GST), a pronounced effect of tobacco smoke on the pulmonary metabolism of xenobiotics and pro-oxidants was found, and the existence of a metabolic phenotype conferring a higher risk of tobacco-associated lung cancer was documented [37].

Polymorphisms of genes coding for some of these toxifying and detoxifying enzymes is of special importance, as shown in the review by NORPPA [23]. The lack of GSTM1

(GSTM1$^{-/-}$) is associated with increased sensitivity to genotoxicity of tobacco smoke, and GSTM1$^{-/-}$ smokers also show an increased frequency of chromosomal aberrations and sister chromatid exchanges. The *N*-acetyltransferase slow acetylation and GSTT1$^{-/-}$ genotypes seem to elevate the baseline level of chromosomal aberrations and sister chromatid exchanges, respectively, possibly because of reduced capacity to detoxify some widespread or endogenous genotoxins. Some evidence exists for an effect of polymorphisms of X-ray repair cross-complementing group 1 (XRCC1) codon 280 and xeroderma pigmentosum group D codon 23 on baseline aberrations, XRCC1 codon 399 on sister chromatid exchange, and methylene tetrahydrofolate reductase codon 677 and methionine synthase reductase on spontaneous micronucleus formation [23].

The effects of tobacco smoke on the DNA repair system has been investigated since the late 1990s; however, the focus has been on lung cancer [38–40]. An effect can also be anticipated for nontumorous lung diseases. Another important mechanism, especially investigated in lung cancer, is gene silencing by methylation. Promoter methylation of several tumour suppressor genes is an early event in tobacco-induced carcinogenesis, which occurs long before dysplastic changes of the epithelium take place, and thus might also influence the development of inflammatory diseases of the lung and remodelling of the architecture [6, 8, 41–44].

Tobacco smoking-induced lung diseases

Habits and changes in the manufacture of cigarettes have changed smoking habits and thereby also the spectrum of lung diseases. Respiratory bronchiolitis was originally described in 1974 [45]. In the 1980s, respiratory bronchiolitis was rarely seen, but an increase in the number of cases has been seen by one of the present authors since 1994. Around the 1970s, filter cigarettes took over, and, in the 1980s, light cigarettes (low tar and low nicotine) were invented. This has changed the composition of tobacco smoke carcinogens as well as their distribution within the airways (see above).

When discussing tobacco-induced lung diseases, the main subject dealt with is cigarette smoking-induced lung diseases, since cigar or pipe smoking usually causes diseases of the oral cavity and the larynx. This type of tobacco smoke is rarely inhaled. Cigarette smoking diseases can be classified into: 1) pulmonary histiocytosis X (HX) or Langerhans' cell (LC) histiocytosis (LCH); 2) respiratory bronchiolitis-combined interstitial lung disease (RB-ILD); 3) combined HX and RB-ILD; 4) desquamative interstitial pneumonia (DIP); and 5) chronic bronchitis with COPD.

HX, currently called LCH, is a granulomatous inflammatory disease caused by a proliferation of LCs and involving the bronchial tree from medium-sized bronchi down to bronchioles and the centroacinar portion of the lung lobules. Infiltration by eosinophils occurs, which is the main cause of bronchiolar destruction (figs 1 and 2). In the early lesion, abundant eosinophilic granulocytes are present in the mucosa, and degranulation of eosinophils can be proven immunohistochemically for basic proteins or simply using Congo red. In later lesions, the granuloma undergoes fibrosis and scarring, and the eosinophils vanish. In these late stages, the lesions acquire a star-like shape, which can also be seen quite characteristically on high-resolution computed tomography (fig. 3).

LCs are part of the antigen-presenting dendritic cell system, and are characterised by their expression of CD1a on the cell surface (fig. 4) and by Birbeck granules, demonstrated electron microscopically (fig. 5) [46]. In addition, LCs are also positive for S100 protein, similar to some alveolar macrophages. LCs can easily be differentiated from macrophages by virtue of their larger ovoid nuclei, finely dispersed chromatin and

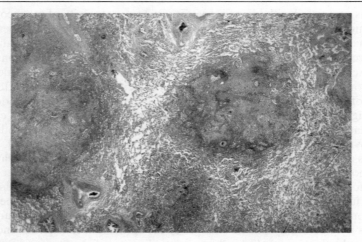

Fig. 1. – Micrograph of histiocytosis X (Langerhans' cell) showing the early bronchocentric granulomatous proliferation of Langerhans' cells and infiltration by eosinophils. The destruction of the bronchioles is clearly visible (haematoxylin and eosin stain).

invisible cell borders. In addition, LCs are negative for CD68, a classic macrophage marker.

The reason for this proliferation of LCs is not entirely clear; however, an excess of inhaled plant antigens, derived from incomplete combustion of tobacco plant proteins, is one of the underlying causes [47]. The disease usually affects young individuals, male as well as female, who can all be characterised as excessive cigarette smokers. Since many more individuals smoke excessively than become diseased, other underlying factors are likely.

Many cytokines have been proven to occur in HX, released from alveolar macrophages and LCs, and predominantly inducing a T-helper cell type 2 reaction, with increased levels of interleukin (IL)-4 and IL-5 [48]. They might be responsible for the eosinophilic infiltration. Eosinophils themselves contain a vast amount of basic proteins, such as major basic protein, which are cytotoxic to the respiratory epithelium.

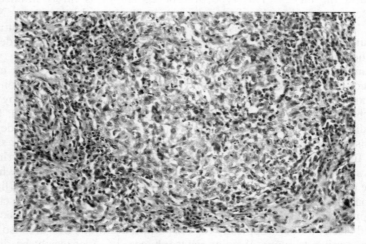

Fig. 2. – High-power view of histiocytosis X showing the Langerhans' cell proliferation and infiltrating eosinophils. Only remnants of the bronchiolar wall remain (haematoxylin and eosin stain).

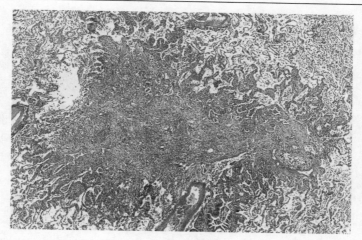

Fig. 3. – Late histiocytosis X. Most of the Langerhans' cell proliferation has been replaced by fibrosis and scarring. The bronchioles are all occluded. The eosinophilic infiltration is gone and scattered lymphocytes prevail (haematoxylin and eosin stain).

Besides pulmonary LCH, a tumour-like classic LCH can be found, involving different organs, such as the skin, bone and lung. This type of LCH usually occurs in a pre-adolescent population and is not related to smoking, whereas pulmonary LCH is associated with smoking. In addition, dendritic cell tumours and sarcomas exist at the malignant end of the spectrum [49]. Whereas the differential diagnosis towards dendritic cell tumours and sarcomas can easily be made, the morphological differentiation of diffuse *versus* tumour-like and tumorous LC proliferations is still not solved. Multi-organ involvement, the absence of cigarette smoke exposure and pre-adolescent age are the most reliable indicators.

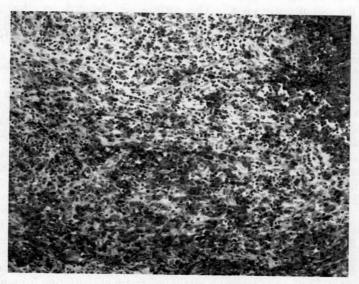

Fig. 4. – CD1a immunohistochemical staining showing the vast numbers of proliferating Langerhans' cells (CD1a antibody; alkaline phosphatase–antialkaline phosphatase development).

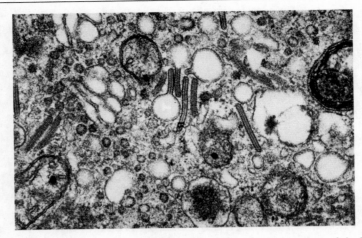

Fig. 5. – Electron micrograph of histiocytosis X showing the tennis racket-like structure of the Birbeck granules, typically found in the Langerhans' cells.

RB-ILD

Similar to HX, RB-ILD is caused by excessive inhalation of cigarette smoke. In contrast to HX, there is usually no reaction and/or proliferation of antigen-presenting cells, but rather a massive accumulation of alveolar macrophages. Similar to HX, the aetiology and pathogenesis of RB-ILD are incompletely understood. It is thought that the disease is caused by excessive inhalation of cigarette smoke, causing an accumulation of waste products, with which the alveolar macrophages cannot cope. This induces an influx of monocytic cells, which differentiate into macrophages. These cells accumulate within the terminal respiratory bronchioles, alveolar ducts and adjacent centroacinar portion of the lobules (figs 6–8). The airflow is reduced by this macrophage accumulation, functionally similarly to bronchiolar obstruction, and reduced airflow in the alveolar region causes decreased gas exchange. Therefore, clinically the disease shows combined obstructive and restrictive ventilatory disturbances.

In later stages, destruction of lung parenchyma occurs and emphysema can result. Most probably, macrophages that have phagocytosed the waste products of cigarette smoke cause their own death by rupture of phagolysosomes, and thus release their toxic enzymes into the surrounding lung [50]. A similar phenomenon was described in the 1950s and 1960s in experimental inhalation experiments. Titanium oxide (TiO_2) was used as a control dust in animal inhalation studies, since it is inert and does not cause disease. However, if the amount of inhaled TiO_2 dust was increased excessively above the threshold that can be removed by the mucus escalator system and the phagocytic capacity of the macrophages, an accumulation of dust-laden macrophages occurred, macrophages died *via* release of their enzymes and a secondary histiocytic and macrophage reaction starts, sometimes evolving into a granulomatous reaction/inflammation [51]. This reaction was called overload phenomenon, and histologically resembled RB-ILD.

However, it should be remembered that RB-ILD is still not a common disease; it is less prevalent in contrast to the millions of heavy smokers in Europe. However, RB-ILD is underestimated clinically; in adjacent lung tissue in patients suffering from lung cancer, it is quite a common finding. Therefore, the aetiology is still not well understood.

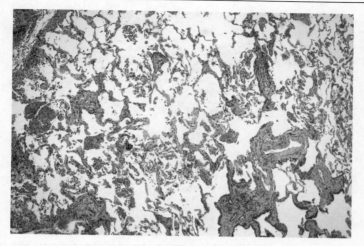

Fig. 6. – Respiratory bronchiolitis. Micrograph showing, to the middle and left-hand side, typical accumulation of alveolar macrophages in the alveoli and a respiratory bronchiole. Most of the lung parenchyma looks normal (haematoxylin and eosin stain).

Combined RB-ILD and HX

A combination of HX and RB-ILD in various parts of the lung is seen with increasing frequency. On diagnostic video-assisted thoracoscopic surgery biopsy, HX granulomas can be seen in one subsegment, but accumulations of macrophages in respiratory bronchioles and centrilobular areas in another (fig. 9). This is not surprising, since patients are usually heavy smokers.

DIP

DIP (figs. 10 and 11) is characterised by an accumulation of alveolar macrophages within the alveolar periphery. Respiratory bronchioles are not involved (figs. 10 and 11).

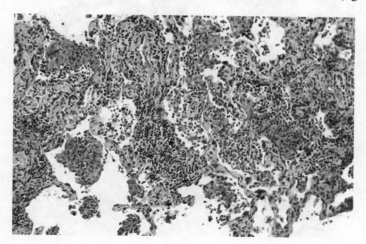

Fig. 7. – Alveolar macrophages nearly completely obstructing three respiratory bronchioles. There is a mild extension of the infiltration into the adjacent parenchyma (haematoxylin and eosin stain).

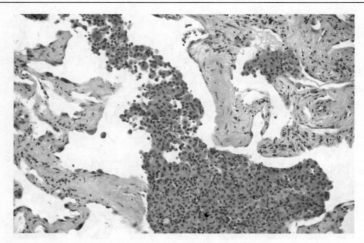

Fig. 8. – High-power view of the obstruction of a respiratory bronchiole by pigmented alveolar macrophages. The dirty greenish brown pigment is quite typical of smokers (haematoxylin and eosin stain).

DIP can mimic a peripheral carcinoma radiologically, since the cellular accumulation is similarly dense, and the cells completely fill the alveoli. Again the aetiology is cigarette smoking in most cases [52–54]. However, it should be noted that cases have been reported that point to inhalation of toxic substances, such as aluminium welding fumes or nylon flock dust [55–59].

DIP, in contrast to RB-ILD, is rare. Indeed, there is no real transition between the two diseases. It is not imaginable where and why accumulations of macrophages should vanish and only concentrate in the alveolar periphery, or how macrophage accumulation

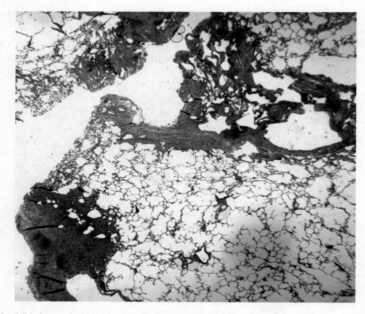

Fig. 9. – Combined histiocytosis X and respiratory bronchiolitis. The proliferation of Langerhans' cells can be seen in one area, and accumulation of alveolar macrophages in other areas (haematoxylin and eosin stain).

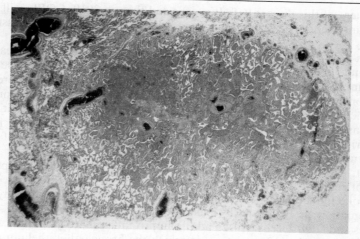

Fig. 10. – Desquamative interstitial pneumonia. The lung parenchyma is completely filled with alveolar macrophages. The patient underwent biopsy because the lesion was diagnosed as cancer. The spaces are a retraction artefact caused by fixation (haematoxylin and eosin stain).

should extend to respiratory bronchioles. In reality, a transition between the two diseases has never been reported. In contrast to RB-ILD, DIP usually induces a restrictive pattern in functional tests.

COPD

COPD is the most frequently occurring smoking-associated disease, with high morbidity and mortality. The development of COPD is >90% directly associated with cigarette smoking, and up to 5–20% of all smokers develop a clinically relevant manifestation of COPD. The fact that a subset of smokers develop COPD without a clear dose–response relationship indicates that there is a genetic susceptibility background to

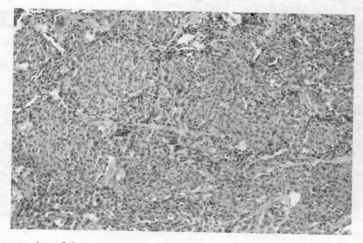

Fig. 11. – High-power view of desquamative interstitial pneumonia showing the dense accumulation of alveolar macrophages within the alveoli. Here, the alveolar lumina are poorly defined (haematoxylin and eosin stain).

the development of this disease [60]. It is expected that, in 2010, COPD will be the third most important cause of death worldwide, and is, therefore, an important issue in human health.

COPD is a heterogeneous manifestation of smoking-induced pathological changes in the airway and parenchyma. The prototypic manifestations of the disease are chronic bronchitis, emphysema and small airways disease, although some authors previously also included bronchiectases [61–63]. Clinically, the most-used distinction for patients is chronic bronchitis and emphysema (fig. 12) [61, 62]. Most patients exhibit overlapping manifestations of airway pathology, as well as parenchymal destruction, in which the relative contribution of both determines the outcome and clinical severity of the resulting airway obstruction.

At present, COPD is generally considered an inflammatory disease. Apart from the toxic effect of cigarette smoke, already described in the first part of the present chapter, cigarette smoke induces specific inflammation in the airways and parenchyma [64, 65]. This inflammation is particularly characterised by the presence of neutrophils, macrophages and CD8 T-cells [66]. In addition, pro-inflammatory changes are observed, involved in inducing the inflammation, in which the bronchial epithelium plays a main role. A surprising and seemingly paradoxical effect of cigarette smoke exposure in COPD is that, on the one hand, airway wall thickening is observed with inflammation and fibrosis, whereas, on the other, in the parenchyma, the inflammation leads to destruction of matrix (*i.e.* the opposite of the fibrotic changes in the bronchial wall) [67, 68]. This indicates that the orchestration and activation of the inflammatory infiltrate in different localisations in the lung, although both induced by cigarette smoke, show differential

a) b)

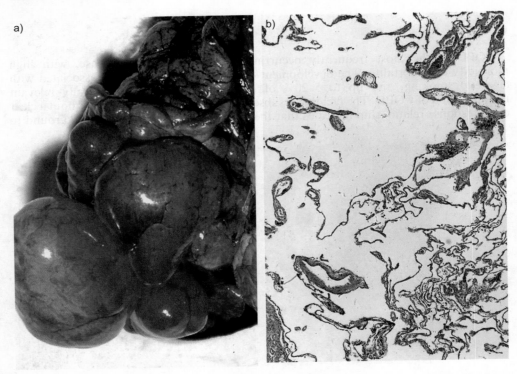

Fig. 12. – a) Bullous emphysema of the lower part of the right lower lobe. b) Micrograph of severe emphysema, showing free-lying segments of alveolar wall and small parenchymal vessels (haematoxylin and eosin stain).

aspects. It seems likely that the bronchial epithelium, and perhaps also the smooth muscle, plays a modulating role with respect to the ultimate effects. The changes in the small airways are rather similar to those found in the larger airways, but quite important differences are found in the effects of inflammation of the parenchyma and peribronchial area [69]. Whereas, in the larger airways, inflammation mainly contributes to an increase in the thickness of the inner airway wall and, thus, to airway narrowing, for the small airways (fig. 13), this is also observed but another factor additionally and importantly contributes to airway narrowing. The inflammation in the parenchyma and peribronchial adventitia leads to loosening of the peribronchial alveolar attachments and, together with direct effects of cigarette smoke, ultimately to emphysematous destruction of these attachments. These effects on alveolar attachments result in gradually increasing loss of elastic recoil, and so are an important factor in small airway narrowing and even collapse.

The inflammatory process is the result of a nonspecific immune response, most probably as a reaction to the irritating effects of cigarette smoke/cigarette smoke particles. As indicated earlier, this leads to epithelial changes that facilitate airway colonisation with microorganisms in patients with COPD [70]. This colonisation is probably a partial explanation for the local inflammation [71, 72]. Whereas, in all smoking patients, increased inflammation is observed, abnormal regulation of this inflammation apparently occurs in patients with COPD. In COPD, there is an increase in the levels of pro-inflammatory mediators of epithelial origin, such as monocyte chemoattractant protein-1, IL-8 and CC chemokine receptor 2 [73], with a decrease in levels of anti-inflammatory mediators, such as secretory component and Clara cell 16-kDa protein [74]. The increase in partially activated T-lymphocyte numbers can be explained by increased expression of CXC chemokine receptor 3 on these T-cells, whereas levels of the ligand interferon-γ-inducible protein 10 are increased in bronchiolar epithelium [75]. The increase in neutrophil granulocyte numbers, especially in small airways, is particularly observed in bronchial glands. It is supposed that these neutrophils may produce factors that contribute to the proliferation and increased mucus production of these glands [76]. In exacerbations of COPD, an increase in eosinophil numbers is

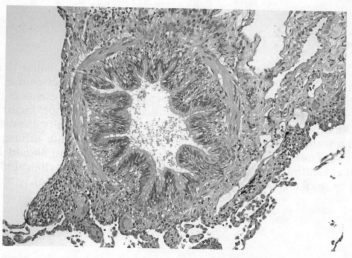

Fig. 13. – Micrograph showing small airway in chronic obstructive pulmonary disease, with a thickened airway wall, caused by inflammation in both the subepithelial area and adventitia, an increase in smooth muscle mass and submucosal and adventitial fibrosis. Only few peribronchial alveolar attachments remain (haematoxylin and eosin stain).

sometimes observed [77, 78]. At present, it is unclear whether this is really eosinophilic inflammation or whether it may be a nonspecific manifestation of an increase in inflammation in general.

In contrast to chronic bronchitis, which is defined by clinical parameters, the definition of emphysema is based on pathological grounds [79, 80]. This definition is that emphysema concerns changes in the lung characterised by an abnormal permanent enlargement of air spaces distal to the terminal bronchioles and accompanied by destruction of alveolar septa without very pronounced fibrosis. Cigarette smoking is particularly associated with the so-called centroacinar form of emphysema. In general, subdivision into the different types of emphysema can only be carried out accurately on *post mortem* specimens fixed under standard pressure, but it is then easy to diagnose. However, this is quite difficult in pathological resection specimens without specific preparation, as is generally often the case in pathology practice.

In the pathogenesis of emphysema, the main hallmark is the destruction of lung parenchyma. Oxidants from cigarette smoke, together with oxidants and proteases from inflammatory cells induced by cigarette smoke, are considered to exert the main destructive effect on lung tissue, with insufficient compensation by antioxidants or antiproteases [61, 81]. More recently, it has been put forward that, in addition to tissue destruction, insufficient tissue repair also occurs in COPD patients [68, 82]. This is more extensively described in another chapter of the present Monograph [83]. The parenchymal inflammation and emphysematous changes contribute to the manifestation of COPD, not only *via* a reduction in diffusion capacity, but also by causing bronchial obstruction. The peribronchial attachments to the small airways are loosened by the local inflammatory process, with increasing uncoupling of parenchymal retraction forces from the small airways. In a later phase, this uncoupling even increases *via* destruction of peribronchial attachments in the case of progressive emphysema [65]. This increasing uncoupling of the lung parenchyma from the airways, in due course, contributes to the progression of lung function loss, with progressive airflow limitation due to increased airway wall thickness, increased production of mucus and loss of peribronchial retracting forces [65, 68].

Conclusion

When encountering an individual patient, it is important to realise that the smoke-induced disease processes, described in the present chapter, are, of course, not mutually exclusive. This means that an individual patient quite often presents clinically with a combination of different reaction patterns caused by the common factor of long-term cigarette smoke exposure. This also affects lung function test results; the disturbances are usually not uniform making clinical differential diagnosis quite difficult. Indeed, all combinations of smoking-related lung diseases described herein should be taken into account when evaluating any individual patient presenting with a clinical picture thought to be related to smoke exposure as an important aetiological factor.

Summary

Smoking is a habit, better called an addiction, which has profound effects upon human health and affects many organ systems. Even without obvious disease, many deleterious effects of (cigarette) smoke exposure are present. Furthermore, whereas the increased risk of (lung) cancer is best known, many other smoke-induced diseases are now known, with some occurring frequently, such as chronic obstructive pulmonary disease, and others with a lower frequency. The present chapter gives an overview of the effects different smoke components have on the cells and compartments of the normal lung, and in what way these factors contribute to increased health risks. It also provides a concise overview of nonmalignant smoking-related diseases in the human lung.

Keywords: Lung, smoking, tobacco-induced lung disease.

References

1. Cooke JP, Bitterman H. Nicotine and angiogenesis: a new paradigm for tobacco-related diseases. *Ann Med* 2004; 36: 33–40.
2. Zhu BQ, Heeschen C, Sievers RE, *et al.* Second hand smoke stimulates tumour angiogenisis and growth. *Cancer Cell* 2003; 4: 191–196.
3. Schick S, Glantz S. Philip Morris toxicological experiments with fresh sidestream smoke: more toxic than mainstream smoke. *Tob Control* 2005; 14: 396–404.
4. Husgafvel-Pursiainen K. Genotoxicity of environmental tobacco smoke: a review. *Mutat Res* 2004; 567: 427–445.
5. Dopp E, Saedler J, Stopper H, Weiss DG, Schiffmann D. Mitotic disturbances and micronucleus induction in Syrian hamster embryo fibroblast cells caused by asbestos fibers. *Environ Health Perspect* 1995; 103: 268–271.
6. Harden SV, Tokumaru Y, Westra WH, *et al.* Gene promoter hypermethylation in tumours and lymph nodes of stage I lung cancer patients. *Clin Cancer Res* 2003; 9: 1370–1375.
7. Lu C, Soria JC, Tang X, *et al.* Prognostic factors in resected stage I non-small-cell lung cancer: a multivariate analysis of six molecular markers. *J Clin Oncol* 2004; 22: 4575–4583.
8. Toyooka S, Maruyama R, Toyooka KO, *et al.* Smoke exposure, histologic type and geography-related differences in the methylation profiles of non-small cell lung cancer. *Int J Cancer* 2003; 103: 153–160.
9. Harke HP, Schuller D, Klimisch JH, Meissner K. Untersuchungen der polyzyklischen aromatischen Kohlenwasserstoffe im Zigarettenrauch. [Investigations of polycyclic aromatic hydrocarbons in cigarette smoke.] *Z Lebensm Unters Forsch* 1976; 162: 291–297.
10. Andrew AS, Warren AJ, Barchowsky A, *et al.* Genomic and proteomic profiling of responses to toxic metals in human lung cells. *Environ Health Perspect* 2003; 111: 825–835.
11. Bachelet M, Pinot F, Polla RI, *et al.* Toxicity of cadmium in tobacco smoke: protection by antioxidants and chelating resins. *Free Radic Res* 2002; 36: 99–106.
12. Waalkes MP. Cadmium carcinogenesis. *Mutat Res* 2003; 533: 107–120.
13. Zaridze DG, Safaev RD, Belitsky GA, Brunnemann KD, Hoffmann D. Carcinogenic substances in Soviet tobacco products. *IARC Sci Publ* 1991; 105: 485–488.
14. Stabbert R, Voncken P, Rustemeier K, *et al.* Toxicological evaluation of an electrically heated cigarette. Part 2: chemical composition of mainstream smoke. *J Appl Toxicol* 2003; 23: 329–339.

15.   International Agency for Research on Cancer. IARC Publications Programme. http://www.iarc.fr/IARCPress/index.php.

16.   Jin Z, Gao F, Flagg T, Deng X. Tobacco-specific nitrosamine NNK promotes functional cooperation of Bcl2 and c-Myc through phosphorylation in regulating cell survival and proliferation. *J Biol Chem* 2004; 279: 40209–40219.

17.   Tsurutani J, Castillo SS, Brognard J, *et al.* Tobacco components stimulate Akt-dependent proliferation and NFκB-dependent survival in lung cancer cells. *Carcinogenesis* 2005; 26: 1182–1195.

18.   Wynder EL, Muscat JE. The changing epidemiology of smoking and lung cancer histology. *Environ Health Perspect* 1995; 103: Suppl. 8, 143–148.

19.   Witschi H. Carcinogenic activity of cigarette smoke gas phase and its modulation by β-carotene and *N*-acetylcysteine. *Toxicol Sci* 2005; 84: 81–87.

20.   White JL, Conner BT, Perfetti TA, *et al.* Effect of pyrolysis temperature on the mutagenicity of tobacco smoke condensate. *Food Chem Toxicol* 2001; 39: 499–505.

21.   Torikai K, Yoshida S, Takahashi H. Effects of temperature, atmosphere and pH on the generation of smoke compounds during tobacco pyrolysis. *Food Chem Toxicol* 2004; 42: 1409–1417.

22.   Knaapen AM, Borm PJ, Albrecht C, Schins RP. Inhaled particles and lung cancer. Part A: mechanisms. *Int J Cancer* 2004; 109: 799–809.

23.   Norppa H. Cytogenetic biomarkers and genetic polymorphisms. *Toxicol Lett* 2004; 149: 309–334.

24.   Wang GF, Lai MD, Yang RR, *et al.* Histological types and significance of bronchial epithelial dysplasia. *Mod Pathol* 2006; 19: 429–437.

25.   Ullmann R, Bongiovanni M, Halbwedl I, *et al.* Bronchiolar columnar cell dysplasia – genetic analysis of a novel preneoplastic lesion of peripheral lung. *Virchows Arch* 2003; 442: 429–436.

26.   Mori M, Rao SK, Popper HH, Cagle PT, Fraire AE. Atypical adenomatous hyperplasia of the lung: a probable forerunner in the development of adenocarcinoma of the lung. *Mod Pathol* 2001; 14: 72–84.

27.   Pilmane M, Luts A, Sundler F. Changes in neuroendocrine elements in bronchial mucosa in chronic lung disease in adults. *Thorax* 1995; 50: 551–554.

28.   Shenberger JS, Shew RL, Johnson DE. Hyperoxia-induced airway remodeling and pulmonary neuroendocrine cell hyperplasia in the weanling rat. *Pediatr Res* 1997; 42: 539–544.

29.   Stevens TP, McBride JT, Peake JL, Pinkerton KE, Stripp BR. Cell proliferation contributes to PNEC hyperplasia after acute airway injury. *Am J Physiol* 1997; 272: L486–L493.

30.   Boers JE, den Brok JL, Koudstaal J, Arends JW, Thunnissen FB. Number and proliferation of neuroendocrine cells in normal human airway epithelium. *Am J Respir Crit Care Med* 1996; 154: 758–763.

31.   Brown MJ, English J, Muller NL. Bronchiolitis obliterans due to neuroendocrine hyperplasia: high-resolution CT–pathologic correlation. *AJR Am J Roentgenol* 1997; 168: 1561–1562.

32.   Miller RR, Muller NL. Neuroendocrine cell hyperplasia and obliterative bronchiolitis in patients with peripheral carcinoid tumours. *Am J Surg Pathol* 1995; 19: 653–658.

33.   Wang H, Tan W, Hao B, *et al.* Substantial reduction in risk of lung adenocarcinoma associated with genetic polymorphism in CYP2A13, the most active cytochrome P450 for the metabolic activation of tobacco-specific carcinogen NNK. *Cancer Res* 2003; 63: 8057–8061.

34.   Paolini M, Perocco P, Canistro D, *et al.* Induction of cytochrome P450, generation of oxidative stress and *in vitro* cell-transforming and DNA-damaging activities by glucoraphanin, the bioprecursor of the chemopreventive agent sulforaphane found in broccoli. *Carcinogenesis* 2004; 25: 61–67.

35.   Kiyohara C, Yoshimasu K, Takayama K, Nakanishi Y. EPHX1 polymorphisms and the risk of lung cancer: a HuGE review. *Epidemiology* 2006; 17: 89–99.

36.   Schabath MB, Spitz MR, Zhang X, Delclos GL, Wu X. Genetic variants of myeloperoxidase and lung cancer risk. *Carcinogenesis* 2000; 21: 1163–1166.

37.   Bartsch H, Petruzzelli S, De Flora S, *et al.* Carcinogen metabolism in human lung tissues and the effect of tobacco smoking: results from a case–control multicenter study on lung cancer patients. *Environ Health Perspect* 1992; 98: 119–124.

38. Hu Z, Ma H, Lu D, *et al.* A promoter polymorphism (-77T>C) of DNA repair gene XRCC1 is associated with risk of lung cancer in relation to tobacco smoking. *Pharmacogenet Genomics* 2005; 15: 457–463.

39. Matullo G, Dunning AM, Guarrera S, *et al.* DNA repair polymorphisms and cancer risk in non-smokers in a cohort study. *Carcinogenesis* 2006; 27: 997–1007.

40. Zienolddiny S, Campa D, Lind H, *et al.* Polymorphisms of DNA repair genes and risk of non-small cell lung cancer. *Carcinogenesis* 2006; 27: 560–567.

41. Forgacs E, Zochbauer-Muller S, Olah E, Minna JD. Molecular genetic abnormalities in the pathogenesis of human lung cancer. *Pathol Oncol Res* 2001; 7: 6–13.

42. He B, You L, Uematsu K, *et al.* SOCS-3 is frequently silenced by hypermethylation and suppresses cell growth in human lung cancer. *Proc Natl Acad Sci USA* 2003; 100: 14133–14138.

43. Lamy A, Sesboue R, Bourguignon J, *et al.* Aberrant methylation of the *CDKN2a/p16INK4a* gene promoter region in preinvasive bronchial lesions: a prospective study in high-risk patients without invasive cancer. *Int J Cancer* 2002; 100: 189–193.

44. Li QL, Kim HR, Kim WJ, *et al.* Transcriptional silencing of the *RUNX3* gene by CpG hypermethylation is associated with lung cancer. *Biochem Biophys Res Commun* 2004; 314: 223–228.

45. Niewöhner DKJ, Rice D. Pathologic changes in peripheral airways of young cigarette smokers. *N Engl J Med* 1974; 291: 755–758.

46. Nezelof C, Basset F. Langerhans cell histiocytosis research. Past, present, and future. *Hematol Oncol Clin North Am* 1998; 12: 385–406.

47. Youkeles LH, Grizzanti JN, Liao Z, Chang CJ, Rosenstreich DL. Decreased tobacco-glycoprotein-induced lymphocyte proliferation *in vitro* in pulmonary eosinophilic granuloma. *Am J Respir Crit Care Med* 1995; 151: 145–150.

48. Egeler RM, Favara BE, van Meurs M, Laman JD, Claassen E. Differential *in situ* cytokine profiles of Langerhans-like cells and T cells in Langerhans cell histiocytosis: abundant expression of cytokines relevant to disease and treatment. *Blood* 1999; 94: 4195–4201.

49. Pileri SA, Grogan TM, Harris NL, *et al.* Tumours of histiocytes and accessory dendritic cells: an immunohistochemical approach to classification from the International Lymphoma Study Group based on 61 cases. *Histopathology* 2002; 41: 1–29.

50. Stachura I, Singh G, Whiteside TL. Mechanisms of tissue injury in desquamative interstitial pneumonitis. *Am J Med* 1980; 68: 733–740.

51. Oberdorster G. Toxicokinetics and effects of fibrous and nonfibrous particles. *Inhal Toxicol* 2002; 14: 29–56.

52. Carrington CB, Gaensler EA, Coutu RE, FitzGerald MX, Gupta RG. Natural history and treated course of usual and desquamative interstitial pneumonia. *N Engl J Med* 1978; 298: 801–809.

53. Liebow AA, Steer A, Billingsley JG. Desquamative interstitial pneumonia. *Am J Med* 1965; 39: 369–404.

54. Ryu JH, Colby TV, Hartman TE, Vassallo R. Smoking-related interstitial lung diseases: a concise review. *Eur Respir J* 2001; 17: 122–132.

55. Abraham JL, Hertzberg MA. Inorganic particulates associated with desquamative interstitial pneumonia. *Chest* 1981; 80: Suppl. 1, 67–70.

56. Freed JA, Miller A, Gordon RE, Fischbein A, Kleinerman J, Langer AM. Desquamative interstitial pneumonia associated with chrysotile asbestos fibres. *Br J Ind Med* 1991; 48: 332–337.

57. Hammar SP, Hallman KO. Localized inflammatory pulmonary disease in subjects occupationally exposed to asbestos. *Chest* 1993; 103: 1792–1799.

58. Herbert A, Sterling G, Abraham J, Corrin B. Desquamative interstitial pneumonia in an aluminum welder. *Hum Pathol* 1982; 13: 694–699.

59. Kern DG, Kuhn C, Ely EW, *et al.* Flock worker's lung: broadening the spectrum of clinicopathology, narrowing the spectrum of suspected etiologies. *Chest* 2000; 117: 251–259.

60. Lomas DA, Silverman EK. The genetics of chronic obstructive pulmonary disease. *Respir Res* 2001; 2: 20–26.

61. Barnes PJ, Shapiro SD, Pauwels RA. Chronic obstructive pulmonary disease: molecular and cellular mechanisms. *Eur Respir J* 2003; 22: 672–688.

62. Calverley PM, Walker P. Chronic obstructive pulmonary disease. *Lancet* 2003; 362: 1053–1061.

63. Thurlbeck WM, Wright JL. Thurlbeck's Chronic Airflow Obstruction. 2nd Edn. Hamilton, ON, B.C. Decker, Inc., 1999.

64. Saetta M, Timens W, Jeffery PK. Pathology. *In:* Postma DS, Siafakas NM, eds. Management of Chronic Obstructive Pulmonary Disease. *Eur Respir Mon* 1998; 7: 92–101.

65. Saetta M, Turato G, Maestrelli P, Mapp CE, Fabbri LM. Cellular and structural bases of chronic obstructive pulmonary disease. *Am J Respir Crit Care Med* 2001; 163: 1304–1309.

66. Saetta M, Di Stefano A, Turato G, *et al.* CD8+ T-lymphocytes in peripheral airways of smokers with chronic obstructive pulmonary disease. *Am J Respir Crit Care Med* 1998; 157: 822–826.

67. Postma DS, Timens W. Remodeling in asthma and chronic obstructive pulmonary disease. *Proc Am Thorac Soc* 2006; 3: 434–439.

68. Van der Geld YM, Van Straaten JFM, Postma DS, Timens W. Role of proteoglycans in development and pathogenesis of emphysema. *In:* Garg HG, Roughley PJ, Hales CA, eds. Proteoglycans in Lung Disease. New York, NY, Marcel Dekker, Inc., 2002; pp. 241–267.

69. Saetta M, Turato G, Baraldo S, *et al.* Goblet cell hyperplasia and epithelial inflammation in peripheral airways of smokers with both symptoms of chronic bronchitis and chronic airflow limitation. *Am J Respir Crit Care Med* 2000; 161: 1016–1021.

70. Sethi S. Bacterial infection and the pathogenesis of COPD. *Chest* 2000; 117: Suppl. 1, 286S–291S.

71. Sethi S, Muscarella K, Evans N, Klingman KL, Grant BJ, Murphy TF. Airway inflammation and etiology of acute exacerbations of chronic bronchitis. *Chest* 2000; 118: 1557–1565.

72. Shapiro SD. End-stage chronic obstructive pulmonary disease: the cigarette is burned out but inflammation rages on. *Am J Respir Crit Care Med* 2001; 164: 339–340.

73. De Boer WI, Sont JK, van Schadewijk A, Stolk J, Van Krieken JH, Hiemstra PS. Monocyte chemoattractant protein 1, interleukin 8, and chronic airways inflammation in COPD. *J Pathol* 2000; 190: 619–626.

74. Pilette C, Godding V, Kiss R, *et al.* Reduced epithelial expression of secretory component in small airways correlates with airflow obstruction in chronic obstructive pulmonary disease. *Am J Respir Crit Care Med* 2001; 163: 185–194.

75. Saetta M, Mariani M, Panina-Bordignon P, *et al.* Increased expression of the chemokine receptor CXCR3 and its ligand CXCL10 in peripheral airways of smokers with chronic obstructive pulmonary disease. *Am J Respir Crit Care Med* 2002; 165: 1404–1409.

76. Saetta M, Turato G, Facchini FM, *et al.* Inflammatory cells in the bronchial glands of smokers with chronic bronchitis. *Am J Respir Crit Care Med* 1997; 156: 1633–1639.

77. Zhu J, Qiu YS, Majumdar S, *et al.* Exacerbations of bronchitis: bronchial eosinophilia and gene expression for interleukin-4, interleukin-5, and eosinophil chemoattractants. *Am J Respir Crit Care Med* 2001; 164: 109–116.

78. Saetta M, Di Stefano A, Maestrelli P, *et al.* Airway eosinophilia in chronic bronchitis during exacerbations. *Am J Respir Crit Care Med* 1994; 150: 1646–1652.

79. American Thoracic Society. Standards for the diagnosis and care of patients with chronic obstructive pulmonary disease (COPD) and asthma. *Am Rev Respir Dis* 1987; 136: 225–244.

80. Siafakas NM, Vermeire P, Pride NB, *et al.* Optimal assessment and management of chronic obstructive pulmonary disease (COPD). The European Respiratory Society Task Force. *Eur Respir J* 1995; 8: 1398–1420.

81. Barnes PJ. Chronic obstructive pulmonary disease. *N Engl J Med* 2000; 343: 269–280.

82. Timens W, Coers W, Van Straaten JFM, Postma DS. Extracellular matrix and inflammation: a role for fibroblast-mediated tissue repair in the pathogenesis of emphysema? *Eur Respir Rev* 1997; 43: 119–123.

83. Wright JL, Kerstjens HAM, Timens W. What is new in chronic obstructive pulmonary disease? *In:* Timens W, Popper HH, eds. Pathology of the Lung. *Eur Respir Mon* 2007; 39: 153–169.

CHAPTER 7

What is new in chronic obstructive pulmonary disease?

J.L. Wright*, H.A.M. Kerstjens#, W. Timens¶

*Dept of Pathology, University of British Columbia, Vancouver, BC, Canada. Depts of #Respiratory Medicine and ¶Pathology, University Medical Centre, University of Groningen, Groningen, the Netherlands.

Correspondence: J.L. Wright, Room GF 164, Dept of Pathology, University Hospital, 2211 Wesbrook Mall, Vancouver BC V6T 2B5, Canada. Fax: 1 6048227104; E-mail: jlwright@interchange.ubc.ca

Until recently, the B-cell has received very little attention in the pathogenesis of chronic obstructive pulmonary disease (COPD). In 1992, BOSKEN et al. [1] analysed the inflammatory pattern of cells in the small airways of patients undergoing resection because of a peripheral tumour. They showed that patients with COPD had more B-lymphocytes in the airway wall than control subjects. Based on their localisation, the B-cells follicles were designated bronchus-associated lymphoid tissue [1]. A more extensive and landmark analysis of inflammation of the small airways was performed by HOGG et al. [2]. The small airways were assessed in surgically resected lung tissue from 159 patients showing a wide range of severity, ranging from stage 0 (at risk) to stage 4 (very severe), according to the classification of the Global Initiative for Chronic Obstructive Lung Disease (GOLD) [3]. The progression of COPD was strongly associated with an increase in the volume of tissue in the wall and the accumulation of inflammatory mucous exudates in the lumen of the small airways. In the more severe stages of disease, a higher percentage of the airways contained neutrophils, macrophages, and CD4 and CD8 cells. Interestingly, there were also a progressive number of airways that contained B-cells. Additionally, similarly to the study of BOSKEN et al. [1], there were again airways that demonstrated lymphoid follicles. The authors suggested that these follicles represent an adaptive immune response that may develop in relation to microbial colonisation and infection occurring in the later stages of COPD [3].

The data regarding involvement of B-cells in small airways in COPD has recently been extended by the observation that numbers of these cells are also increased in biopsy specimens from the bronchi of patients with increasing severity by GOLD classification [4]. Additionally, it has also recently been shown that the B-cell follicles that were mainly found localised in the small airways in the studies of BOSHEN et al. [2] and HOGG et al. [1], are also present in the parenchyma (fig. 1) [5]. These parenchymal follicular B-cells in human COPD patients were shown to be of oligoclonal origin. Interestingly, the same authors found similar B-cell follicles in their smoking mouse model in parallel with the development of airspace enlargement [5].

Thus the presence of B-cell follicles has now been demonstrated in human and murine lung tissue in association with emphysema, and in both the airway wall and lung parenchyma. The important question that arises from these findings is the potential role of these B-cells in the development of emphysema. The observed ongoing mutations in clonally related B-cells within the lymphoid follicles suggest an antigen-driven selection process. At present, it is unclear against which antigen(s) this B-cell proliferation is directed. In addition to the microbial nature suggested by HOGG et al. [2], there are at

Eur Respir Mon, 2007, 39, 153–169. Printed in UK - all rights reserved. Copyright ERS Journals Ltd 2007; European Respiratory Monograph; ISSN 1025-448x.

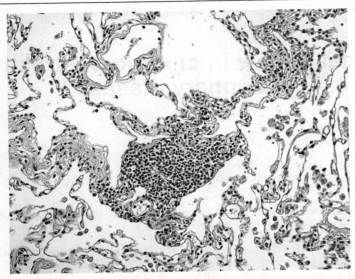

Fig. 1. – Small lymphoid follicle in parenchyma of lung of a chronic obstructive pulmonary disease patient (haematoxylin and eosin stain).

least two alternative potential sources of antigens that should be considered, cigarette smoke components or derivatives and degradation products of extracellular matrix (ECM). However, in the smoking mouse model mentioned above [5], the littermate control mice were exposed to the same housing and (sham) handling, but did not develop these follicles. Additionally, no evidence was found of Mycoplasma, Chlamydia, adenovirus or *Pneumocystis jiroveci*, nor of specific bacterial pathogens. The second source of antigens that could theoretically cause specific B-cell proliferation is cigarette smoke. Cigarette smoke contains ~4,500 different compounds [6], some of which are potentially immunogenic [7]. Some of these compounds precipitate in the lung, possibly bind to the ECM and may elicit an antibody response. Alternatively, reactive components from smoke can react with proteins in the tissue to form new immunogenic adducts [8]. Subsequently, immune complex formation may occur, eliciting an inflammatory response and subsequently tissue degradation. Whether this mechanism indeed occurs, remains to be shown.

Finally, the ECM itself may be a source of antigens. Previous studies have demonstrated that breakdown products of several ECM proteins, such as hyaluronic acid, elastin and collagen, exert chemotactic and activating effects on neutrophils and macrophages, resulting in the release of oxidants and proteases that are detrimental to the ECM [9, 10]. Additionally, hyaluronic acid causes activation and proliferation of B-cells [11]. Apart from this general chemotactic and activating role, it can be hypothesised that cigarette smoke-induced breakdown products of the ECM might be immunogenic and trigger the specific B-cell reaction in a T-cell-dependent or -independent fashion. The induced anti-ECM antibodies may subsequently bind to ECM fragments or intact ECM, causing further degradation of ECM by phagocytes. ECM products contain proteins, and also polysaccharides. The response to poly-saccharides is often T-cell-independent in mice, in particular related to the B1 B-cell, which is an immunoglobulin (Ig) M-positive and IgD-negative CD5 B-cell subset, whereas, in humans, it involves the (spleen-based) marginal zone B-cell, which is IgM-positive and IgD-negative, strongly CD21-positive and CD5-negative.

The present authors have found preliminary evidence that the lung B-cells in the B-cell follicles were CD5-negative and weakly CD21-positive in humans, and also CD5-negative in mice (unpublished results). The absence of IgD may thus indicate an activated state of lung B-cells, but does not indicate a specific origin or nature. Moreover, the fact that it was already known that, in COPD, CD8 and CD4 T-cells are prominent permits the suggestion that CD4 cells, in particular, may not only result from nonspecific activation or provide specific help to cytotoxic CD8 cells but also provide help for T-cell-dependent B-cell responses. Although the option of an ECM-directed B-cell reaction is speculative as far as the lung is concerned, this option is supported by the presence of similar B-cell follicles in the inflamed synovia and the humoral response against ECM fragments that has been documented in rheumatoid arthritis [12–14]. It is conceivable that viral or bacterial infection or colonisation, as frequently seen in COPD, could lead to the breakdown of tolerance, facilitating such a reaction against self antigens. Such events are also thought to play a role in the initial phase and during exacerbations of several autoimmune diseases [15].

Exacerbations in COPD

To date, it has been very difficult to adequately define what an (acute) exacerbation of COPD is. Nevertheless, it is clear that exacerbations define the clinical course of COPD. With increasing severity of the disease, patients are prone to increasing rates of exacerbation. Although these exacerbations are mild at first, they later require more intensive treatment with systemic steroids and antibiotics. Finally, patients need to be hospitalised for these exacerbations. A third of patients hospitalised for acute exacerbations of COPD die within 1 yr and half within 3 yrs [16]. It has been suggested, from the East London cohort, that recovery from exacerbations is incomplete in that lung function is not fully restored, and, therefore, that the rate of disease progression is related to the occurrence of exacerbations [17].

Given the importance of exacerbations in this disease, it is sobering to realise how little is known about the histopathology of exacerbations. Only a few groups have studied bronchial biopsy specimens taken during exacerbations [18–20]. The pathology of the (peri)bronchiolar area and alveolar walls has never been investigated. A more detailed analysis of the histopathology of exacerbations is hampered by the invasive nature of the diagnostic approach required. More recently, there has been a large surge in the examination of sputum from patients with, usually rather mild-to-moderate, exacerbations of COPD. Much insight has been gained from the study of WEDZICHA and DONALDSON [21], in which a cohort of patients was followed up for a prolonged period of time and repeated sputum samples were collected, during both the stable phase and exacerbations. Exacerbations of COPD are characterised above all by marked recruitment of neutrophils, with the associated increase in mediators, cytokines and chemokines, such as myeloperoxidase, interleukin (IL)-8 and tumour necrosis factor (TNF)-α. More recently, it has also become more clearly appreciated that exacerbations of COPD are associated with increased numbers of eosinophils [22, 23]. This eosinophilia is associated with the response to corticosteroid treatment [24, 25]. Nevertheless, the response to treatment remains poor and further elucidation of both the aetiology of COPD exacerbations and the pathology of the inflammatory cascade are crucial in helping to discover new therapeutic interventions [26]. Additionally, since it is difficult to bring about clinical changes in COPD in a short time, novel therapies will increasingly be tested in proof-of-principle studies that use sputum or even biopsy specimens to provide evidence of effect [27, 28].

ECM changes in COPD

COPD is a heterogeneous disease, which means that the pathological changes that can be observed in an individual patient may vary greatly. Within a specific compartment of the lung that is involved in the disease, characteristic changes may be observed. With respect to ECM changes in COPD, a specific difference has already been observed between airway changes and parenchymal changes. In airways, in general, an increase in ECM is observed, which is supposed to contribute to increased stiffening of the airways and which may involve the inner subepithelial as well as the outer adventitial part of the airways (fig. 2). In contrast, in the parenchyma (including the peribronchial attachments), destruction of matrix is observed with loss of lung tissue, ultimately resulting in emphysema of varying severity. In the following section, the most characteristic ECM changes and possible pathogenetic factors are discussed in respect of the large and small airways and of parenchyma and peribronchial attachments.

ECM changes in large and small airways

Apart from the many other airway changes contributing to the increase in airway wall thickness, airway fibrosis had also already been described in early reports [29], in smokers as well as in COPD [30, 31]. Although such fibrotic changes are also supposed to be present in larger airways, most studies have focused on the small airways. Whereas, in large airways in asthma, there is a clear fibrotic change in the marked and even thickening of the reticular basement membrane, this is not always that obvious in COPD, and this is often used as the critical difference between asthma and COPD [32–34]. Nevertheless, in COPD, considerable fibrosis can often be observed in the subepithelial area, the pattern of which is often different from that observed in asthma.

In general, there is very uneven deposition of collagen directly apposing the reticular basement membrane, although, in some cases, a very even distribution can also be seen,

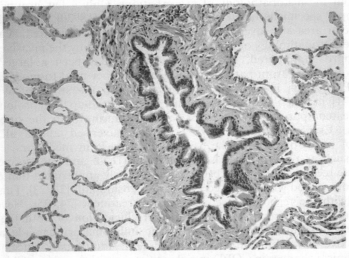

Fig. 2. – Lung of a chronic obstructive pulmonary disease patient with thickened airway wall and fibrosis of the inner subepithelial, as well as the outer adventitial part of the small airway (haematoxylin and eosin stain; scale bar=100 µm).

very much resembling the even reticular basement membrane thickening observed in asthma. Fibrotic changes can also be observed in small airways. Most changes in the small and large airways are supposed to reflect a reactive process as a consequence of local damage by cigarette smoke and the chronic inflammatory changes induced by this smoke [35–37]. Consequently, the local matrix changes are, in general, considered to reflect similar changes to those observed in wound healing [34].

As a reflection of early events observed after (ongoing) damage, in patients with COPD, increased levels of hyaluronan were found in induced sputum [38]. Furthermore, deposition of collagens I and III is observed in the subepithelial area, as well as the peribronchial adventitia. When comparing the composition of the ECM between control subjects and patients with mild and severe emphysema, there were no very obvious differences in the presence of collagen or fibronectin in small airways [39]. A clearer finding was the different expression of proteoglycans in the airway adventitia, which was clearly diminished for decorin (fig. 3) and biglycan, in particular, in the lung tissue of patients with severe COPD compared with control subjects and patients with mild COPD [39, 40]. This means that, although there may be airway wall thickening with, for the large part, characteristics seemingly similar to scar tissue after wound healing, in a specific subset of patients, a clear difference in proteoglycan expression occurs. Proteoglycans have important functions as a component of the ECM. These glycoproteins interconnect collagen fibres, and thus the number of connections determines the rigidity of the fibrous tissue. This implies that, when there is too much loss of proteoglycans, this leads to a loosening of tissue despite the fact that, at first sight, fibrosis may be present. In particular, in the area of the peribronchiolar attachments, despite the increase in airway wall thickness, this may lead to too much loosening of alveolar attachments, loss of elastic recoil, and, in due course, breaking and loss of attachments [40]. Another main feature of proteoglycans is that these can bind several important regulatory chemokines, cytokines and growth factors [40, 41]. This also implies that, with loss of proteoglycans, a local abnormal environment may develop with respect to normal regulation of inflammation and remodelling processes.

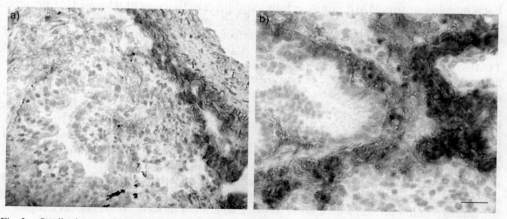

Fig. 3. – Small airway with accompanying arteriole in lung of a) a chronic obstructive pulmonary disease (COPD) patient, and b) a healthy control, stained for the small proteoglycan decorin. The adventitias of the arterioles (right-hand side) show clear decorin expression (red-brown) in both, whereas, around the bronchiole (left-hand side), expression is lacking in COPD (a) and clearly present in normal lung (b; immunoperoxidase staining; scale bar=50 µm).

ECM changes in pulmonary emphysema

The structural alterations in pulmonary emphysema, such as the loss of lung tissue and disordered architecture of the lung tissue can be considered the consequence of quantitative and qualitative changes in the composition of the local ECM. As indicated above, changes in the ECM can affect the structural integrity of the tissue, as well as the binding, release or regulation of locally bound mediators such as cytokines, in this way affecting remodelling and inflammatory processes.

Pulmonary emphysema has been reported to be associated with decreased elastin content [42], disrupted elastin sheaths [43], relatively increased collagen content [42, 44] and disorganised collagen fibrils [43]. Furthermore, a decreased hyaluronic acid and chondroitin sulphate content has been described [45, 46]. In addition, a loss of heparin sulphate proteoglycans has been found in alveolar tissue, although this was not specific for emphysema, but was also found in many other diseases showing destruction of lung architecture [39]. With respect to the breakdown of connective tissue components, elastin, in particular, has been considered a main critical component in the pathogenesis of emphysema. Elastin is an important target for proteolytic enzymes and loss of elastin consequently results in loss of elasticity, and, in due course, destruction of lung parenchyma.

Changes in the ECM in COPD are considered to be the net result of the balance between matrix-degrading and matrix-stimulating effects. Many of the matrix-degrading influences are counterbalanced by mechanisms designed to reduce this harmful effect. With respect to the effects of cigarette smoke, oxidants and proteases are the main degrading effectors. Oxidants are present in cigarette smoke itself, and are produced by the increased numbers of neutrophils and macrophages, whose increased presence is also induced by cigarette smoke components. The effects of these damaging oxidants are reduced by the protective effects of intra- and extracellular antioxidant defence systems [47]. The other main damaging mechanism is caused by proteases, which are mainly produced by epithelial and inflammatory cells, induced by cigarette smoke. In a similar way to the case for oxidants, the effect of proteases is counterbalanced by local production of antiproteases [48–50].

Several of these proteases belong to the group of matrix metalloproteinases (MMPs). Each member of this MMP family exhibits certain selectivity as to which ECM proteins can be degraded. The MMPs are inactivated by the presence of so-called tissue inhibitors of metalloproteinases (TIMPs), and the net effect of MMPs is caused by the presence of activated MMPs not inhibited by TIMPs. A dysbalance between certain MMPs and TIMPs, in COPD, is considered to play an important role in the pathogenesis of the disease [51], and, in particular, of emphysema. The real relevance of these findings is difficult to determine since many MMPs can be present with overlapping functions. In addition, in tissue, it is often very difficult to ascertain whether a certain MMP that has been detected is indeed active and, as such, capable of local degradation of the matrix [52]. In particular, increased concentrations of MMP-1 (collagenase) and MMP-9 (gelatinase-B) have been found in bronchoalveolar lavage fluid [53, 54] and sputum [55–58] from patients with COPD. In addition, MMP-1 expression has been found to be increased in the lungs of patients with emphysema, in particular in type-II pneumocytes [59]. MMP-9 expression is increased in alveolar macrophages from smokers, and this is surpassed by the expression in patients with COPD [60–62]. In animal models, MMP-12 (macrophage elastase) is supposed to play an important role in the development of COPD, since cigarette smoke-induced emphysema is not found in mice lacking MMP-12 [63]. In humans a role for MMP-12 is far less clear, although associations with polymorphisms of the MMP-12 gene have been found [64]. In humans, MMP-9 seems to be of greater importance, in particular by virtue of its capacity to activate transforming growth factor (TGF)-β (see below) [65, 66].

Basic fibroblast growth factor and TGF-β are main and central regulators in tissue repair. In particular, TGF-β has been the subject of several investigations in relation to the pathogenesis of COPD [67–70]. The presence of TGF-β is required for normal tissue repair, whereas increased levels result in fibrosis. TGF-β is activated by MMP-9, and this is one of the explanations as to why increased MMP-9 levels may be responsible for elastolytic activity in the lung parenchyma, and, by activation of TGF-β in the airways at the same time, would lead to airway wall fibrosis [71]. Another explanation would be that, by virtue of the decrease in decorin in the airway wall, there is reduced binding capacity for the increased TGF-β production, possibly leading to local fibrosis (in particular in the subepithelial area, since bronchial epithelial cells are main producers of TGF-β), whereas, with respect to peribronchial attachments, too little bound TGF-β is present for instant release after local matrix damage.

The effects of TGF-β are mediated by the Smad pathway [72, 73]. Recent studies have shown that aberrant levels of certain Smad proteins, in particular the inhibiting Smad-7, are found in COPD [74], which may be responsible for the local enhanced effects of TGF-β, even when its concentration would be considered reduced compared with normal subjects.

In conclusion, as is clear from the above, the regulation of the integrity of the ECM in the lung in COPD is the result of a very complex interaction between different components with mutual and many counterbalancing effects, in order to maintain tissue homeostasis. As a result of these complex interrelationships, it is quite clear that determination of aberrant expression of single components of this complex interplay will not identify a main individual mechanism responsible for the core effect in the pathogenesis of COPD [75]. The careful unravelling of the different components with an eye as to how these molecules interrelate will gradually lead to increased understanding of the complex ECM changes.

What is new in animal models of COPD

Since the mid-1990s, there has been a resurgence of interest in animal models for determining the mechanisms involved in the destruction and remodelling of the lung parenchyma, airways and pulmonary vasculature found in COPD.

Lung parenchymal destruction: emphysema

Role of proteolysis: antiproteolysis

A large body of evidence has been gathered to support the proteolysis–antiproteolysis theory of emphysema, but the details of this process have turned out to be much more complicated than the original belief in neutrophils and neutrophil elastase as the effectors of matrix destruction. It is now quite clear that inflammation, and the release of a wide variety of proteases, results in matrix degradation and emphysematous airspace enlargement. Indeed, it appears that serine proteases and MMPs work in concert, with neutrophil elastase required for activation of MMP-12, and each elastase is apparently able to inactivate the endogenous inhibitor of the other [76]. Furthermore, MMP-12 is required to liberate TNF-α from the macrophage surface, thus permitting it to recruit neutrophils, which then release elastases [77, 78]. Neutrophil-elastase-deficient mice experience ~60% protection from smoke-induced airspace enlargement [76], whereas those that were MMP-12-deficient experienced 100% protection [63].

There are many examples of mice with genetic defects, and genetically modified mice have been developed to investigate the pathophysiological mechanisms involved in emphysema (reviewed in [79, 80]). Models of interferon (IFN)-γ and IL-13 over-expression both result in emphysema, but probably act through increased MMP-12 production [65, 78, 81]. However, overexpression of MMP-1 [82, 83] also results in emphysema, and this is specifically related to destruction of collagen III, thus suggesting that alterations to the alveolar matrix in general are important, data which are supported by the tight-skin and blotchy mice, both characterised by abnormal matrix.

Inflammatory cells can potentially be recruited, or their actions induced, by a wide variety of the compounds present in cigarette smoke. Thus animals showing increased sensitivity to oxidants [84], or with a pro-inflammatory phenotype [85], might prove to be more susceptible to cigarette smoke. The above studies are important in that they provide a possible explanation as to why only a subset of human cigarette smokers develop emphysema.

These data imply that anti-inflammatory or antiprotease therapy would prove efficacious. Indeed, a phosphodiesterase 4 inhibitor was able to reduce the number of smoke-recruited neutrophils and macrophages in bronchoalveolar lavage fluid from acutely exposed mice, and decreased tissue macrophage density and prevented smoke-induced airspace enlargement after chronic exposure [86]. Since phosphodiesterase 4 is known to reduce release of TNF-α [87], these results may be due to alterations in the TNF-α-dependent inflammatory cascade (see above). Administration of the neutrophil elastase inhibitors ZD0892 [88] or α₁-antitrypsin [89] ameliorated, but did not completely ablate, cigarette smoke-induced emphysema, whereas administration of metalloprotease inhibitors appeared to exhibit a greater effect (reviewed in [75]).

Alteration in lung maintenance and repair

Lung maintenance and repair depends upon a complex system involving apoptosis, apoptotic cell removal and cellular replacement in order to maintain homeostasis. Failure of this mechanism could result from overinduction of apoptosis and/or blockade of the cell replacement process [90], with the ultimate production of emphysematous alveolar destruction [91]. The role of caspases in apoptosis is well established. When mice were given intraperitoneal caspase-3 combined with a Chariot protein transfection system [92], increased alveolar epithelial cell apoptosis with airspace enlargement and morphometric evidence of alveolar wall destruction were present within 2 h of treatment. The apoptosis disappeared after 6 h, and, although the airspace enlargement was present at 15 days, it was less than that at 6 h, suggesting the possibility of repair.

However, there also appears to be interaction between apoptosis and survival factors such as vascular endothelial growth factor (VEGF). In human emphysema, there is both increased apoptosis and a decrease in levels of VEGF and VEGF receptor (VEGFR) 2 [93]. In animals, when VEGFR-2 is blocked, there is increased alveolar septal apoptosis and airspace enlargement; administration of a caspase inhibitor prevented both the apoptosis and the airspace enlargement [94]. Proliferating cell nuclear antigen immunohistochemistry showed that blockade did not inhibit cell proliferation, and thus it was concluded that the airspace enlargement was secondary to the induced apoptosis. Oxidative stress appears to be integral to the relationship between apoptosis and cell maintenance; high levels of oxidants trigger apoptosis, whereas low levels mediate cell growth signalling. The cycle is further complicated by the fact that cells undergoing apoptosis also show increased oxidative stress. For example, when

VEGFR-2 is blocked, oxidative stress induces apoptosis that can be blocked by superoxide dismutase mimetics, and inhibition of apoptosis by caspase inhibitors reduces oxidative stress [95].

Ceramide appears to be an upstream regulator of apoptosis, oxidative stress and proteolysis, and provides a translational link with human disease, since ceramide levels are increased in the lungs in cigarette-associated emphysema [96]. VEGFR-2 blockade increased alveolar septal cell ceramide levels and induced apoptosis and airspace enlargement in mice. When ceramide synthesis was blocked, there was no VEGFR-2-blockade-induced increase in alveolar size, and, conversely, when ceramide was administered intratracheally, there was increased apoptosis and airspace enlargement, which could be blocked using caspase-3 inhibitors.

In a very intriguing perspective, TUDER et al. [97] drew analogies between the processes involved in the development of emphysema and ageing, suggesting that both are a response to injury and repair. They suggested that failure of the lung maintenance and repair system results from an integrated action among genes, environment and intrinsic defects, and thus, in emphysema, there is significant and sustained lung injury induced by cigarette smoke. This concept is supported by work demonstrating that cigarette smoke induces changes in the alveolar epithelium identical to those found in senescent cells [98].

TUDER et al. [97] further suggest that, rather than being a primary response to injury, inflammation represents a response to these unrepaired cellular and molecular alterations.

Against this portion of the theory is the apparent linkage of apoptosis as a downstream event in type-1 T-helper cell/cytotoxic T-cell cytokine-induced emphysema [99]. In this study, mice were genetically modified with a doxycycline-inducible IFN-γ linked to a Clara cell 10-kDa protein promoter. Some were crossed into a caspase-3-null construct, whereas other animals received intraperitoneally administered caspase inhibitor. The IFN-γ mice developed emphysema with inflammation, increased cathepsin and MMP levels, and increased apoptosis. Both caspase inhibitor and the caspase-3-null crosses caused decreased inflammation, MMP-9 mRNA level and apoptosis, and decreased, but did not abrogate, the IFN-γ-induced emphysema.

The lung as an immunological target

It is possible that failure of the lung maintenance and repair system results in the development of an immune inflammatory reaction [100]. Under homeostatic conditions, macrophages clear apoptotic cells from the tissue, preventing cell lysis and the release of toxic or immunogenic components, and leading instead to secretion of growth and survival factors, such as VEGF [101], and anti-inflammatory mediators, such as prostaglandin E_2 and IL-10. However, it is important to remember that the same macrophage receptors that permit recognition of the apoptotic cells are also involved in the innate immune system [100]. Cells undergoing apoptosis lose phospholipid symmetry, but this same loss of symmetry could also facilitate the exposure of other recognition domains since such sites contain many of the proteins known to induce antibody production in autoimmune disease. Furthermore, oxidants produced during apoptosis are able to generate these types of membrane lipid, which can then act as antigens [102]. Another possibility is that engulfment of necrotic cells by dendritic cells induces maturation of the dendritic cells and activates T-lymphocytes (reviewed in [100]).

The role of autoimmunity in the genesis of emphysema has been supported by the development of emphysema in immunocompetent rats 3 weeks after the intraperitoneal injection of xenogeneic endothelial cells [103]. The injected rats produced antibodies directed against endothelial cells, specifically VEGFR-2, leading to increased septal cell apoptosis and increased activity of metalloproteinases MMP-9 and MMP-2. These data suggest that an immune reaction can dysregulate the lung maintenance and repair system and lead to apoptosis, which, in turn, could lead to amplification of the immune effects upon the lung. In a possible translational link to human emphysema [104], the injected rats showed increased numbers of lung CD4 T-cells, and injection of spleen-derived CD4 T-cells also induced emphysema.

Another idea that has been proposed is that cigarette smoke itself either contains antigenic substances or modifies normal human proteins, perhaps through oxidative damage, in such a way as to make them immunogenic [105].

Airway remodelling

Perhaps surprisingly, there are very few animal-based experimental data relating to the effects of cigarette smoke on the airways. Mucin gene upregulation is induced by smoke [106, 107], and, although there are considerable differences between rodent species, secretory cell metaplasia can be found in the central and peripheral airways [84, 106–108] and is reduced upon smoking cessation [109].

The role of inflammatory cell cytokines in mucin production was suggested by studies showing induced expression of mucin genes by IL-1β and TNF-α [110, 111], the latter perhaps working through activation of TNF-α-converting enzyme [112]. There may be a role for the type-2 T-helper cell inflammatory pathway in secretory cell metaplasia, since mice genetically modified to express doxycyclin-inducible IL-13 showed an increased number of secretory cells in the small airways [71], a process which was independent of MMP-9 and -12. Supporting a role for inflammatory cells are data demonstrating upregulation of mucin 5 subtypes A and C by metalloproteinases [113] and neutrophil elastase [114], the latter accompanied by mucous cell metaplasia [115].

Airway wall remodelling was found in IL-6 and -11 transgenic mice, and was characterised by increased airway inflammation and increased levels of airway wall collagen, with collagen deposition out of proportion to airway size, and associated with increased airway responsiveness in the IL-11 mice, but with increased bronchiolar diameter in the IL-6 mice [116]. Although the above models are developmental rather than inducible, they suggest a potential role for the inflammatory process in airway remodelling.

In human smokers, there is considerable structural reorganisation of the airway wall with increases in submucosal fibrous tissue [117]. These changes can be modelled in rat tracheal explants. When the explants were exposed to smoke, there was an increase in pro-collagen gene expression, associated with an increase in hydroxyproline level, indicative of collagen synthesis [118], and there was upregulation of TGF-β1, its downstream signalling molecule phospho-Smad2 and connective tissue growth factor, a mediator of TGF-β effects [119]. The process was independent of inflammatory cells, and could be abolished by antioxidants, suggesting that smoke has a direct effect on airway remodelling *via* induction of fibrogenic growth factors.

Vascular remodelling

There are now increasing data demonstrating that vascular remodelling occurs, with extension of muscle into the usually poorly muscularised arteries, in the lungs of guinea pigs chronically exposed to cigarette smoke [120], a finding that mimics the human condition [121]. Recent work has clarified the mechanisms behind this finding, clearly demonstrating increased gene expression and immunohistochemically identified production of vasoactive mediators (endothelin and VEGF) in both animal [122, 123] and human vessels [124, 125]. Thus it appears that cigarette smoke can directly affect the lung vessels, altering the balance of vasoactive mediators and inducing cell proliferation, factors which ultimately result in vascular remodelling and increased pulmonary arterial pressure. It has been suggested that some of the proliferating cells are acquired from circulating progenitor cells derived from the bone marrow (J. Barbera, University of Barcelona, Barcelona, Spain; personal communication). Although these cells may enter as a part of a VEGF-mediated repair reaction, they may, in addition to proliferation of the resident myofibroblasts and smooth muscle cells, also be a component of the increased muscularisation found in these vessels.

Conclusions

COPD is the result of a large number of different, and often inter-related, processes. Satisfactory treatment strategies can only be developed when it is possible to understand, first, the pathophysiological mechanisms involved in the genesis of abnormalities in the various lung compartments, and, secondly, how these abnormalities can be manifested clinically.

Summary

There has been a resurgence of interest in the pathophysiological mechanisms involved in chronic obstructive pulmonary disease since the early 1990s. The present chapter presents an overview of new information in two important areas in human disease, namely the role of the lymphocyte and exacerbations. The role of the extracellular matrix is much more important, and more complicated, than early work suggested. This is followed by an analysis of new data in both humans and animals. Finally, new information gleaned from animal studies is described and discussed.

Keywords: Emphysema, immunity, matrix, remodelling.

References

1. Bosken CH, Hards J, Gatter K, Hogg JC. Characterization of the inflammatory reaction in the peripheral airways of cigarette smokers using immunocytochemistry. *Am Rev Respir Dis* 1992; 145: 911–917.
2. Hogg JC, Chu F, Utokaparch S, *et al.* The nature of small-airway obstruction in chronic obstructive pulmonary disease. *N Engl J Med* 2004; 350: 2645–2653.
3. National Heart Lung and Blood Institute, World Health Organization. Global Initiative for Chronic Obstructive Lung Disease. Global Strategy for Diagnosis, Management, and Prevention of Chronic Obstructive Pulmonary Disease. 2004 Update. Bethesda, MD, National Institutes of Health, 2004.
4. Gosman MM, Willemse BW, Jansen DF, *et al.* Increased number of B-cells in bronchial biopsies in COPD. *Eur Respir J* 2006; 27: 60–64.
5. van der Strate BW, Postma DS, Brandsma CA, *et al.* Cigarette smoke-induced emphysema: a role for the B cell? *Am J Respir Crit Care Med* 2006; 173: 751–758.

6. Sopori M. Effects of cigarette smoke on the immune system. *Nat Rev Immunol* 2002; 2: 372–377.

7. Becker CG, Dubin T. Activation of factor XII by tobacco glycoprotein. *J Exp Med* 1977; 146: 457–467.

8. Phillips DH. Smoking-related DNA and protein adducts in human tissues. *Carcinogenesis* 2002; 23: 1979–2004.

9. Horton MR, Shapiro S, Bao C, Lowenstein CJ, Noble PW. Induction and regulation of macrophage metalloelastase by hyaluronan fragments in mouse macrophages. *J Immunol* 1999; 162: 4171–4176.

10. McKee CM, Penno MB, Cowman M, *et al.* Hyaluronan (HA) fragments induce chemokine gene expression in alveolar macrophages. The role of HA size and CD44. *J Clin Invest* 1996; 98: 2403–2413.

11. Rafi A, Nagarkatti M, Nagarkatti PS. Hyaluronate–CD44 interactions can induce murine B-cell activation. *Blood* 1997; 89: 2901–2908.

12. Magalhaes R, Stiehl P, Morawietz L, Berek C, Krenn V. Morphological and molecular pathology of the B cell response in synovitis of rheumatoid arthritis. *Virchows Arch* 2002; 441: 415–427.

13. Berg L, Ronnelid J, Sanjeevi CB, Lampa J, Klareskog L. Interferon-γ production in response to *in vitro* stimulation with collagen type II in rheumatoid arthritis is associated with HLA-DRB1*0401 and HLA-DQ8. *Arthritis Res* 2000; 2: 75–84.

14. Souto-Carneiro MM, Burkhardt H, Muller EC, *et al.* Human monoclonal rheumatoid synovial B lymphocyte hybridoma with a new disease-related specificity for cartilage oligomeric matrix protein. *J Immunol* 2001; 166: 4202–4208.

15. Strassburg CP, Vogel A, Manns MP. Autoimmunity and hepatitis C. *Autoimmun Rev* 2003; 2: 322–331.

16. Gunen H, Hacievliyagil SS, Kosar F, *et al.* Factors affecting survival of hospitalised patients with COPD. *Eur Respir J* 2005; 26: 234–241.

17. Donaldson GC, Seemungal TA, Bhowmik A, Wedzicha JA. Relationship between exacerbation frequency and lung function decline in chronic obstructive pulmonary disease. *Thorax* 2002; 57: 847–852.

18. Sohy C, Pilette C, Niederman MS, Sibille Y. Acute exacerbation of chronic obstructive pulmonary disease and antibiotics: what studies are still needed? *Eur Respir J* 2002; 19: 966–975.

19. Maestrelli P, Saetta M, Di Stefano A, *et al.* Comparison of leukocyte counts in sputum, bronchial biopsies, and bronchoalveolar lavage. *Am J Respir Crit Care Med* 1995; 152: 1926–1931.

20. Qiu Y, Zhu J, Bandi V, *et al.* Biopsy neutrophilia, neutrophil chemokine and receptor gene expression in severe exacerbations of chronic obstructive pulmonary disease. *Am J Respir Crit Care Med* 2003; 168: 968–975.

21. Wedzicha JA, Donaldson GC. Exacerbations of chronic obstructive pulmonary disease. *Respir Care* 2003; 48: 1204–1213.

22. Saetta M, Di Stefano A, Maestrelli P, *et al.* Airway eosinophilia in chronic bronchitis during exacerbations. *Am J Respir Crit Care Med* 1994; 150: 1646–1652.

23. Fujimoto K, Yasuo M, Urushibata K, Hanaoka M, Koizumi T, Kubo K. Airway inflammation during stable and acutely exacerbated chronic obstructive pulmonary disease. *Eur Respir J* 2005; 25: 640–646.

24. Pizzichini E, Pizzichini MM, Gibson P, *et al.* Sputum eosinophilia predicts benefit from prednisone in smokers with chronic obstructive bronchitis. *Am J Respir Crit Care Med* 1998; 158: 1511–1517.

25. Brightling CE, Monteiro W, Ward R, *et al.* Sputum eosinophilia and short-term response to prednisolone in chronic obstructive pulmonary disease: a randomised controlled trial. *Lancet* 2000; 356: 1480–1485.

26. Barnes PJ, Shapiro SD, Pauwels RA. Chronic obstructive pulmonary disease: molecular and cellular mechanisms. *Eur Respir J* 2003; 22: 672–688.

27. Gamble E, Grootendorst DC, Brightling CE, *et al.* Anti-inflammatory effects of the phosphodiesterase 4 inhibitor cilomilast (Ariflo) in COPD. *Am J Respir Crit Care Med* 2003; 168: 976–982.

28. Barnes NC, Qiu YS, Pavord ID, *et al.* Antiinflammatory effects of salmeterol/fluticasone propionate in chronic obstructive lung disease. *Am J Respir Crit Care Med* 2006; 173: 736–743.

29. Niewoehner DE, Kleinerman J, Rice DB. Pathologic changes in the peripheral airways of young cigarette smokers. *N Engl J Med* 1974; 291: 755–758.

30. Wright JL, Lawson LM, Pare PD, Wiggs BJ, Kennedy S, Hogg JC. Morphology of peripheral airways in current smokers and ex-smokers. *Am Rev Respir Dis* 1983; 127: 474–477.

31. Wright JL, Hobson J, Wiggs BR, Pare PD, Hogg JC. Effect of cigarette smoking on structure of the small airways. *Lung* 1987; 165: 91–100.

32. Jeffery PK. Structural and inflammatory changes in COPD: a comparison with asthma. *Thorax* 1998; 53: 129–136.

33. Jeffery PK. Comparison of the structural and inflammatory features of COPD and asthma. Giles F. Filley Lecture. *Chest* 2000; 117: Suppl. 1, 251S–260S.

34. Jeffery PK. Remodeling in asthma and chronic obstructive lung disease. *Am J Respir Crit Care Med* 2001; 164: S28–S38.

35. Jeffery PK. Morphology of the airway wall in asthma and in chronic obstructive pulmonary disease. *Am Rev Respir Dis* 1991; 143: 1152–1158.

36. Saetta M, Timens W, Jeffery PK. Pathology. *In:* Postma DS, Siafakas NM, eds. Management of Chronic Obstructive Pulmonary Disease. *Eur Respir Mon* 1998; 7: 92–101.

37. Saetta M, Turato G, Maestrelli P, Mapp CE, Fabbri LM. Cellular and structural bases of chronic obstructive pulmonary disease. *Am J Respir Crit Care Med* 2001; 163: 1304–1309.

38. Dentener MA, Vernooy JH, Hendriks S, Wouters EF. Enhanced levels of hyaluronan in lungs of patients with COPD: relationship with lung function and local inflammation. *Thorax* 2005; 60: 114–119.

39. Van Straaten JFM, Coers W, Noordhoek J, *et al.* Proteoglycan changes in the extracellular matrix of lung tissue from patients with pulmonary emphysema. *Mod Pathol* 1999; 12: 697–705.

40. Van der Geld YM, Van Straaten JFM, Postma DS, Timens W. Role of proteoglycans in development and pathogenesis of emphysema. *In:* Garg HG, Roughley PJ, Hales CA, eds. Proteoglycans in Lung Disease. New York, Marcel Dekker, 2002; pp. 241–267.

41. Timens W, Coers W, Van Straaten JFM, Postma DS. Extracellular matrix and inflammation: a role for fibroblast-mediated tissue repair in the pathogenesis of emphysema? *Eur Respir Rev* 1997; 7: 119–123.

42. Cardoso WV, Sekhon HS, Hyde DM, Thurlbeck WM. Collagen and elastin in human pulmonary emphysema. *Am Rev Respir Dis* 1993; 147: 975–981.

43. Finlay GA, O'Donnell MD, O'Connor CM, Hayes JP, FitzGerald MX. Elastin and collagen remodeling in emphysema – a scanning electron microscopy study. *Am J Pathol* 1996; 149: 1405–1415.

44. Lang MR, Fiaux GW, Gillooly M, Stewart JA, Hulmes DJS, Lamb D. Collagen content of alveolar wall tissue in emphysematous and non-emphysematous lungs. *Thorax* 1994; 49: 319–326.

45. Konno K, Arai H, Motomiya M, *et al.* A biochemical study on glycosaminoglycans (mucopolysaccharides) in emphysematous and in aged lungs. *Am Rev Respir Dis* 1982; 126: 797–801.

46. Laros CD, Kuyper CMA, Janssen HMJ. The chemical composition of fresh human lung parenchyma. *Respiration* 1972; 29: 458–467.

47. MacNee W. Pathogenesis of chronic obstructive pulmonary disease. *Proc Am Thorac Soc* 2005; 2: 258–266.

48. Shapiro SD. Evolving concepts in the pathogenesis of chronic obstructive pulmonary disease. *Clin Chest Med* 2000; 21: 621–632.

49. Parks WC, Shapiro SD. Matrix metalloproteinases in lung biology. *Respir Res* 2001; 2: 10–19.

50. Shapiro SD, Ingenito EP. The pathogenesis of chronic obstructive pulmonary disease: advances in the past 100 years. *Am J Respir Cell Mol Biol* 2005; 32: 367–372.

51. Cataldo DD, Gueders MM, Rocks N, *et al.* Pathogenic role of matrix metalloproteases and their inhibitors in asthma and chronic obstructive pulmonary disease and therapeutic relevance of matrix metalloproteases inhibitors. *Cell Mol Biol (Noisy-le-grand)* 2003; 49: 875–884.

52. Ohbayashi H. Matrix metalloproteinases in lung diseases. *Curr Protein Pept Sci* 2002; 3: 409–421.

53. Finlay GA, Russell KJ, McMahon KJ, *et al.* Elevated levels of matrix metalloproteinases in bronchoalveolar lavage fluid of emphysematous patients. *Thorax* 1997; 52: 502–506.

54. Culpitt SV, Maziak W, Loukidis S, Nightingale JA, Matthews JL, Barnes PJ. Effect of high dose inhaled steroid on cells, cytokines, and proteases in induced sputum in chronic obstructive pulmonary disease. *Am J Respir Crit Care Med* 1999; 160: 1635–1639.

55. Beeh KM, Beier J, Kornmann O, Buhl R. Sputum matrix metalloproteinase-9, tissue inhibitor of metalloprotinease-1, and their molar ratio in patients with chronic obstructive pulmonary disease, idiopathic pulmonary fibrosis and healthy subjects. *Respir Med* 2003; 97: 634–639.

56. Mercer PF, Shute JK, Bhowmik A, Donaldson GC, Wedzicha JA, Warner JA. MMP-9, TIMP-1 and inflammatory cells in sputum from COPD patients during exacerbation. *Respir Res* 2005; 6: 151.

57. Culpitt SV, Rogers DF, Traves SL, Barnes PJ, Donnelly LE. Sputum matrix metalloproteases: comparison between chronic obstructive pulmonary disease and asthma. *Respir Med* 2005; 99: 703–710.

58. Vignola AM, Riccobono L, Mirabella A, *et al.* Sputum metalloproteinase-9/tissue inhibitor of metalloproteinase-1 ratio correlates with airflow obstruction in asthma and chronic bronchitis. *Am J Respir Crit Care Med* 1998; 158: 1945–1950.

59. Imai K, Dalal SS, Chen ES, *et al.* Human collagenase (matrix metalloproteinase-1) expression in the lungs of patients with emphysema. *Am J Respir Crit Care Med* 2001; 163: 786–791.

60. Russell RE, Culpitt SV, DeMatos C, *et al.* Release and activity of matrix metalloproteinase-9 and tissue inhibitor of metalloproteinase-1 by alveolar macrophages from patients with chronic obstructive pulmonary disease. *Am J Respir Cell Mol Biol* 2002; 26: 602–609.

61. Russell RE, Thorley A, Culpitt SV, *et al.* Alveolar macrophage-mediated elastolysis: roles of matrix metalloproteinases, cysteine, and serine proteases. *Am J Physiol Lung Cell Mol Physiol* 2002; 283: L867–L873.

62. Lim S, Roche N, Oliver BG, Mattos W, Barnes PJ, Chung KF. Balance of matrix metalloprotease-9 and tissue inhibitor of metalloprotease-1 from alveolar macrophages in cigarette smokers. Regulation by interleukin-10. *Am J Respir Crit Care Med* 2000; 162: 1355–1360.

63. Hautamaki RD, Kobayashi DK, Senior RM, Shapiro SD. Requirement for macrophage elastase for cigarette smoke-induced emphysema in mice. *Science* 1997; 277: 2002–2004.

64. Wallace AM, Sandford AJ. Genetic polymorphisms of matrix metalloproteinases: functional importance in the development of chronic obstructive pulmonary disease? *Am J Pharmacogenomics* 2002; 2: 167–175.

65. Zheng T, Zhu Z, Wang Z, *et al.* Inducible targeting of IL-13 to the adult lung causes matrix metalloproteinase- and cathepsin-dependent emphysema. *J Clin Invest* 2000; 106: 1081–1093.

66. Atkinson JJ, Senior RM. Matrix metalloproteinase-9 in lung remodeling. *Am J Respir Cell Mol Biol* 2003; 28: 12–24.

67. Takizawa H, Tanaka M, Takami K, *et al.* Increased expression of transforming growth factor-β1 in small airway epithelium from tobacco smokers and patients with chronic obstructive pulmonary disease (COPD). *Am J Respir Crit Care Med* 2001; 163: 1476–1483.

68. De Boer WI, van Schadewijk A, Sont JK, *et al.* Transforming growth factor β1 and recruitment of macrophages and mast cells in airways in chronic obstructive pulmonary disease. *Am J Respir Crit Care Med* 1998; 158: 1951–1957.

69. Baraldo S, Bazzan E, Turato G, *et al.* Decreased expression of TGF-β type II receptor in bronchial glands of smokers with COPD. *Thorax* 2005; 60: 998–1002.

70. Pons AR, Sauleda J, Noguera A, *et al.* Decreased macrophage release of TGF-β and TIMP-1 in chronic obstructive pulmonary disease. *Eur Respir J* 2005; 26: 60–66.

71. Lanone S, Zheng T, Zhu Z, *et al.* Overlapping and enzyme-specific contributions of matrix metalloproteinases-9 and -12 in IL-13-induced inflammation and remodeling. *J Clin Invest* 2002; 110: 463–474.

72. Camoretti-Mercado B, Solway J. Transforming growth factor-β1 and disorders of the lung. *Cell Biochem Biophys* 2005; 43: 131–148.

73. Groneberg DA, Witt H, Adcock IM, Hansen G, Springer J. Smads as intracellular mediators of airway inflammation. *Exp Lung Res* 2004; 30: 223–250.

74. Springer J, Scholz FR, Peiser C, Groneberg DA, Fischer A. Smad-signaling in chronic obstructive pulmonary disease: transcriptional down-regulation of inhibitory Smad 6 and 7 by cigarette smoke. *Biol Chem* 2004; 385: 649–653.

75. Churg A, Wright JL. Proteases and emphysema. *Curr Opin Pulm Med* 2005; 11: 153–159.

76. Shapiro SD, Goldstein NM, Houghton AM, Kobasyashi DK, Kelley D, Belaaouaj A. Neutrophil elastase contributes to cigarette smoke-induced emphysema in mice. *Am J Pathol* 2003; 163: 2329–2335.

77. Churg A, Zay K, Shay S, *et al.* Acute cigarette smoke induced connective tissue breakdown requires both neutrophils and macrophage metalloelastase in mice. *Am J Respir Cell Mol Biol* 2002; 27: 368–374.

78. Churg A, Wang RD, Tai H, *et al.* Macrophage metalloelastase mediates acute cigarette smoke-induced inflammation *via* tumor necrosis factor-α release. *Am J Respir Crit Care Med* 2003; 167: 1083–1089.

79. Mahadeva R, Shapiro SD. Chronic obstructive pulmonary disease*3: experimental animal models of pulmonary emphysema. *Thorax* 2002; 57: 908–914.

80. Tuder RM, McGrath S, Neptune E. The pathobiological mechanisms of emphysema models: what do they have in common? *Pulm Pharmacol Ther* 2003; 16: 67–78.

81. Wang Z, Zheng T, Zhu Z, *et al.* Interferon γ induction of pulmonary emphysema in the adult murine lung. *J Exp Med* 2000; 192: 1587–1599.

82. Foronjy RF, Okada Y, Cole R, D'Armiento J. Progressive adult-onset emphysema in transgenic mice expressing human MMP-1 in the lung. *J Appl Physiol* 2003; 284: L727–L737.

83. Shiomi T, Okada Y, Foronjy R, *et al.* Emphysematous changes are caused by degradation of type III collagen in transgenic mice expressing MMP-1. *Exp Lung Res* 2003; 29: 1–15.

84. Bartalesi B, Cavarra E, Fineschi S, *et al.* Different lung responses to cigarette smoke in two strains of mice sensitive to oxidants. *Eur Respir J* 2005; 25: 15–22.

85. Guerassimov A, Hoshino M, Takubo Y, *et al.* The development of emphysema in cigarette smoke-exposed mice is strain dependent. *Am J Respir Crit Care Med* 2005; 170: 974–980.

86. Martorana PA, Beume R, Lucattelli M, Wollin L, Lungarella G. Roflumilast fully prevents emphysema in mice chronically exposed to cigarette smoke. *Am J Respir Crit Care Med* 2005; 172: 848–853.

87. Hatzelmann A, Schudt C. Anti-inflammatory and immunomodulatory potential of the novel PDE4 inhibitor roflumilast *in vitro. J Pharmacol Exp Ther* 2001; 297: 267–279.

88. Wright JL, Farmer SG, Churg A. Synthetic serine elastase inhibitor reduces cigarette smoke induced emphysema in guinea pigs. *Am J Respir Crit Care Med* 2002; 166: 954–960.

89. Churg A, Wang RD, Xie C, Wright JL. α-1-Antitrypsin ameliorates cigarette smoke-induced emphysema in the mouse. *Am J Respir Crit Care Med* 2003; 168: 199–207.

90. Tuder RM, Petrache I, Elias JA, Voelkel NF, Henson PM. Apoptosis and emphysema: the missing link. *Am J Respir Cell Mol Biol* 2003; 28: 551–554.

91. Yokohori A, Aoshiba K, Nagai A. Increased levels of cell death and proliferation in alveolar wall cells in patients with pulmonary emphysema. *Chest* 2004; 125: 626–632.

92. Aoshiba K, Yokohori N, Nagai A. Alveolar wall apoptosis causes lung destruction and emphysematous changes. *Am J Respir Cell Mol Biol* 2003; 28: 555–562.

93. Kasahara Y, Tuder RM, Cool CD, Lynch DA, Flores SC, Voelkel NF. Endothelial cell death and decreased expression of vascular endothelial growth factor and vascular endothelial growth factor receptor 2 in emphysema. *Am J Respir Crit Care Med* 2001; 163: 737–744.

94. Kasahara Y, Tuder RM, Taraseviciene-Stewart L, *et al.* Inhibition of VEGF receptors causes lung cell apoptosis and emphysema. *J Clin Invest* 2000; 106: 1311–1319.

95. Tuder RM, Zhen L, Cho CY, *et al.* Oxidative stress and apoptosis interact and cause emphysema due to vascular endothelial growth factor receptor blockade. *Am J Respir Cell Mol Biol* 2003; 29: 88–97.

96. Petrache I, Natarajan V, Zhen L, *et al.* Ceramide upregulation causes pulmonary cell apoptosis and emphysema-like disease in mice. *Nature Med* 2005; 11: 491–498.

97. Tuder RM, Yoshida T, Arap W, Pasqualini R, Petrache I. State of the art. Cellular and molecular mechanisms of alveolar destruction in emphysema: an evolutionary perspective. *Proc Am Thorac Soc* 2006; 3: 503–511.

98. Tsuji T, Aoshiba K, Nagai A. Cigarette smoke induces senescence in alveolar epithelial cells. *Am J Respir Cell Mol Biol* 2004; 31: 643–649.

99. Zheng T, Kang MJ, Crothers K, *et al.* Role of cathepsin S-dependent epithelial cell apoptosis in IFN-γ-induced alveolar remodeling and pulmonary emphysema. *J Immunol* 2005; 174: 8106–8115.

100. Fadok VA, Bratton DL, Henson PM. Phagocyte receptors for apoptotic cells: recognition, uptake, and consequences. *J Clin Invest* 2001; 108: 957–962.

101. Golpon HA, Fadok VA, Taraseviene-Stewart L, *et al.* Life after corpse engulfment: phagocytosis of apoptotic cells leads to VEGF secretion and cell growth. *FASEB J* 2004; 18: 1716–1728.

102. Bratton DL, Henson PM. Autoimmunity and apoptosis: refusing to go quietly. *Nat Med* 2005; 11: 26–27.

103. Taraseviciene-Stewart L, Scerbavicius R, Choe KH, *et al.* An animal model of autoimmune emphysema. *Am J Respir Crit Care Med* 2005; 171: 734–742.

104. Sullivan AL, Simonian PL, Falta MT, *et al.* Oligoclonal CD4+ T cells in the lungs of patients with severe emphysema. *Am J Respir Crit Care Med* 2005; 172: 590–596.

105. Agusti A, MacNee W, Donaldson K, Cosio M. Hypothesis: does COPD have an autoimmune component? *Thorax* 2003; 58: 832–834.

106. Takeyama K, Jung B, Shim JJ, *et al.* Activation of epidermal growth factor receptors is responsible for mucin synthesis induced by cigarette smoke. *Am J Physiol* 2002; 280: L165–L172.

107. Lee SY, Kang EJ, Hur GY, *et al.* The inhibitory effects of rebamipide on cigarette smoke-induced airway mucin production. *Respir Med* 2005; 100: 503–511.

108. Leikauf GD, Borchers MT, Prows DR, Simpson LG. Mucin apoprotein expression in COPD. *Chest* 2002; 121: Suppl. 5, 166S–182S.

109. Wright JL, Churg A. Smoking cessation decreases the number of metaplastic secretory cells in the small airways of the guinea pig. *Inhal Toxicol* 2002; 14: 101–107.

110. Gray T, Coakley R, Hirsh A, *et al.* Regulation of MUC5AC mucin secretion and airway surface liquid metabolism by IL-1β in human bronchial epithelia. *Am J Physiol* 2004; 286: L320–L330.

111. Koo JS, Kim YD, Jetten AM, Belloni P, Nettesheim P. Overexpression of mucin genes induced by interleukin-1β, tumor necrosis factor-α, lipopolysaccharide, and neutrophil elastase is inhibited by a retinoic acid receptor α antagonist. *Exp Lung Res* 2002; 28: 315–332.

112. Shao MXG, Nakanaga T, Nadel JA. Cigarette smoke induces MUC5AC mucin overproduction *via* tumor necrosis factor-α-converting enzyme in human airway epithelial (NCI-H292) cells. *Am J Physiol* 2004; 287: L420–L427.

113. Deshmukh HS, Case LM, Wesselkamper SC, *et al.* Metalloproteinases mediate mucin 5AC expression by epidermal growth factor receptor activation. *Am J Respir Crit Care Med* 2005; 171: 305–314.

114. Fischer BM, Voynow JA. Neutrophil elastase induces MUC5AC gene expression in airway epithelium *via* a pathway involving reactive oxygen species. *Am J Respir Cell Mol Biol* 2002; 26: 447–452.

115. Voynow JA, Fischer BM, Malarkey DE, *et al.* Neutrophil elastase induces mucus cell metaplasia in mouse lung. *Am J Physiol* 2004; 287: L1293–L1302.

116. Kuhn C, Homer RJ, Zhu Z, *et al.* Airway hyperresponsiveness and airway obstruction in transgenic mice: morphologic correlates in mice overexpressing interleukin (IL)-11 and IL-6 in the lung. *Am J Respir Cell Mol Biol* 2000; 22: 289–295.

117. McParland BE, Macklem PT, Pare PD. Airway wall remodeling: friend or foe? *J Appl Physiol* 2003; 95: 426–434.

118. Wang RD, Tai H, Xie C, Wang X, Wright JL, Churg A. Cigarette smoke produces airway wall remodeling in rat tracheal explants. *Am J Respir Crit Care Med* 2003; 168: 1232–1236.

119. Wang RD, Wright JL, Churg A. Transforming growth factor-β1 drives airway remodeling in cigarette smoke-exposed tracheal explants. *Am J Respir Cell Mol Biol* 2005; 33: 387–393.

120. Wright JL, Farmer SG, Churg A. A neutrophil elastase inhibitor reduces cigarette smoke-induced remodelling of lung vessels. *Eur Respir J* 2003; 22: 77–81.

121. Wright JL, Levy RD, Churg A. Pulmonary hypertension in chronic obstructive pulmonary disease: current theories of pathogenesis and their implications for treatment. *Thorax* 2005; 60: 605–609.

122. Wright JL, Tai H, Dai J, Churg A. Cigarette smoke induces rapid changes in gene expression in pulmonary arteries. *Lab Invest* 2002; 82: 1391–1398.

123. Wright JL, Tai H, Churg A. Vasoactive mediators and pulmonary hypertension after cigarette smoke exposure in the guinea pig. *J Appl Physiol* 2006; 100: 672–676.

124. Santos S, Peinado VI, Ramirez J, *et al.* Enhanced expression of vascular endothelial growth factor in pulmonary arteries of smokers and patients with moderate chronic obstructive pulmonary disease. *Am J Respir Crit Care Med* 2003; 167: 1250–1256.

125. Kranenburg AR, de Boer WI, Alagappan VKT, Sterk PJ, Sharma HS. Enhanced bronchial expression of vascular endothelial growth factor and receptors (Flk-1 and Flt-1) in patients with chronic obstructive pulmonary disease. *Thorax* 2005; 60: 106–113.

CHAPTER 8

Idiopathic interstitial pneumonia and connective tissue disorder-related interstitial lung disease

O.A. Harari*, P.S. Hasleton[#]

*Dept of Rheumatology, Hammersmith Hospital, Imperial College London, London, and [#]Dept of Histopathology, Clinical Sciences Block, Manchester Royal Infirmary, Manchester, UK.

Correspondence: P.S. Hasleton, Dept of Histopathology, Clinical Sciences Block, Manchester Royal Infirmary, Oxford Road, Manchester, M13 9WL, UK. Fax: 44 1612766348; E-mail: philip.hasleton@manchester.ac.uk

Background

Idiopathic interstitial pneumonia (IIP)/interstitial lung disease (ILD) has multiple causes, which can be found in standard papers [1]. History is often essential in diagnosis, since there are relatively few causes which manifest with such obvious pathology that a microscope slide will give the diagnosis. The following provide immediate clues as to a diagnosis: viral pneumonias with typical inclusions; Langerhans' cell histiocytosis; drugs, such as busulphan, with gross cytological atypia; and rheumatoid disease, with rheumatoid nodules (fig. 1) or a rheumatoid pleurisy (fig. 2). However, the most common histological pattern is usual interstitial pneumonia (UIP), and, in the absence of identifiable secondary causes, this is diagnostic of cryptogenic fibrosing alveolitis (CFA)/idiopathic pulmonary fibrosis (IPF; fig. 3). The incidence and prevalence of ILD are poorly documented. This is due in part to difficulties in diagnosis. Estimates have been given at 11 males and seven females per $100,000 \cdot yr^{-1}$ in New Mexico (USA), whilst in Nottingham (UK) a prevalence estimate of six cases per 100,000 was reported [2]. Recent reports have suggested that the prevalence rates are 5–10 times higher than previously reported, i.e. 20.2 and 13.2 cases per 100,000 persons per year for males and females, respectively [3].

The majority of deaths attributed to ILD occur in patients aged >55 yrs. In a British Thoracic Society study of nearly 600 cases, the mean age at presentation was 67.4 yrs. These patients have usually been symptomatic with breathlessness and cough for ~1 yr. There may be basal inspiratory crackles, bilateral radiographic shadowing predominant in the lower zones and restrictive lung function abnormalities. Connective tissue diseases (CTDs) can present their lung manifestations in a disease-specific manner (table 1). Rheumatoid arthritis (RA) may present in advance of joint symptoms with lung nodules. Systemic lupus erythematosus (SLE) can present as adult respiratory distress syndrome (ARDS) or pleurisy. The diagnostic gold standard, as alluded to above, is still lung biopsy, although clear-cut cases of CFA/IPF may have a confident diagnosis by using a high-resolution computed tomography (HRCT) scan. HRCT is also useful for selecting the site of a lung biopsy. If possible, this should be taken from the advancing edge of disease, rather than areas with established fibrosis. The American Thoracic Society (ATS)/European Respiratory Society (ERS) recently stated that in >50% of cases suspected of having CFA/IPF, the presence of typical clinical and HRCT features of this

Eur Respir Mon, 2007, 39, 170–188. Printed in UK - all rights reserved. Copyright ERS Journals Ltd 2007; European Respiratory Monograph; ISSN 1025-448x.

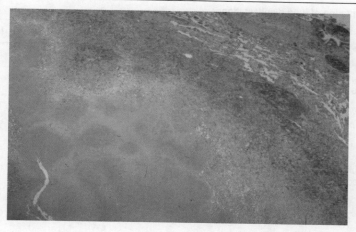

Fig. 1. – Rheumatoid nodule showing a large area of acellular necrosis with some peripheral collapsed alveolar tissue.

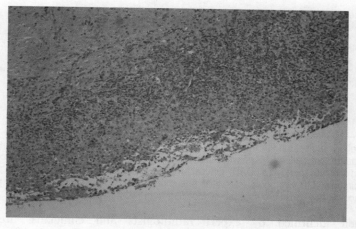

Fig. 2. – Rheumatoid pleurisy with a marked chronic inflammatory reaction and underlying fibrosis. The histological findings are nonspecific and there is no typical pallisading of histiocytes.

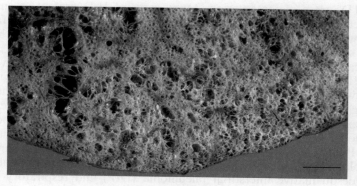

Fig. 3. – Lower lobe interstitial pulmonary fibrosis. Scale bar=10 mm.

Table 1. – Presentation of lung manifestations

CTD	RA	SLE	SSc	DM/PM	SS	MCTD	AS
Pleural lesions							
Pleuritis	+	+	+	+	+	+	+
Spontaneous pneumothorax	+	-	-	+	-	-	+
Interstitial disease							
DAD	+	+	+	+	-	+	-
UIP	+	+	+	+	+	+	-
OP	+	+	+	+	+	+	-
LIP	+	-	-	-	+	+	-
NSIP	+	+	+	+	+	+	-
Amyloid	+	-	-	-	+	-	+
Atypical fibrobullous disease	+	-	+	-	-	+	+
Rheumatoid nodules	+	-	-	-	-	+	-
Airway lesions							
RB	+	-	-	-	-	+	-
Bronchiectasis	+	+	-	-	-	+	-
Alveolar lesions							
Pulmonary haemorrhage	+	+	+	+	-	+	-
Eosinophilic pneumonia	+	-	-	-	-	+	-
Vascular lesions							
Vasculitis	-	+	+	+	+	+	
Pulmonary hypertension	+	+	+	+	+	+	-
Thromboembolism	-	+	-	-	-	-	-
Indirect effects							
Thoracic cage immobility	+	-	-	+	-	+	-
Cricoarytenoid arthritis	+	+	-	-	-	-	+
Diaphragmatic dysfunction	-	-	+	-	-	+	-
Shrinking atelectasis	-	+	-	-	-	-	-
Xerotrachea	-	-	-	-	+	-	-
Neoplasia							
Lung cancer	-	-	+	+	-	+	+
Lymphoma	-	-	-	-	+	+	-

CTD: connective tissue disease; RA: rheumatoid arthritis; SLE: systemic lupus erythematosus; SSc: systemic sclerosis; DM: dermatomyositis; PM: polymyositis; SS: Sjogren's syndrome; MCTD: mixed connective tissue disease; AS: ankylosing spondylitis; DAD: diffuse alveolar damage; UIP: usual interstitial pneumonia; OP: organising pneumonia; LIP: lymphoid interstitial pneumonia; NSIP: nonspecific interstitial pneumonia; RB: respiratory bronchiolitis; +: positive; -: negative. Modified from [4], with permission.

disease, when identified by expert radiologists and clinicians, are sufficiently characteristic for a confident diagnosis, in the absence of a surgical lung biopsy [5]. One of these was by bi-basilar, reticular abnormalities with minimal ground-glass opacities on HRCT. However, exclusion criteria of other known causes of ILD, including CTD, are a major criterion. Many cases of ILD present as end-stage lung disease. Patients often present late on with established disease due to the fact that they feel that "slowing up" is part of a normal ageing. Patients in their 60s may be taking less exercise and so breathlessness only manifests on exercise.

Pathological diagnosis is an opinion. Recently, the presence of interobserver pathology variation in ILD has been highlighted. NICHOLSON et al. [6] showed a 50% interobserver variation between nonspecific interstitial pneumonia (NSIP) and UIP. Pathologists were good at diagnosing sarcoidosis and organising pneumonia (OP), but were poorer at diagnosing extrinsic allergic alveolitis and NSIP. HRCT showed good agreement between regional teaching centres [6]. HRCT was least discriminating with NSIP and poor with OP and smoking-related interstitial disease, but better with sarcoidosis and allergic alveolitis. Histology in ILD relates to outcome. Response to treatment was more frequent in desquamative interstitial pneumonia (DIP) and respiratory bronchiolitis (RB)-ILD than in NSIP or UIP [7].

Ultrastructure and pathogenesis in IIP/ILD

Defining a temporal sequence of histopathological change in ILD has been problematic. Many papers state that macrophage alveolitis, referred to as DIP pattern, characterises the early stages of the lung lesion [8]. NAGAO *et al.* [9] suggested that UIP pattern, in the CTD context, as opposed to CFA/IPF, has fewer alveolar macrophages, but rather lymphocytosis (lymphocytic interstitial pneumonia). However, in that paper, there were only nine CTD cases, other than six systemic sclerosis (SSc) cases. In this small series totalling 31 cases, it is obviously difficult to base firm conclusions. This is a recurring problem, as few centres have a vast experience of the histopathology of CTD-ILD.

Some cases of IIP/ILD and CTD-ILD may present with ARDS or acute interstitial pneumonia (AIP). This is usually associated with the histological pattern of diffuse alveolar damage (DAD), but a localised form of the process of regional alveolar damage has been described in 10% of adult autopsies [10]. It is postulated that this process, in a microscopic form, may be the initiating event in the alveolar wall. It is well known that ARDS/AIP may progress to established ILD and, therefore, this is a good model for consideration of the pathogenesis of the disease. Ultrastructural studies of ARDS in humans, for obvious reasons, are not well described [11]. A series of patients who had open lung biopsies before and after cardiopulmonary bypass for coronary artery disease were examined. This is a well-known potential cause of ARDS. No cases had hyaline membranes or an active neutrophilic infiltration in pulmonary capillaries or alveolar walls on light or electron microscopy. The changes tended to be more severe post-bypass and consisted of damage to type I pneumocytes (fig. 4) with the formation of papillary processes, enlargement of the cell, increase in mitochondrial size and separation from the basement membrane. Type II pneumocyte damage, oedema of the basement membrane and focal endothelial damage were also found (fig. 5). One patient with sickle cell trait developed frank ARDS, which resulted in death [12]. No other patient in the series died or suffered pulmonary complications, despite the electron microscopic changes.

KATZENSTEIN [13] studied seven cases of progressive AIP. These cases were further advanced than those studied by the current authors, in that the changes were cytoplasmic oedema and loss of type I epithelium, with focal-to-extensive denudation of alveolar epithelial cell membranes, cytoplasmic oedema and necrosis of type II cells, and

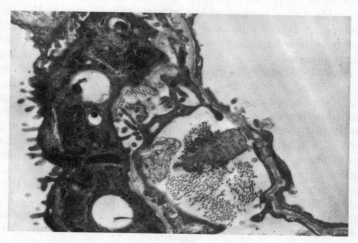

Fig. 4. – Ultrastructure of the alveolar wall post-bypass with loss of type I pneumocyte cytoplasm on the right-hand side and papillary foci in the same cells on the left-hand side.

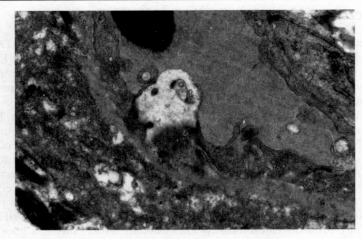

Fig. 5. – Early adult respiratory distress syndrome with fibrin lining a denuded alveolar cell and focal electron lucency in an endothelial cell.

sloughing of capillary endothelial cells. Cell debris, admixed with fibrin, erythrocytes and surfactant-like material, was often layered along the alveolar surfaces, most prominently in the cases in which hyaline membranes were seen by light microscopy. Such hyaline membranes were not present in the current chapter. In addition, these authors found scattered inflammatory cells, usually macrophages, lymphocytes and plasma cells within alveolar spaces. Similar cells, as well as fibroblasts and scattered difficult to classify primitive mesenchymal cells, were also identified in the interstitium. The cells were usually separated by an oedematous stroma, which also contained various amounts of collagen and elastin. However, the paper described two other main observations: 1) collapse and apposition of alveolar septa; and 2) incorporation of intra-alveolar exudates into the alveolar septa. Figures 4 and 5 show partial collapse, which affected numerous alveoli in all cases. This was usually in areas in which the epithelial basal lamina was denuded. There was folding of epithelial basal lamina upon themselves, with a formation of deep clefts that extended into the alveolar septa. This collapse and apposition probably occurs because of loss of surfactant from type II cells. This means that there is no "nonwettable" material to keep the alveolar walls apart. Some of the involved alveolar septa were oedematous, containing few cells and occasional collagen bundles. Others possessed more numerous fibroblasts, inflammatory cells and collagen bundles. As type II pneumocytes proliferated to re-epithelialise the denuded basal lamina, the cytoplasm often covered the surfaces of the infolded clefts, rather than extending into them. Therefore, as part of the normal reparative process, a portion of the alveolus remained permanently collapsed. This led to the light microscopic appearance of a thickened or fibrotic alveolar septum. In some areas, a tangle of basal lamina was found beneath the epithelium, as if part of the alveolar wall had contracted upon itself following the initial loss of lining cells. Occasionally, entire alveoli had collapsed but this change was less frequent than partial collapse. In addition to these changes, loose basement membrane fragmentation that varied in length was found deep within the interstitium, unattached to the surface. These membranes do not appear to be related to endothelial cells, fibroblasts or inflammatory cells. It was thought that most membranes represented remnants of basal laminae and previous incorporated portions of alveolar walls. Some may have come from destroyed capillaries. The other process that was part of AIP/DAD was incorporation of intra-alveolar exudates into alveolar septa. This can be seen in any OP, whatever the cause, and is also present in established UIP, where fibroblastic foci become incorporated into the established interstitial fibrosis. This phenomenon of incorporation of intra-alveolar exudates is more difficult to demonstrate ultrastructurally in alveolar collapse. However, it can be seen clearly by light microscopy.

Part of the progressive nature of IPF is due to the loss of subepithelial basement membrane integrity [14]. The likelihood is that the loss of the alveolar epithelium due to cell death causes an absence of the protective barrier. Exposure of the underlying basement membrane to various oxidative injuries causes degradation of some of the key constituents. Epithelial cell regeneration probably occurs as a resort of failure of these cells to attach to the underlying basement membrane and provides signals to stop epithelial cell proliferation.

Cytokines and type II pneumocyte apoptosis

Type II cell injury may be an important early feature in the pathogenesis of ILD. Electron microscopic studies have shown injury and apoptosis to these cells in lung biopsies from patients with CFA/IPF [10, 15–17]. There was increased expression of pro-apoptotic proteins in alveolar epithelial cells and bronchoalveolar lavage (BAL) cells in CFA/IPF. There is strong suggestion of increased oxidative stress in the alveolar epithelium in patients with CFA/IPF [14, 18]. Fibroblasts from cases of IPF may produce angiotensin-like peptides that promote epithelial apoptosis [19]. A key factor in fibrosis is transforming growth factor (TGF)-β, which also promotes epithelial cell apoptosis [20]. TGF-β is not the only pro-fibrotic cytokine, but it appears to be the most potent [21]. The repair fibrotic cytokines include platelet-derived growth factor (PDGF), insulin-like growth factor-1, basic fibroblast growth factor, interleukin (IL)-10 and IL-13.

TGF-β is a member of a family of growth differentiation factors, including bone morphogenetic proteins. It effects proliferation and differentiation in many cell types and acts both as a growth inhibitor and stimulator. It also induces synthesis of extracellular matrix proteins, modulates the expression of matrix proteases and protease inhibitors, increases integrin expression, causing enhanced cell adhesion and plays an important part in the wound healing [21]. It produces mesenchymal differentiation and is a potent chemotactic agent for various cell types, including fibroblasts. It causes progressive deposition of collagens, elastin, proteoglycans and fibronectin. There are three mammalian isoforms of TGF-β (1–3), each of which is encoded by a separate gene [22]. TGF-β1 is released by activated macrophages, lymphocytes and platelets. The recruitment of mesenchymal cells, including myofibroblasts, is induced by TGF-β, as well as PDGF. These two cytokines are potent chemotactic factors for fibroblasts. There is polymorphism in the TGF-β1 gene. It has been shown that TGF-β1 genotype has prognostic significance in transplant patients. Patients requiring lung transplantation for fibrotic lung conditions had an increase in the frequency of the TGF-β1 allele associated with a high production of TGF-β1 (codon 25 arginine-proline). This allele was significantly associated with pre-transplant fibrotic pathology, when compared with controls (p<0.02) and with pre-transplant nonfibrotic pathology (p<0.004) [23]. Further study is required in the various forms of ILD.

Another cytokine, which has received attention in pulmonary fibrosis, is tumour necrosis factor (TNF)-α. The TNF-α gene is located on the short arm of chromosome 6, being closely linked to the major histocompatibility complex. The principal cellular sources of TNF-α are blood monocytes and tissue macrophages. It is an important mediator of acute lung injury, which can be seen alongside areas of established interstitial pulmonary fibrosis. In ARDS, TNF-α may be orchestrating the inflammatory response by activating pro-inflammatory cytokine genes, such as IL-1 and IL-6, as well as its own production. TNF-α promotes apoptosis in alveolar epithelial cells [24]. TNF-α expression is increased in type II cells in patients with CFA/IPF [25].

CTD-ILD: the role of auto-immunity

ILD is established as a clinical corollary across the spectrum of CTDs, with an overall incidence estimated at 15% [26]. The CTD group of rheumatic diseases includes RA, SLE, SSc, dermatomyositis (DM)/polymyositis (PM), mixed CTD (MCTD) and Sjogren's syndrome (SS). Rates of ILD differ between these diseases. Using HRCT to detect ILD in CTD patient cohorts (cohort sizes ranging 21–156), prevalence varies from 19% in RA to 67 and 85% in MCTD and diffuse SSc, respectively [27–30]. Intermediate prevalence in the range 23–38% is found in SLE and DM/PM [31–33]. These rheumatic diseases are grouped together under the heading of CTD for several reasons. First, clinical manifestations are often similar between CTDs (*e.g.* articular synovitis or Raynaud's phenomenon). Secondly, although the individual diseases have specific classification criteria applicable to the majority of clinical cases, a significant number of patients present with features that overlap from one entity to another (*i.e.* MCTD), or alternatively there are those in which one CTD evolves into another over the course of several years. Thirdly, the pathology of involved tissue invariably evinces a greater or lesser degree of chronic inflammation. Fourthly, there is aetiological evidence for dysregulated immunity driving inflammation in these diseases, for instance in the generation of limited repertoires of specific auto-antibodies and autoreactive T-lymphocytes [34]. In the CTD context, the occurrence of ILD represents one facet of the multisystem nature of these disorders. Therefore, it seems reasonable to postulate an inflammatory/immune aetiology for CTD-ILD. Furthermore, for many years, it was assumed that IIP/ILD shared this immune aetiology with CTD-ILD. Research findings in either of these entities were considered applicable to both. However, this has been questioned more recently, due in large to the improved recognition of histopathological subtypes of ILD [5, 35]. This has permitted a clear distinction to be drawn between UIP and other patterns, such as cellular NSIP, RB and OP. It has been suggested that while the UIP pattern predominates in idiopathic ILD, it only accounts for a minority of cases in CTD-ILD [36]. Therefore, it seems possible that these are substantially different diseases, with UIP a nonimmune-mediated pattern predominantly found in IIP/ILD, and non-UIP patterns, which are immune mediated and found in CTD-ILD. However, the current authors question whether the evidence that is presently available allows for this simplistic approach.

Making a distinction between CTD-ILD and IIP/ILD

CTD-ILD and IIP/ILD look like two different conditions. Most of the current literature draws distinctions between them in terms of the frequency of associated histological pattern, natural history and response to treatment. ILD case series for which histology is available evince ~60% UIP and 20% NSIP, while the (significantly smaller) series of CTD-ILD show 5% UIP and 40% NSIP [36–39]. UIP in both IIP/ILD and CTD-ILD carries a 5-yr survival rate of ~40%, whilst 5-yr survival for NSIP is much higher at 90–100% [7, 36, 37, 40–42]. Therapeutic response to corticosteroids in one series of IIP/ILD was 17% for UIP and 40% for NSIP [37]. Comparable data for CTD-ILD are lacking. Taken together, these data would suggest that IIP/ILD and CTD-ILD are indeed different diseases. Furthermore, overall prognosis in CTD-ILD appears to be superior to that in IIP/ILD, as has been suggested [26, 32, 43]. However, the largest study designed to formally compare outcome in these two groups unexpectedly showed that there was no difference in mortality, and pointed to confounding variables that can account for apparent differences in prognosis [44]. First are the confounding effects of diagnosis. CTD precedes ILD in most cases and, therefore, patients are already under close surveillance prior to development of ILD. They are more likely to participate in case-finding investigations such as HRCT and pulmonary function testing. As a result, ILD is detected earlier, which will improve time-delineated outcome. Secondly, there are confounding effects of variations in medical management. CTD patients are less likely to undergo biopsy and more likely to receive aggressive immunotherapy than their ILD counterparts, which might also make outcome appear intrinsically better. Finally, there are confounding effects of variations in patient population, with CTD patients more likely to be female and younger [45]. Smoking rates are likely to also differ [44]. However, it is important to bear in mind that all-cause mortality in CTD-ILD will also include nonrespiratory deaths due to the CTD itself.

In summary, it is not possible at present to be conclusive on whether CTD-ILD is the same as or different to idiopathic ILD. This is because of the lack of comparative studies with large enough numbers in the CTD-ILD group. Certainly IIP/ILD is a heterogeneous disease, with diverse potential triggers (infections, environmental exposures) and diverse disease patterns (UIP, NSIP, etc.). Auto-immunity will surely be the initiating factor in some patients, and these are likely to resemble those with CTD-ILD (in that they are more likely to have NSIP than UIP, for example) [46, 47]. Furthermore, some IIP/ILD patients are actually CTD patients whose ILD precedes the onset of CTD. Conversely, the majority of CTD-ILD is likely to be immune mediated. Nevertheless, a significant subset of these patients will have other triggers, such as infection or drug toxicity. This nonimmune-mediated subset of CTD-ILD may more closely resemble nonimmune-mediated idiopathic ILD, and may correlate with the small UIP subset in CTD-ILD. Research in this area is hampered by the lack of reliable clinical markers that allow for distinction between immune-mediated and other cases.

Histological disease patterns in CTD-ILD

How successfully have the ATS/ERS classification criteria been applied to the patterns of lung histology in CTD-ILD? This question is important as current thinking seeks to infer mechanistic hypotheses in the different histological patterns. For example, the different histological patterns may represent a range of possible, mutually independent, disease outcomes. Some authors, according to this view, seek a correlation between the various causative triggers and the histological end-points. Others posit that outcome is independent of trigger, and is either stochastic or related to other, unidentified genetic or environmental factors. Alternatively, there is the view that the patterns are related to one another and represent different stages of the same pathological process, with DIP or DAD progressing to UIP or fibrotic NSIP, and eventually to end-stage lung disease. Clearly, as a basis for further research, accurate prevalence rates for the different patterns in CTD-ILD are required. Detailed descriptions of the pathology of CTD-ILD are given in a recent review article [48]. There is much crossover in the microscopic pattern seen in CTD-ILD between the various CTDs; this is shown in table 1. Several studies have described the aforementioned predominance of NSIP over UIP in CTD-ILD [38]. The largest is a series of 39 cases, which showed that NSIP was the most common overall pattern in patients with RA, DM/PM, SLE and SS [36]. These authors found that DM/PM commonly showed OP, whereas rheumatoid disease showed follicular bronchiolitis and SS showed chronic bronchiolitis. Only four patients showed a pattern of UIP: two with RA and one each with DM/PM and SLE. Nevertheless, these trends were nonsignificant due to small individual CTD sample sizes. Other patterns described in review articles of SLE are vasculitis (fig. 6), which may involve the alveolar capillaries (fig. 7). SSc was not included in the aforementioned series as the authors reported 80 biopsies from SSc-ILD patients separately [43]. Again, the majority of patients showed NSIP (78%) with only six UIP patients. In addition, SSc may present as pulmonary hypertension (fig. 8) with intimal fibrosis in pulmonary arteries and arterioles. In some cases, this may take on the same onion-skin pattern as seen in the kidney in this disease.

The apparent clinico-pathological association between CTD-ILD and NSIP must be

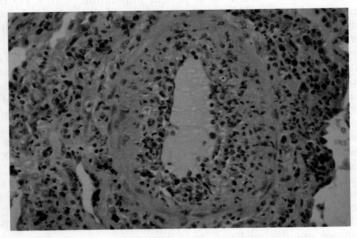

Fig. 6. – Systemic lupus erythematosus with a neutrophilic infiltrate in a muscular pulmonary arterial wall (vasculitis). There is no inflammation in the adjacent lung, excluding a pneumonic process as the cause of the capillaritis.

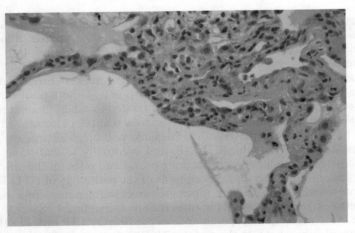

Fig. 7. – Systemic lupus erythematosus with a neutrophilic infiltrate in capillary walls. There is no inflammation in the adjacent lung, excluding a pneumonic process as the cause of the capillaritis.

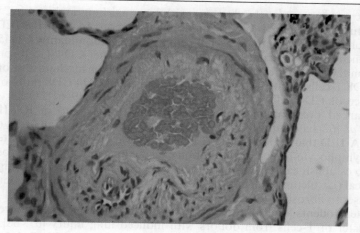

Fig. 8. – Scleroderma with muscular and intimal thickening of the vascular wall.

interpreted with caution. Sample sizes are too small to allow for accurate prevalence rates for the different patterns, particularly in analyses of individual CTD-ILDs. Indeed, a series of 18 RA-ILD biopsies showed that UIP was the most frequent pattern (n=10) with NSIP (n=6) and OP (n=2) in the minority [41]. These discrepancies may reflect geographical variation (*i.e.* Korean *versus* UK study populations). However, other points to consider are as follows. First, interobserver variability in assigning histological pattern is not particularly high, with kappa coefficients in the range of 0.6–0.8 [7]. Secondly, many patients (55% in the largest combined series) have findings of more than one histological pattern in different lung areas [49, 50]. These factors compound the problem of small sample size. At this point, one can only be cautious in one's conclusions. It appears that any interstitial pneumonia pattern can occur in any individual CTD. It also appears that NSIP is the most common pattern, but this is only really convincing in the disease with the highest rate of ILD and, therefore, the largest sample sizes, *i.e.* SSc [43, 51]. In contrast, the evidence for the predominance of NSIP is conflicting in RA-ILD and weak in DM/PM-ILD. Furthermore, at this stage, it appears that DAD is a consistent feature in a minority of patients with DM/PM who present clinically with AIP [33, 52, 53]. In summary, one cannot readily generalise findings in one CTD to another, due to apparent differences in individual pattern prevalence and overall rate of ILD in each CTD. Therefore, the clinical evidence that any individual interstitial pneumonia pattern (in this case NSIP) is strongly linked, by its association with CTD, to a putative auto-immune aetiology is currently insufficient. Any histological pattern may be linked to auto-immunity, but the probability for such an association at this point appears to be greater for NSIP than for UIP.

Immunopathogenesis of ILD

Histological analysis of the cellular inflammation

Lymphocytes are rarely found in the interstitium of the normal lung. Therefore, it is striking that the predominant infiltrating inflammatory cell in ILD is the lymphocyte. This observation holds true whether the pattern is UIP or NSIP [5, 54–56]. The presence of lymphocytes suggests that an antigen-specific immune process occurs. It is not clear whether that process causes the damage to the normal lung architecture, which is the cardinal feature of ILD, or is merely an epiphenomenon. In both IIP/ILD and CTD-ILD, T-lymphocytes predominate over B-cells and are predominantly CD45RO positive (antigen primed) [57, 58]. Data are conflicting over whether CD4 T-cells predominately facilitate monocyte (T-helper (Th)1) or B-cell (Th2) effector mechanisms, or the directly cytotoxic CD8 T-cells. Some studies have shown an equal CD4/CD8 ratio, or a moderate predominance of CD4 cells in idiopathic UIP and NSIP [59–61]. Other studies have shown a marked predominance of CD8 cells in IIP/ILD and in RA-ILD [62, 63]. TURESSON *et al.* [62] have reported that the lymphocytic infiltrate is an order of magnitude greater in RA-ILD than in idiopathic ILD, irrespective of whether the pattern is UIP or NSIP. Is T-lymphocyte-driven inflammation causing lung damage and fibrosis in ILD? It is difficult to establish causality from human studies. This has been investigated in mice using chemical (*i.e.* bleomycin), particle (*i.e.* silica) or radiation-induced acute lung injury that progresses to fibrosis. Fibrosis has been shown to be inhibited in T-cell-deficient and T-cell-depleted rodents [64–66]. Furthermore, lung fibrosis has been induced in mice by passive transfer of T-cells from donors with induced lung injury [67, 68]. Conversely, several studies have shown fibrosis to be entirely independent of T-cells [69–73]. Thus, at this stage, it is equally feasible that the lymphocytic infiltrate in ILD is a response to alveolar damage or its cause.

T-lymphocytes cannot mount an antigen-driven immune response without interaction with antigen-presenting cells. In spite of their importance, professional antigen-presenting cells, termed dendritic cells, are relatively understudied, both generally and in ILD. One study in IIP/ILD using S-100 as a marker of dendritic cells showed that UIP and NSIP could be clearly differentiated in a way that lymphocyte studies have been unable to achieve. S-100 dendritic cells were abundant in NSIP but uniformly absent in UIP. Furthermore, in NSIP, dendritic cells were surrounded by T-lymphocytes, and specifically in fibrotic areas, these T-cell aggregates were predominantly CD8 cells [63]. Further work is required to establish whether dendritic cell activation is driving a CD8 T-cell response and subsequent fibrosis.

Immunohistochemical analysis of cytokines in ILD

If interstitial lung inflammation and fibrosis is driven by an immune response, there will be an increase in inflammatory/immune-signalling cytokines in the lung interstitium. Furthermore, one would expect the cytokine profile to be skewed according to the profile of one of the two CD4 T-cell subsets, Th1 and Th2. Several studies have confirmed an increase in cytokine production in lung biopsies from ILD compared with those from nondiseased lung. These studies consistently show Th2 predominance [59, 74]. This is the case in idiopathic NSIP, CFA/IPF (UIP pattern disease) and SSc-ILD. In keeping with the idea that UIP is a noninflammatory process, cytokine levels in UIP are considerably lower than those found in other interstitial pneumonia patterns [59, 75]. However, in contradiction to the "noninflammatory UIP" hypothesis, cytokine levels in UIP, albeit lower than in NSIP or SSc-ILD, are even more skewed towards Th2 than in NSIP or SSc-ILD [76]. Furthermore, a study on cytokine receptors showed that key Th2 cytokine receptor α-chains, IL13Rα and IL4Rα, are expressed considerably more in UIP than in either NSIP or RB-ILD [77]. Also, it appears that IL-4 levels increase progressively during the course of CFA/IPF [78]. Similar findings have been reported in studies on BAL cells, although there is uncertainty as to the degree of correlation between BAL findings and histological analysis [57, 60, 61, 79]. Consistent with these observations of Th2 cytokine predominance in ILD are data on chemokine and chemokine receptor expression. Again, Th2-chemoattractant chemokine–chemokine ligand pairs are preferentially expressed in both UIP and SSc-ILD (CCR4 and CCL22, for instance) [76, 79]. In summary, studies on cytokine expression suggest that the inflammatory cells present in the lung interstitium in ILD are activated and produce a cytokine milieu that is permissive for an immune effector response, which could then lead to tissue damage. No cytokine studies convincingly differentiate between IIP/ILD and CTD-ILD, or between UIP and NSIP. In all of these situations, the conditions required for an effective local immune response are present.

The role of humoral immunity in ILD

T-cells and T-cell-derived cytokines are not the only immune components detected in lung biopsies in ILD. B-cells are also present and were found to comprise 27% of total mononuclear cells in a study on NSIP [59]. Furthermore, a study on CFA/IPF showed that not only are B-lymphocytes present, but that they organise into aggregates similar to mucosal-associated lymphoid tissue and, in a minority of cases, germinal centres were observed [80]. This suggests that conditions required for a local humoral immune response are present in ILD. Therefore, what is the evidence for auto-antibody production? It is that clear differences emerge between IIP/ILD and CTD-ILD. There is a large body of evidence indicating that CTD-ILD is associated with the presence of auto-antibodies in a way that IIP/ILD is not. These auto-antibodies are associated with the underlying CTD with a high specificity and, furthermore, are often markers for increased frequency of ILD as a manifestation. In PM, the Jo-1 antibody is found in 11–30% of cases [81, 82]. If ILD is also present, the Jo-1 positivity rate increases to 40–70% [33, 52, 83–85]. Jo-1 is directed against histidyl-tRNA synthetase, which catalyses the binding of the histidine to its cognate tRNA during protein synthesis. Jo-1 is the most common of a family of anti-synthetase auto-antibodies. The other anti-synthetase antibodies (PL-7: anti-threonyl-tRNA synthetase; PL-12: anti-alanyl-tRNA synthetase; anti-KS: anti-asparagyl-tRNA synthetase; anti-OJ: anti-isoleucyl-tRNA synthetase) have been described recently, and prevalence rates are lower (<1–2%) [81, 86]. Intriguingly, small-number case series with the minor anti-synthetase antibodies consistently showed that the ILD rate is extremely high (90–100%) [87]. Furthermore, some cases evince ILD without PM [88, 89]. This has prompted the notion that anti-synthetase syndrome is an overlap CTD entity in its own right, with a stronger association to ILD than to other features, such as myositis and inflammatory arthritis [81, 86].

The second auto-antibody group, strongly associated with CTD-ILD, is found in patients with SSc. In total, 10–20% of diffuse cutaneous scleroderma cases are positive for Scl-70, which is an antibody against DNA topoisomerase I. The presence of the antibody is a marker for the development of lung disease, therefore, the Scl-70 positivity rate in SSc-ILD is 50% [90]. Anti-centromere antibodies are a marker of the localised cutaneous form of SSc, which is present in 60% of cases. In contrast to Scl-70, this auto-antibody is negatively associated with CTD-ILD, and anti-centromere-positive patients are more likely to develop primary pulmonary hypertension in the absence of ILD (fig. 8) [91]. The third auto-antibody group associated with CTD-ILD is found in patients with CTD overlap syndromes. These antibodies include anti-U1-ribonucleoprotein (RNP) and PM-Scl (Rrna-processing exosome complex) [92]. Both of these are markers of overlap disease in which ILD is frequently a feature, with anti-U1-RNP-associated CTD known as MCTD [86, 93, 94]. There are other CTD-related auto-antibodies, such as rheumatoid factor and anti-citrullinated peptide in RA, and anti-Sm and anti-dsDNA in SLE; however, these antibodies have not been shown to be significantly associated with the development of ILD in those conditions.

Thus, CTD-ILD can be seen to be frequently associated with the generation of an auto-antibody response, which is highly CTD specific. The same can not be said for IIP/ILD. In this disease group, a high frequency of up to 40% of auto-antibodies has been reported in early studies [95, 96]. However, the range of antigen specificities is wide. A small sample of reported target auto-antigens includes vimentin, IL-1α, cytokeratins 18 and 19, topoisomerase II, collagen and ribonucleoprotein [95, 97–101]. Furthermore, the sensitivities of each individual candidate auto-antibody, and their specificity for IIP/ILD, have not been high enough to deem them as true clinical markers. For the same reason, it is not likely that the auto-immune response against any one of these antigens will play a significant pathogenetic role in ILD. However, generally speaking, the generation of auto-antibodies is a feature seen in both IIP/ILD and CTD-ILD. How are these antibodies generated? The Jo-1 antibody provides a good example of function in this area [81]. The target antigen, histidyl-tRNA synthetase, has an intracellular function, and has been localised in cytoplasm, nucleus and nucleolus. Therefore, it is protected from exposure to the immune system. It has been suggested that an immune response to RNA from picornavirus generates Jo-1 antibody, which then binds to its auto-antigenic target *via* molecular mimicry [102]. Another possibility is that apoptotic cells, or blebs, express caspase- or granzyme B-modified forms of Jo-1 antigen on the cell surface. These neoantigens are not recognised as self and trigger an antibody response. A third possibility arises from the observation that cleaved tRNA can be secreted and can bind to chemokine receptors, leading to the recruitment of immune and inflammatory cells [103]. Finally, recombinant fragments of Jo-1 antigen have been shown to drive T-cell proliferation in the presence of antigen presenting cells. However, this process is independent of whether the T-cell donor was a healthy control or a Jo-1-positive patient [104]. What is the direct evidence that auto-antibodies can participate in lung injury? A histological and ultrastructural study, including 42 biopsies from IIP/ILD and CTD-ILD, found no evidence of antigen-antibody complex deposition within alveolar hyaline membranes [105]. The single exception was one case of SLE-ILD, in which immunoglobulin and complement was detected in alveolar capillary walls and the alveolar hyaline membrane. Therefore, in some, but not all, SLE-ILD cases, the auto-antibodies target their cognate antigens and form circulating immune complexes, which subsequently deposit in the lung parenchyma where they fix complement and trigger an inflammatory process. However, this pathogenic mechanism does not account for the majority of cases of IIP/ILD or CTD-ILD. In conclusion, a humoral response occurs in ILD and represents a possible pathogenic mechanism; however, it could equally arise as a result or epiphenomenon of the disease process [106].

Conclusions

The association of ILD with underlying CTD suggests that immunopathogenetic mechanisms are involved in interstitial pneumonia. An auto-immune process is one of many potential aetiologies, which can cause injury to cellular elements of the lung parenchyma. It is not clear whether this process is directed against one or several defined lung-specific auto-antigens, or whether immune-mediated inflammation localises to the lung for other, unidentified reasons. The result of this cellular injury is a loss of pneumocytes and alveolar collapse. As repair processes are induced, there probably follows a range of divergent pathways, giving rise to different histological patterns of interstitial pneumonia and different clinical outcomes. This diversity may be determined in part by genetic or environmental factors affecting expression and function of fibrogenic mediators such as TGF-β and, in part, by the nature of the initiating injury. The inflammatory milieu that either accompanies or instigates this process is likely to be characterised by Th2 lymphocyte-derived cytokines. Alongside this, auto-antibodies can be elaborated but the evidence for their direct pathogenicity is lacking. Immune-mediated interstitial pneumonia may well result in more cellular patterns of lung injury, with temporally heterogeneous fibrogenesis, in contrast to nonimmune-mediated disease in which a UIP outcome is more likely.

Keynote messages

1) CTDs strongly associate with the development of ILD.
2) Immune-mediated inflammation is one of the causes of ILD.
3) The diverse histological patterns of interstitial pneumonia may represent stages in the evolution of the disease or a range of possible outcomes.
4) Injury to cellular elements of lung parenchyma and alveolar collapse are followed by varying degrees of organising inflammation and fibrogenesis.
5) The cytokine milieu is likely to inform this process and is characterised by Th2 and pro-fibrotic cytokines.
6) CTD-ILD differs from IIP in that association with specific auto-antibodies is strong.
7) In contrast to IIP, in CTD-ILD the histological pattern of UIP appears to be unusual.

Summary

Interstitial lung diseases are heterogeneous, encompassing a variety of aetiological factors. There is considerable variability in histological appearance over time in an individual patient and across the patient population. Light and electron microscopy reveal common themes, such as injury and apoptosis of the cellular elements of the lung parenchyma, basement membrane fragmentation, alveolar collapse and hyaline membrane formation. Organising inflammation and fibrogenesis are more variable features.

The different histological patterns may represent a temporal sequence of changes within the evolution of disease, with focal or diffuse alveolar damage, as seen in adult respiratory distress syndrome or acute interstitial pneumonia. Alternatively, they represent a range of possible end-points, perhaps reflecting different aetiological factors. For instance, usual interstitial pneumonia is seen as a nonimmune-mediated process. This range of outcome is also informed by genetic or other variation in expression and function of pro-fibrotic mediators. The strong clinical association between interstitial lung disease and connective tissue diseases provides a clear argument for a role for auto-immunity in the pathogenesis of some interstitial pneumonia. Clear differentiation of immune interstitial pneumonia from other types has not been achieved, due to both inherent and sampling variability.

There is considerable evidence for an activation of the adaptive immune system in interstitial lung disease, and also for the generation of auto-antibodies. However, the precise role of immune dysregulation in the pathogenesis of this disease remains unknown.

Keywords: Adult respiratory distress syndrome, immunopathogenesis, interstitial lung disease.

References

1. Hasleton PS. Fibrosing alveolitis. *In:* Hasleton PS, ed. Spencer's Pathology of the Lung. 5th Edn. New York, McGraw Hill, 1996; p. 402.

2. Johnston IDA, Prescott RJ, Chalmers JC, Rudd RM. British Thoracic Society study of cryptogenic fibrosing alveolitis: current presentation and initial management. *Thorax* 1997; 52: 38–44.

3. Coultas DB, Zumwalt IE, Black WC, Sobonya RE. The epidemiology of interstitial lung diseases. *Am J Respir Crit Care Med* 1994; 150: 967–972.

4. Colby T, Lombard C, Yousem S, Kitaichi M. Atlas of pulmonary surgical pathology. *In:* Bordin G, ed. Atlases in Diagnostic Surgical Pathology. Philadelphia, WB Saunders, 1991; p. 380.

5. American Thoracic Society. European Respiratory Society. American Thoracic Society/European Respiratory Society International Multidisciplinary Consensus Classification of the Idiopathic Interstitial Pneumonias. *Am J Respir Crit Care Med* 2002; 165: 277–304.

6. Nicholson AG, Colby TV, Dubois RM, Hansell DM, Wells U. The prognostic significance of the histologic pattern of interstitial pneumonia in patients presenting with a clinical entity of cryptogenic fibrosing alveolitis. *Am J Respir Crit Care Med* 2000; 162: 2213–2217.

7. Aziz ZA, Wells AU, Hansell DM, *et al.* HRCT diagnosis of diffuse parenchymal lung disease: inter-observer variation. *Thorax* 2004; 59: 5006–5011.

8. Lynch JP 3rd, Hunninghake GW. Pulmonary complications of collagen vascular disease. *Annu Rev Med* 1992; 43: 17–35.

9. Nagao T, Nagai S, Kitaichi M, *et al.* Usual interstitial pneumonia: idiopathic pulmonary fibrosis *versus* collagen vascular diseases. *Respiration* 2001; 68: 151–159.

10. Yazdy AM, Tomashefski JF Jr, Yagan R, Kleinerman J. Regional alveolar damage (RAD): a localised counterpart of diffuse alveolar damage. *Am J Clin Pathol* 1989; 92: 10–15.

11. Hasleton PS. Adult respiratory distress syndrome: a review. *Histopathology* 1983; 7: 307–332.

12. Hasleton PS, Orr K, Webster A, Lawson RAM. Evolution of acute chest syndrome in sickle cell trait: an ultrastructural and light microscopic study. *Thorax* 1989; 44: 1057–1058.

13. Katzenstein LA. "Pathogenesis of fibrosis" in interstitial pneumonia: an electron microscopic study. *Hum Pathol* 1985; 16: 1015–1024.

14. Kuwano K, Hagimoto N, Maeyama T, *et al.* Mitochondria-mediated apoptosis of lung epithelial cells in idiopathic interstitial pneumonias. *Lab Invest* 2002; 82: 1695–1706.

15. Kuwano K, Hagimoto N, Tanaka T, *et al.* Expression of apoptosis-regulatory genes in epithelial cells in pulmonary fibrosis in mice. *J Pathol* 2000; 190: 221–229.

16. Kuwano K, Kawasaki M, Maeyama T, *et al.* Soluble form of fas and fas ligand in BAL fluid from patients with pulmonary fibrosis and bronchiolitis obliterans organising pneumonia. *Chest* 2000; 118: 451–458.

17. Kuwano K, Nakashima N, Inoshima I, *et al.* Oxidative stress in lung epithelial cells from patients with idiopathic interstitial pneumonia. *Eur Respir J* 2003; 21: 232–240.

18. Wang R, Ibarra-Sunga O, Verlinski I, *et al.* Aborogation or bleomycin-induced epithelial apoptosis and lung fibrosis by captopril or caspase inhibiter. *Am J Physiol Lung Cell Mol Physiol* 2000; 279: L143–L151.

19. Hagimoto N, Kuwano K, Inoshima I, *et al.* TGF-beta 1 as an enhancer of Fas-mediated apoptosis of lung epithelial cells. *J Immunol* 2002; 168: 6470–6478.

20. Hasleton PS, Roberts TE. Adult respiratory distress syndrome: an update. *Histopathology* 1999; 34: 285–294.

21. Beck LS, DeGuzman L, Lee WP, *et al.* One systemic administration of transforming growth factor-beta 1 reverses age or glucocorticoid-impaired wound healing. *J Clin Invest* 1993; 92: 2841–2849.

22. Derynck R, Lindquist PB, Lee A, *et al.* A new type of transforming factor-beta, TGF beta 3. *EMBO J* 1988; 7: 3737–3743.

23. Awad MR, El-Gamel A, Hasleton P, Turner DM, Sinnott PJ, Hutchinson IV. Genotypic variation in the transforming growth factor-beta 1 gene in association with transforming growth factor

beta 1 production, fibrotic disease and graft fibrosis after lung transplantation. *Transplantation* 1998; 66: 1014–1020.

24. Wang R, Alam G, Zagarya A, *et al.* Apoptosis of lung epithelial cells in response to TNF-alpha requires angiotensin II generation *de novo. J Cell Physiol* 2000; 185: 253–259.

25. Zhang Y, Lee TC, Guillemin B, *et al.* Enhanced IL-1 beta and tumour necrosis factor-alpha release and messenger RNA expression in macrophages from idiopathic pulmonary fibrosis of after asbestosis exposure. *J Immunol* 1993; 150: 4188–4196.

26. Jindal SK, Agarwal R. Autoimmunity and interstitial lung disease. *Curr Opin Pulm Med* 2005; 11: 438–446.

27. Devenyi K, Czirjak L. High resolution computed tomography for the evaluation of lung involvement in 101 patients with scleroderma. *Clin Rheumatol* 1995; 14: 633–640.

28. Bodolay E, Szekanecz Z, Devenyi K, *et al.* Evaluation of interstitial lung disease in mixed connective tissue disease (MCTD). *Rheumatology (Oxford)* 2005; 44: 656–661.

29. Dawson JK, Fewins HE, Desmond J, Lynch MP, Graham DR. Fibrosing alveolitis in patients with rheumatoid arthritis as assessed by high resolution computed tomography, chest radiography, and pulmonary function tests. *Thorax* 2001; 56: 622–627.

30. Saito Y, Terada M, Takada T, *et al.* Pulmonary involvement in mixed connective tissue disease: comparison with other collagen vascular diseases using high resolution CT. *J Comput Assist Tomogr* 2002; 26: 349–357.

31. Sant SM, Doran M, Fenelon HM, Breatnach ES. Pleuropulmonary abnormalities in patients with systemic lupus erythematosus: assessment with high resolution computed tomography, chest radiography and pulmonary function tests. *Clin Exp Rheumatol* 1997; 15: 507–513.

32. Schnabel A, Reuter M, Biederer J, Richter C, Gross WL. Interstitial lung disease in polymyositis and dermatomyositis: clinical course and response to treatment. *Semin Arthritis Rheum* 2003; 32: 273–284.

33. Marie I, Hachulla E, Cherin P, *et al.* Interstitial lung disease in polymyositis and dermatomyositis. *Arthritis Rheum* 2002; 47: 614–622.

34. Isomaki P, Clark JM, Panesar M, Cope AP. Pathways of T cell activation and terminal differentiation in chronic inflammation. *Curr Drug Targets Inflamm Allergy* 2005; 4: 287–293.

35. Selman M, Thannickal VJ, Pardo A, Zisman DA, Martinez FJ, Lynch JP 3rd. Idiopathic pulmonary fibrosis: pathogenesis and therapeutic approaches. *Drugs* 2004; 64: 405–430.

36. Tansey D, Wells AU, Colby TV, *et al.* Variations in histological patterns of interstitial pneumonia between connective tissue disorders and their relationship to prognosis. *Histopathology* 2004; 44: 585–596.

37. Travis WD, Matsui K, Moss J, Ferrans VJ. Idiopathic nonspecific interstitial pneumonia: prognostic significance of cellular and fibrosing patterns: survival comparison with usual interstitial pneumonia and desquamative interstitial pneumonia. *Am J Surg Pathol* 2000; 24: 19–33.

38. Nakamura Y, Chida K, Suda T, *et al.* Nonspecific interstitial pneumonia in collagen vascular diseases: comparison of the clinical characteristics and prognostic significance with usual interstitial pneumonia. *Sarcoidosis Vasc Diffuse Lung Dis* 2003; 20: 235–241.

39. Ito I, Nagai S, Kitaichi M, *et al.* Pulmonary manifestations of primary Sjogren's syndrome: a clinical, radiologic, and pathologic study. *Am J Respir Crit Care Med* 2005; 171: 632–638.

40. Daniil ZD, Gilchrist FC, Nicholson AG, *et al.* A histologic pattern of nonspecific interstitial pneumonia is associated with a better prognosis than usual interstitial pneumonia in patients with cryptogenic fibrosing alveolitis. *Am J Respir Crit Care Med* 1999; 160: 899–905.

41. Lee HK, Kim DS, Yoo B, *et al.* Histopathologic pattern and clinical features of rheumatoid arthritis-associated interstitial lung disease. *Chest* 2005; 127: 2019–2027.

42. Monaghan H, Wells AU, Colby TV, du Bois RM, Hansell DM, Nicholson AG. Prognostic implications of histologic patterns in multiple surgical lung biopsies from patients with idiopathic interstitial pneumonias. *Chest* 2004; 125: 522–526.

43. Bouros D, Wells AU, Nicholson AG, *et al.* Histopathologic subsets of fibrosing alveolitis in

patients with systemic sclerosis and their relationship to outcome. *Am J Respir Crit Care Med* 2002; 165: 1581–1586.

44. Kocheril SV, Appleton BE, Somers EC, *et al.* Comparison of disease progression and mortality of connective tissue disease-related interstitial lung disease and idiopathic interstitial pneumonia. *Arthritis Rheum* 2005; 53: 549–557.

45. Ishioka S, Nakamura K, Maeda A, *et al.* Clinical evaluation of idiopathic interstitial pneumonia and interstitial pneumonia associated with collagen vascular disease using logistic regression analysis. *Intern Med* 2000; 39: 213–219.

46. Sato T, Fujita J, Yamadori I, *et al.* Non-specific interstitial pneumonia; as the first clinical presentation of various collagen vascular disorders. *Rheumatol Int* 2005: 1–5.

47. Fujita J, Ohtsuki Y, Yoshinouchi T, *et al.* Idiopathic non-specific interstitial pneumonia: as an "autoimmune interstitial pneumonia". *Respir Med* 2005; 99: 234–240.

48. Leslie KO. Pathology of interstitial lung disease. *Clin Chest Med* 2004; 25: 657–703, vi.

49. Nicholson AG, Wells AU. Nonspecific interstitial pneumonia-nobody said it's perfect. *Am J Respir Crit Care Med* 2001; 164: 1553–1554.

50. Flaherty KR, Travis WD, Colby TV, *et al.* Histopathologic variability in usual and nonspecific interstitial pneumonias. *Am J Respir Crit Care Med* 2001; 164: 1722–1727.

51. Kim DS, Yoo B, Lee JS, *et al.* The major histopathologic pattern of pulmonary fibrosis in scleroderma is nonspecific interstitial pneumonia. *Sarcoidosis Vasc Diffuse Lung Dis* 2002; 19: 121–127.

52. Douglas WW, Tazelaar HD, Hartman TE, *et al.* Polymyositis-dermatomyositis-associated interstitial lung disease. *Am J Respir Crit Care Med* 2001; 164: 1182–1185.

53. Kang EH, Lee EB, Shin KC, *et al.* Interstitial lung disease in patients with polymyositis, dermatomyositis and amyopathic dermatomyositis. *Rheumatology (Oxford)* 2005; 44: 1282–1286.

54. Katzenstein AL, Zisman DA, Litzky LA, Nguyen BT, Kotloff RM. Usual interstitial pneumonia: histologic study of biopsy and explant specimens. *Am J Surg Pathol* 2002; 26: 1567–1577.

55. Kradin RL, Divertie MB, Colvin RB, *et al.* Usual interstitial pneumonitis is a T-cell alveolitis. *Clin Immunol Immunopathol* 1986; 40: 224–235.

56. White ES, Lazar MH, Thannickal VJ. Pathogenetic mechanisms in usual interstitial pneumonia/idiopathic pulmonary fibrosis. *J Pathol* 2003; 201: 343–354.

57. Papiris SA, Kollintza A, Kitsanta P, *et al.* Relationship of BAL and lung tissue CD4+ and CD8+ T lymphocytes, and their ratio in idiopathic pulmonary fibrosis. *Chest* 2005; 128: 2971–2977.

58. Wells AU, Lorimer S, Majumdar S, *et al.* Fibrosing alveolitis in systemic sclerosis: increase in memory T-cells in lung interstitium. *Eur Respir J* 1995; 8: 266–271.

59. Keogh KA, Limper AH. Characterization of lymphocyte populations in nonspecific interstitial pneumonia. *Respir Res* 2005; 6: 137.

60. Yamadori I, Fujita J, Kajitani H, *et al.* Lymphocyte subsets in lung tissues of non-specific interstitial pneumonia and pulmonary fibrosis associated with collagen vascular disorders: correlation with CD4/CD8 ratio in bronchoalveolar lavage. *Lung* 2000; 178: 361–370.

61. Yamadori I, Fujita J, Kajitani H, *et al.* Lymphocyte subsets in lung tissues of interstitial pneumonia associated with untreated polymyositis/dermatomyositis. *Rheumatol Int* 2001; 21: 89–93.

62. Turesson C, Matteson EL, Colby TV, *et al.* Increased CD4+ T cell infiltrates in rheumatoid arthritis-associated interstitial pneumonitis compared with idiopathic interstitial pneumonitis. *Arthritis Rheum* 2005; 52: 73–79.

63. Shimizu S, Yoshinouchi T, Ohtsuki Y, *et al.* The appearance of S-100 protein-positive dendritic cells and the distribution of lymphocyte subsets in idiopathic nonspecific interstitial pneumonia. *Respir Med* 2002; 96: 770–776.

64. Sharma SK, MacLean JA, Pinto C, Kradin RL. The effect of an anti-CD3 monoclonal antibody on bleomycin-induced lymphokine production and lung injury. *Am J Respir Crit Care Med* 1996; 154: 193–200.

65. Suzuki N, Ohta K, Horiuchi T, *et al.* T lymphocytes and silica-induced pulmonary inflammation and fibrosis in mice. *Thorax* 1996; 51: 1036–1042.

66. Westermann W, Schobl R, Rieber EP, Frank KH. Th2 cells as effectors in postirradiation pulmonary damage preceding fibrosis in the rat. *Int J Radiat Biol* 1999; 75: 629–638.

67. Stein-Streilein J, Salter-Cid L, Roberts B, Altman NH. Persistent pulmonary interstitial fibrosis, induced by immune response to TNP, is associated with altered mRNA procollagen type I:III ratio. *Reg Immunol* 1992; 4: 391–400.

68. Hu H, Stein-Streilein J. Hapten-immune pulmonary interstitial fibrosis (HIPIF) in mice requires both CD4+ and CD8+ T lymphocytes. *J Leukoc Biol* 1993; 54: 414–422.

69. Christensen PJ, Goodman RE, Pastoriza L, Moore B, Toews GB. Induction of lung fibrosis in the mouse by intratracheal instillation of fluorescein isothiocyanate is not T-cell-dependent. *Am J Pathol* 1999; 155: 1773–1779.

70. Denis M, Cormier Y, Laviolette M, Ghadirian E. T cells in hypersensitivity pneumonitis: effects of *in vivo* depletion of T cells in a mouse model. *Am J Respir Cell Mol Biol* 1992; 6: 183–189.

71. Helene M, Lake-Bullock V, Zhu J, Hao H, Cohen DA, Kaplan AM. T cell independence of bleomycin-induced pulmonary fibrosis. *J Leukoc Biol* 1999; 65: 187–195.

72. Janick-Buckner D, Ranges GE, Hacker MP. Effect of cytotoxic monoclonal antibody depletion of T-lymphocyte subpopulations on bleomycin-induced lung damage in C57BL/6J mice. *Toxicol Appl Pharmacol* 1989; 100: 474–484.

73. Szapiel SV, Elson NA, Fulmer JD, Hunninghake GW, Crystal RG. Bleomycin-induced interstitial pulmonary disease in the nude, athymic mouse. *Am Rev Respir Dis* 1979; 120: 893–899.

74. Wallace WA, Howie SE. Immunoreactive interleukin 4 and interferon-gamma expression by type II alveolar epithelial cells in interstitial lung disease. *J Pathol* 1999; 187: 475–480.

75. Majumdar S, Li D, Ansari T, *et al.* Different cytokine profiles in cryptogenic fibrosing alveolitis and fibrosing alveolitis associated with systemic sclerosis: a quantitative study of open lung biopsies. *Eur Respir J* 1999; 14: 251–257.

76. Choi ES, Jakubzick C, Carpenter KJ, *et al.* Enhanced monocyte chemoattractant protein-3/CC chemokine ligand-7 in usual interstitial pneumonia. *Am J Respir Crit Care Med* 2004; 170: 508–515.

77. Jakubzick C, Choi ES, Kunkel SL, *et al.* Augmented pulmonary IL-4 and IL-13 receptor subunit expression in idiopathic interstitial pneumonia. *J Clin Pathol* 2004; 57: 477–486.

78. Ando M, Miyazaki E, Fukami T, Kumamoto T, Tsuda T. Interleukin-4-producing cells in idiopathic pulmonary fibrosis: an immunohistochemical study. *Respirology* 1999; 4: 383–391.

79. Luzina IG, Atamas SP, Wise R, Wigley FM, Xiao HQ, White B. Gene expression in bronchoalveolar lavage cells from scleroderma patients. *Am J Respir Cell Mol Biol* 2002; 26: 549–557.

80. Wallace WA, Howie SE, Krajewski AS, Lamb D. The immunological architecture of B-lymphocyte aggregates in cryptogenic fibrosing alveolitis. *J Pathol* 1996; 178: 323–329.

81. Hengstman GJ, van Engelen BG, van Venrooij WJ. Myositis specific autoantibodies: changing insights in pathophysiology and clinical associations. *Curr Opin Rheumatol* 2004; 16: 692–699.

82. Zampieri S, Ghirardello A, Iaccarino L, Tarricone E, Gambari PF, Doria A. Anti-Jo-1 antibodies. *Autoimmunity* 2005; 38: 73–78.

83. Fathi M, Dastmalchi M, Rasmussen E, Lundberg IE, Tornling G. Interstitial lung disease: a common manifestation of newly diagnosed polymyositis and dermatomyositis. *Ann Rheum Dis* 2004; 63: 297–301.

84. Hochberg MC, Feldman D, Stevens MB, Arnett FC, Reichlin M. Antibody to Jo-1 in polymyositis/dermatomyositis: association with interstitial pulmonary disease. *J Rheumatol* 1984; 11: 663–665.

85. Grau JM, Miro O, Pedrol E, *et al.* Interstitial lung disease related to dermatomyositis. Comparative study with patients without lung involvement. *J Rheumatol* 1996; 23: 1921–1926.

86. Targoff IN. Update on myositis-specific and myositis-associated autoantibodies. *Curr Opin Rheumatol* 2000; 12: 475–481.

87. Sato S, Hirakata M, Kuwana M, *et al.* Clinical characteristics of Japanese patients with anti-PL-7 (anti-threonyl-tRNA synthetase) autoantibodies. *Clin Exp Rheumatol* 2005; 23: 609–615.

88. Hirakata M, Suwa A, Nagai S, *et al.* Anti-KS: identification of autoantibodies to asparaginyl-transfer RNA synthetase associated with interstitial lung disease. *J Immunol* 1999; 162: 2315–2320.

89. Friedman AW, Targoff IN, Arnett FC. Interstitial lung disease with autoantibodies against aminoacyl-tRNA synthetases in the absence of clinically apparent myositis. *Semin Arthritis Rheum* 1996; 26: 459–467.

90. Reveille JD, Solomon DH. Evidence-based guidelines for the use of immunologic tests: anticentromere, Scl-70, and nucleolar antibodies. *Arthritis Rheum* 2003; 49: 399–412.

91. Mitri GM, Lucas M, Fertig N, Steen VD, Medsger TA Jr. A comparison between anti-Th/To- and anticentromere antibody-positive systemic sclerosis patients with limited cutaneous involvement. *Arthritis Rheum* 2003; 48: 203–209.

92. Mahler M, Bluthner M, Pollard KM. Advances in B-cell epitope analysis of autoantigens in connective tissue diseases. *Clin Immunol* 2003; 107: 65–79.

93. Steen VD. Autoantibodies in systemic sclerosis. *Semin Arthritis Rheum* 2005; 35: 35–42.

94. Marguerie C, Bunn CC, Copier J, *et al.* The clinical and immunogenetic features of patients with autoantibodies to the nucleolar antigen PM-Scl. *Medicine (Baltimore)* 1992; 71: 327–236.

95. Chapman JR, Charles PJ, Venables PJ, *et al.* Definition and clinical relevance of antibodies to nuclear ribonucleoprotein and other nuclear antigens in patients with cryptogenic fibrosing alveolitis. *Am Rev Respir Dis* 1984; 130: 439–443.

96. Turner-Warwick M, Doniach D. Auto-antibody studies in interstitial pulmonary fibrosis. *BMJ* 1965; 5439: 886–891.

97. Nakos G, Adams A, Andriopoulos N. Antibodies to collagen in patients with idiopathic pulmonary fibrosis. *Chest* 1993; 103: 1051–1058.

98. Meliconi R, Bestagno M, Sturani C, *et al.* Autoantibodies to DNA topoisomerase II in cryptogenic fibrosing alveolitis and connective tissue disease. *Clin Exp Immunol* 1989; 76: 184–189.

99. Fujita J, Dobashi N, Ohtsuki Y, *et al.* Elevation of anti-cytokeratin 19 antibody in sera of the patients with idiopathic pulmonary fibrosis and pulmonary fibrosis associated with collagen vascular disorders. *Lung* 1999; 177: 311–319.

100. Dobashi N, Fujita J, Murota M, *et al.* Elevation of anti-cytokeratin 18 antibody and circulating cytokeratin 18: anti-cytokeratin 18 antibody immune complexes in sera of patients with idiopathic pulmonary fibrosis. *Lung* 2000; 178: 171–179.

101. Yang Y, Fujita J, Bandoh S, *et al.* Detection of antivimentin antibody in sera of patients with idiopathic pulmonary fibrosis and non-specific interstitial pneumonia. *Clin Exp Immunol* 2002; 128: 169–174.

102. Walker EJ, Jeffrey PD. Sequence homology between encephalomyocarditis virus protein VPI and histidyl-tRNA synthetase supports a hypothesis of molecular mimicry in polymyositis. *Med Hypotheses* 1988; 25: 21–25.

103. Howard OM, Dong HF, Yang D, *et al.* Histidyl-tRNA synthetase and asparaginyl-tRNA synthetase, autoantigens in myositis, activate chemokine receptors on T lymphocytes and immature dendritic cells. *J Exp Med* 2002; 196: 781–791.

104. Ascherman DP, Oriss TB, Oddis CV, Wright TM. Critical requirement for professional APCs in eliciting T cell responses to novel fragments of histidyl-tRNA synthetase (Jo-1) in Jo-1 antibody-positive polymyositis. *J Immunol* 2002; 169: 7127–7134.

105. Endo Y, Matsushita H, Matsuya S, Hara M. A study of human interstitial lung diseases with special reference to immune complexes and hyaline membrane. *Acta Pathol Jpn* 1990; 40: 239–248.

106. Fritzler MJ. Autoantibodies: diagnostic fingerprints and etiologic perplexities. *Clin Invest Med* 1997; 20: 50–66.

CHAPTER 9

Chronic hypersensitivity pneumonitis and its differential diagnosis

A. Churg*, N.L. Müller#, J. Flint*, J.L. Wright*

Depts of *Pathology and #Radiology, University of British Columbia, Vancouver, BC, Canada.

Correspondence: A. Churg, Dept of Pathology, University of British Columbia, 2211 Wesbrook Mall, Vancouver, BC, V6T 2B5 Canada. Fax: 1 6048227635; E-mail: achurg@interchange.ubc.ca

Background and clinical features

Hypersensitivity pneumonitis (HP), also known as extrinsic allergic alveolitis, is a form of allergic interstitial lung disease caused by inhalation of an organic (and occasionally inorganic chemical) sensitising agent that serves as an antigen. Classic examples include farmers' lung, where the usual agent is *Thermophilic actinomyces* found in mouldy hay, grain and silage, and bird fanciers' lung, which is caused by sensitisation to avian proteins in droppings or feathers. There are numerous different occupations in which HP develops, which are often named by the job or antigen [1]. HP may also be seen in patients with subtle environmental exposures, typically to fungi or bacteria that colonise households or ventilation and water systems [1].

HP is usually divided on clinical grounds into three different forms [2–4]. Acute HP is seen in patients with previous sensitisation and high-level exposure to the offending antigen, with resulting fever, chills and cough developing within 4–8 h and resolving over 24–48 h [2, 3]. However, most cases of HP diagnosed clinically and pathologically are of the subacute form, in which the patient is exposed either continuously or intermittently to much lower doses of the antigen. Patients with subacute HP characteristically present with slowly developing shortness of breath unrelated to any obvious episodes of exposure. Clinically subacute HP appears like an interstitial lung disease with restrictive pulmonary function abnormalities and interstitial markings on plain chest films. In the classic case, a high-resolution computed tomography (HRCT) scan shows poorly defined centrilobular nodules or ground-glass opacities [5, 6]. Most importantly, the majority of cases of subacute HP respond well to removal from antigen exposure and treatment with steroids [7].

Chronic HP is also believed to develop from low-level long-term exposure to an antigen, but differs from subacute HP as patients with chronic HP have radiological evidence of fibrosis. Such patients also present with the insidious onset of shortness of breath, which is typically slowly progressive, and patients may develop very marked functional abnormalities. The prognosis of chronic HP is not well defined in the literature, but such patients appear to have a worse outcome than those with subacute HP [7–10].

Pathological features of chronic HP

The differing prognoses of the various forms of HP make accurate pathological diagnosis important. Patients with acute-stage HP are rarely biopsied and the

Eur Respir Mon, 2007, 39, 189–198. Printed in UK - all rights reserved. Copyright ERS Journals Ltd 2007; European Respiratory Monograph; ISSN 1025-448x.

pathological findings are unclear. The pathological features of subacute HP are, however, well defined and widely known. In classic cases, there is a relatively mild chronic interstitial inflammatory infiltrate, which is centred around the bronchioles; the infiltrate may involve the wall of the bronchiole as well. In most cases (70% according to the literature [11]), isolated interstitial giant cells or poorly formed granulomas are found; however, their absence does not alter the diagnosis.

In some instances, subacute HP has a much more homogeneous distribution of the interstitial inflammatory infiltrate through the pulmonary lobule. Such cases are indistinguishable from cellular forms of nonspecific interstitial pneumonia (NSIP) [12]. The presence of giant cells or granulomas suggests the correct diagnosis, but, to reiterate, giant cells and granulomas are not always present [12].

Few papers have been written about the pathological features of chronic HP, and some of the published descriptions originate from older literature and so are hard to interpret in light of the present classification of interstitial pneumonias. However, it is clear from the original reports of SEAL *et al.* [13] that chronic HP grossly can show honeycombing, which is sometimes in the upper zone (fig. 1a), a diagnostically useful finding when present, since relatively few forms of fibrotic lung disease are predominantly upper zonal. SEAL *et al.* [13] also noted the presence of what they termed linear fibrosis (possibly equivalent to fibrotic NSIP), along with peribronchiolar fibrosis.

More recently, the current authors described 13 new cases of chronic HP and found several different patterns as follows [14]. 1) Predominantly peripheral fibrosis in a patchy pattern was found, resembling the changes seen in usual interstitial pneumonia

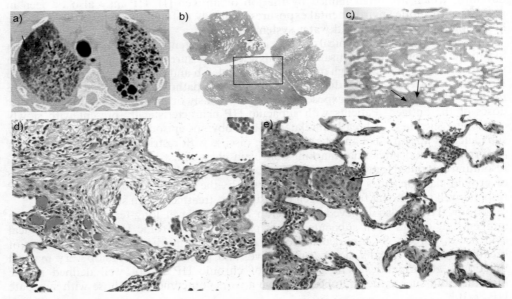

Fig. 1. – Chronic hypersensitivity pneumonitis (HP) caused by household mould exposure. a) High-resolution computed tomography scan showing severe upper zone fibrosis consistent with severe chronic HP in a female with long-term household mould exposure. Upper zone fibrosis is seen in some cases of chronic HP. Note the few centrilobular nodules (arrows), a finding suggesting underlying subacute HP. b) Low-power view of several sections from the patient's biopsy showing several fibrosis with honeycombing. The boxed area shows patchy usual interstitial pneumonia (UIP)-like pattern of involvement. c) Low-power view of another section demonstrating patchy irregular fibrosis in a UIP-like pattern. Note the presence of peribronchiolar fibrosis (arrows), a finding seen in chronic HP and not in UIP. d) High-power view of a fibroblast focus. e) An area of subacute HP. Note the poorly formed granuloma (arrow).

(UIP; figs 1 and 2). The peripheral fibrosis was always associated with fibroblast foci (figs 1d and 2d). 2) Homogeneous linear fibrosis (fig. 3) was observed which was very similar to that found in fibrotic NSIP. 3) Peribronchiolar fibrosis was also found, which often extended to the periphery of the lobule in an irregular fashion (fig. 2c). The pattern

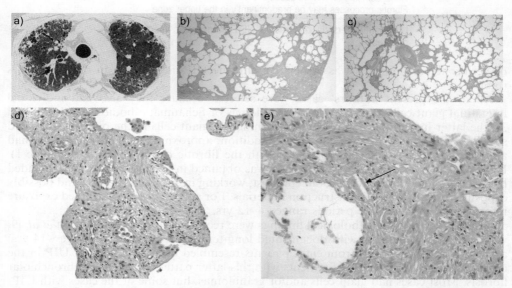

Fig. 2. – Chronic hypersensitivity pneumonitis (HP) of unknown aetiology. a) High-resolution computed tomography scan showing peripheral reticulation, honeycombing and traction bronchiectasis. This image is identical to that of usual interstitial pneumonia (UIP). b) Low-power view of a biopsy showing UIP-like pattern with patchy irregular dense fibrosis and peripheral architectural distortion. c) Irregular dense fibrosis around the airway and pulmonary artery branch in the centre of the lobule. This finding should suggest chronic HP and not UIP as the correct diagnosis. d) Fibroblast focus found in an area of irregular peripheral fibrosis. e) Isolated interstitial giant cell in an area of irregular peripheral fibrosis (arrow).

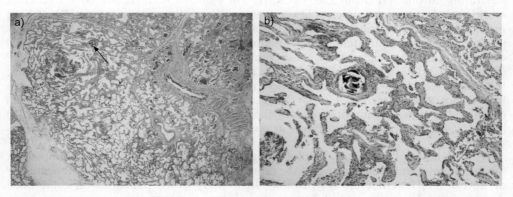

Fig. 3. – Chronic hypersensitivity pneumonia (HP) in a 12-yr-old male exposed to pigeons nearly since birth. A chest radiograph showed diffuse reticular opacities with sparing of the bases. a) Low-power view of a biopsy showing fairly homogeneous linear fibrosis in a pattern suggestive of fibrotic nonspecific interstitial pneumonia (NSIP). A Schaumann body (arrow) is a marker of an old granuloma and indicates chronic HP should be the first choice of pathological diagnosis. b) High-power view of the region around the Schaumann body illustrating the NSIP-like pattern of fibrosis.

Table 1. – Pathological features of chronic hypersensitivity pneumonitis (HP)

Interstitial giant cells, granulomas or Schaumann bodies
UIP-like areas or fibrotic NSIP-like areas
Peribronchiolar fibrosis
Areas of subacute HP
Honeycombing (in severe cases)
Fibrotic processes may be predominantly in the upper zone

UIP: usual interstitial pneumonia; NSIP: nonspecific interstitial pneumonia.

of peribronchiolar fibrosis was associated with the UIP-like pattern in most instances (table 1).

All of the present authors' cases were selected because they also had individual interstitial giant cells, poorly formed granulomas or Schaumann bodies (figs 1e, 2e and 3), the latter indicating the presence of granulomas/giant cells in the past, *i.e.* they had some features typical of subacute HP. In addition, approximately half of the cases had areas of actual subacute HP combined with the fibrotic component (fig. 1e; table 1). History of exposure to a sensitising agent was obtained in 10 of the cases, and included birds, household mould, mushroom compost, working in a plastics factory, and possibly exposure to wood dust or construction materials. For six patients with detailed exposure information, the exposure periods ranged 4–12 yrs.

Remarkably similar pathological findings were recently described by OHTANI *et al.* [9] who reported 19 patients with documented long-term bird exposure (average ~14 yrs) and chronic HP. Biopsies from eight patients resembled fibrotic NSIP and UIP in the other 11. Of note, a number of patients with this latter pattern also had peribronchiolar fibrosis. Most cases had giant cells and/or granulomas, but some of the cases with UIP-like features apparently did not.

Radiological features of chronic HP

Radiological features are often helpful in the diagnosis of chronic HP and in separating chronic HP from UIP or NSIP. On plain films, there are coarse reticular markings, which may be upper or lower zonal in distribution. Studies using HRCT have provided more diagnostic detail. Reticulation, which indicates the presence of fibrosis, is present, sometimes in a patchy, quite random distribution, but sometimes in a peripheral distribution and associated with honeycombing, a feature similar to that seen in UIP (figs 1a and 2a). Ground-glass opacities are common and typically much more extensive than those seen in UIP. In addition, there may be mosaic perfusion or air trapping, a feature not usually seen in UIP or NSIP. The fibrotic process may be upper zonal (fig. 1a), but more commonly involves the middle or lower zones; however, in such instances, there is sparing of the bases, as opposed to UIP, which almost always involves the bases.

While radiology is frequently helpful in suggesting the correct diagnosis, it is important for the pathologist to remember that the radiological separation of chronic HP from UIP or fibrotic NSIP is not always possible. In a study of 60 patients with established diagnoses of UIP or chronic HP, LYNCH *et al.* [15] made a confident separation based on the radiological findings in only 62% of cases, and not all of the cases labelled confidently as UIP or chronic HP on the CT scan were in fact diagnosed correctly. Similarly, HARTMAN *et al.* [16] reviewed 50 patients with NSIP and found that in 20% the CT findings were indistinguishable from those of HP.

Pathological differential diagnosis of chronic HP

It is clear that radiological information and clinical information, particularly exposure history or immunological evidence of exposure [7, 10], are important in obtaining a diagnosis of HP. The limitations of radiology in separating chronic HP from UIP and NSIP have been discussed. It is also important to realise that in many patients with (classical) pathologically diagnosed HP, a clear history of exposure cannot be obtained. VOURLEKIS *et al.* [7] reported 72 patients with pathological HP on biopsy, a history of exposure could be found in 62%. Similarly, COLEMAN and COLBY [17] described 27 cases of typical subacute HP diagnosed *via* biopsy; a history of exposure was obtained in only 37%. Thus, in many instances, the diagnosis depends on interpretation of the findings at biopsy. The pathological features of chronic HP compared with UIP and fibrotic NSIP are shown in table 2.

Chronic HP needs to be separated from several different general types of interstitial lung disease, which are: 1) idiopathic interstitial pneumonias, UIP and NSIP; 2) sarcoidosis; and 3) several newly described forms of airway-centred interstitial fibrosis.

Depending on the pathological pattern in a given biopsy, separation from UIP or NSIP may be very difficult. One helpful finding is the presence of predominantly upper zone fibrosis, since UIP almost always shows predominantly lower zone fibrosis, and NSIP also tends to follow this distribution. However, as mentioned previously, many cases of chronic HP have a mid-to-lower zonal distribution. Consultation with the radiologist is extremely valuable here, because the distribution is quite obviously radiological, but, even with several biopsies from different sites, may not be obvious pathologically.

Microscopically, there is considerable overlap between some forms of chronic HP and UIP. Giant cells, granulomas, Schaumann bodies or classic subacute HP are features of HP and not UIP. The combination of peripheral fibrosis with architectural distortion/honeycombing and fibroblast foci can be seen in both chronic HP and UIP, but the presence of peribronchiolar fibrosis should suggest the diagnosis of chronic HP. However, the combination of UIP and peribronchiolar fibrosis may also be seen in patients with collagen vascular disease, particularly rheumatoid arthritis. A history of exposure, evidence of precipitating antibodies or lymphocyte blast transformation [18] against known sensitising antigens, and serological examination for collagen vascular disease are useful pieces of information in arriving at the proper diagnosis in this situation.

Similar problems apply when separating chronic HP from fibrotic NSIP, since the basic morphological patterns of linear fibrosis are indistinguishable. Poorly defined granulomas and giant cells were a part of the original description of NSIP by KATZENSTEIN and FIORELLI [19], and these authors raised the possibility that some of their cases were actually HP. The current authors suggest that any process which looks like NSIP (fibrotic or cellular) with giant cells or granulomas should be viewed as HP until proven otherwise. It is better in this context to raise the question of HP than to simply make a diagnosis of NSIP, because removal from antigen exposure is important in

Table 2. – Pathological features of chronic hypersensitivity pneumonia (HP) compared with usual interstitial pneumonia (UIP) and fibrotic nonspecific interstitial pneumonia (NSIP)

	GC/Gran/SB	Peripheral fibrosis with architectural distortion	Fibroblast foci	Linear fibrosis	Zone of lung involved
Chronic HP	Yes (usually)	Can be present	Can be present	Can be present	Upper or lower
UIP	No	Yes	Yes	No	Lower
NSIP	Occasional	No	No	Yes	Lower

GC: giant cells; Gran: granulomas; SB: Schaumann bodies.

treating HP, and it is unlikely that the clinician involved will look for an antigen if the biopsy is reported as NSIP.

It has been reported that giant cells and granulomas tend to disappear from the lung over time, particularly if exposure to the antigen has ceased [13]. Schaumann bodies can serve as a substitute for giant cells and granulomas, but in the current authors' experience they are relatively uncommon in both subacute and chronic HP. Also, roughly a third of cases of otherwise typical subacute HP do not have giant cells or granulomas to begin with [11]. These observations raise the difficult question of whether some cases that appear, pathologically, to be UIP or fibrotic NSIP without giant cells, *etc.*, are really chronic HP. This question has been partially answered by VOURLEKIS *et al.* [7], who reported six patients with documented sensitising exposures, but a pathological picture on biopsy of cellular or fibrotic NSIP without any giant cells or granulomas. Thus, it is clear that some cases of morphological NSIP will turn out to be HP. The findings of OHTANI *et al.* [9], who, as noted previously, did not observe giant cells/granulomas in ~25% of their cases with a UIP-like pattern, raise the question of how many cases diagnosed as UIP pathologically and radiologically are actually chronic HP, and the even more important issue of whether this distinction has any prognostic importance.

The presence of fibrosis and granulomas also raises sarcoidosis as a differential diagnosis. In general, the granulomas of sarcoid are much better defined than those of HP, and often have a distinct hyalinised rim. Acute forms of sarcoid do not, as a rule, have an interstitial inflammatory infiltrate. As sarcoid scars, it most commonly produces progressively hyalinised nodules with granulomas around the periphery. These are distinctly different from the findings in chronic HP, as are the radiological manifestations of sarcoid. However, sarcoid can produce upper zone honeycombing and, thus, there is some potential for confusion.

One of the features of chronic HP is peribronchiolar fibrosis. There are three recent descriptions of new forms of interstitial lung characterised by fibrosis around and extending away from the bronchioles: 1) airway-centred interstitial fibrosis [20] (fig. 4); 2) idiopathic bronchiolocentric interstitial pneumonia [21]; and 3) peribronchiolar metaplasia [22]. In all three conditions, the bronchioles are visibly damaged and fibrotic, and sometimes, but not always, inflamed. The fibrosing process appears to radiate from the bronchioles through the interstitium in a linear fashion, sometimes reaching the pleura (fig. 4a), but without significantly disturbing the underlying architecture. Characteristically, there is bronchiolar metaplasia over the fibrotic interstitium (fig. 4b). In the reports of

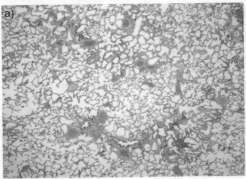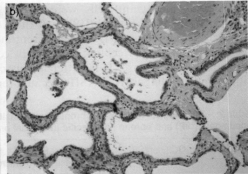

Fig. 4. – Airway-centred interstitial fibrosis in a male with clinical interstitial lung disease and positive precipitins against avian proteins. a) Low-power view showing patches of dense linear fibrosis extending around bronchioles. b) High-power view showing typical linear fibrosis with areas of overlying metaplastic bronchiolar epithelium.

CHURG *et al.* [20] and YOUSEM and DACIC [21], no giant cells or granulomas were seen, but occasional small granulomas were present in three out of the 15 cases reported by FUKUOKA *et al.* [22].

In the current authors' opinion, these are probably all variants of the same lesion, but, as noted by FUKUOKA *et al.* [22], the diagnosis (whichever name one picks) should only be applied to cases in which there is clinical interstitial lung disease and no other morphological finding to account for it, since minor degrees of peribronchiolar fibrosis with bronchiolar metaplasia are common in lungs with some other interstitial or even neoplastic process (fig. 5).

The nature of this lesion(s) remains obscure. In all three series, the authors queried the possibility that these conditions were variants of chronic HP. The morphological findings are not typical of chronic HP, as described above, and the constant finding of bronchiolar metaplasia over the areas of fibrosis is not seen in typical chronic HP. In addition, the pattern of peribronchiolar fibrosis (fig. 5) is considerably more regular than is seen in typical chronic HP cases (fig. 2c).

The cases reported by CHURG *et al.* [20] are from a respiratory centre in Mexico City (Central America) with a great deal of experience in the diagnosis of HP [8], but there was no serological finding to support this diagnosis in any patient, although two out of 12 did have a history of bird exposure. One of 15 patients reported by FUKUOKA *et al.* [22] was also exposed to pigeons, but again there were no supporting serological data. The patient whose biopsy is illustrated in figure 4 was employed on a farm and had serum precipitins against avian proteins, but this is the only case of airway-centred fibrosis the present authors have encountered in which there is serological evidence to suggest chronic HP.

Therapy and prognosis of chronic HP

The approach to treating HP is removal from antigen exposure, where exposure can be identified, and therapy with steroids. Patients with subacute HP on biopsy generally

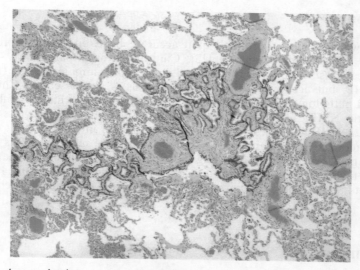

Fig. 5. – Airway damage showing a pattern of airway-centred peribronchiolar fibrosis with airway scarring and extensive bronchiolar metaplasia. This was an incidental finding in a patient with Wegener's granulomatosis and should not be reported as airway-centred interstitial fibrosis. The latter term is reserved for patients with airway-centred interstitial fibrosis, clinical interstitial lung disease and no other lesion to explain the interstitial lung disease.

appear to respond favourably to this regime [7], but the prognosis for those with chronic HP is considerably worse. PEREZ-PADILLA *et al.* [8] reported 78 patients with HP and exposure to pigeons. The overall 5-yr survival was 71%, but the presence of fibrosis was an important prognostic factor. When patients were separated into those whose biopsies showed >50% fibrosis (unfortunately not defined in any specific anatomic sense) and those whose biopsies showed <50%, the 4-yr survival was 37 and 75%, respectively. The figure of 37% was comparable to the survival in a control series of patients with UIP.

The biopsies in the 72 cases of HP reported by VOURLEKIS *et al.* [7] were further subdivided by extent of fibrosis and presence or absence of honeycombing; patients were labelled fibroid if their biopsy showed interstitial fibrosis in >5% of the parenchyma or honeycombing was present. Patients falling into the fibrotic category, *i.e.* those with chronic HP, had a median survival of 7.1 yrs, compared with >20 yrs for those without fibrosis.

In the study by OHTANI *et al.* [9], only one out of seven patients with a pattern of fibrotic NSIP stabilised with treatment, one was deteriorating and the other five had died at the time of writing. Out of nine patients with a UIP-like pattern, one improved and two stabilised on treatment, but the other six died. The median survival for both patterns was ~60 months (as interpreted from fig. 5 [9]).

In the current authors' series of cases [14], five patients improved, but the follow-up times were very short (3–12 months), whereas two died of their disease at 9 months and 5 yrs. Both of the patients that died had a UIP-like pattern on biopsy, while three patients who improved had a UIP-like picture and two a fibrotic NSIP-like picture.

It is difficult to draw firm conclusions about survival in chronic HP from these limited data, but the presence of fibrosis generally appears to have an adverse effect and the greater the amount of fibrosis the worse the prognosis. However, again judging from very limited data, the overall survival is probably better in chronic HP than in UIP, thus, it is worthwhile pursuing criteria to make this diagnostic separation. There are simply too few data to indicate whether the pathological pattern of fibrosis has any effect on survival.

Conclusion

There is a widespread, and probably quite accurate, belief on the part of respirologists that chronic HP is underdiagnosed [23]. Clinical features, particularly evidence of immunological sensitisation and radiological studies, play a major role in the diagnosis of chronic HP, but accurate pathological diagnosis is also essential. Chronic HP is characterised pathologically by a variety of patterns, some of which resemble UIP and others fibrotic NSIP. The presence of peribronchiolar fibrosis suggests the correct diagnosis in the UIP-like cases. However, the presence of interstitial giant cells, poorly formed granulomas, Schaumann bodies or areas of typical subacute HP is required for definitive diagnosis on the basis of a lung biopsy. It is clear from clinical data that some cases of fibrotic NSIP without these latter features are, nonetheless, chronic HP. Whether some patients who appear to have UIP actually have chronic HP remains to be determined.

Keynote messages

Chronic HP is defined by the presence of fibrosis on radiological or pathological examination in a patient with HP. Radiologically, a number of features suggest chronic HP, but there is a radiological overlap with UIP and NSIP. Pathologically, chronic HP shows three different patterns: 1) a UIP-like pattern with peripheral architectural distortion and fibroblast foci; 2) a fibrotic NSIP-like pattern; and 3) a pattern of irregular peribronchiolar fibrosis. The presence of giant cells, poorly formed granulomas, Schaumann bodies or areas of accompanying subacute HP is required for the diagnosis, but the literature implies that some cases of chronic HP will lack these features. Chronic HP has a considerably worse prognosis than subacute HP.

Summary

Chronic hypersensitivity pneumonitis (HP) is defined as HP with radiological evidence of fibrosis. Pathologically a variety of patterns are seen, including those which resemble usual interstitial pneumonia (UIP), fibrotic nonspecific interstitial pneumonia (NSIP) and peribronchiolar fibrosis. Cases of chronic HP typically show poorly formed granulomas, individual giant cells or Schaumann bodies, which are all crucial clues to the correct diagnosis. Areas of subacute HP (purely cellular infiltrates, usually in a centrilobular pattern) are also frequently present. It is unknown what proportions of chronic HP cases do not show any of these identifying features and, thus, are pathologically indistinguishable from UIP or fibrotic NSIP. Chronic HP has a distinctly worse prognosis than subacute HP, but whether the specific patterns of fibrosis impact on survival is not yet known.

Keywords: Airway-centred interstitial fibrosis, hypersensitivity pneumonitis, nonspecific interstitial pneumonia, peribronchiolar fibrosis, usual interstitial pneumonia.

References

1. Myers JL. Idiopathic interstitial pneumonias. *In*: Churg AM, Myers JL, Tazelaar HD, Wright JL, eds. Thurlbecks Pathology of the Lung. 3rd Edn. New York, Thieme Medical Publishers, 2005; pp. 563–600.

2. Bourke SJ, Dalphin JC, Boyd G, McSharry C, Baldwin CI, Calvert JE. Hypersensitivity pneumonitis: current concepts. *Eur Respir J* 2001; 18: Suppl. 32, 81s–92s.

3. Wild LG, Lopez M. Hypersensitivity pneumonitis: a comprehensive review. *J Investig Allergol Clin Immunol* 2001; 11: 3–15.

4. Yi ES. Hypersensitivity pneumonitis. *Crit Rev Clin Lab Sci* 2002; 39: 581–629.

5. Hansell DM, Moskovic E. High-resolution computed tomography in extrinsic allergic alveolitis. *Clin Radiol* 1991; 43: 8–12.

6. Remy-Jardin M, Remy J, Wallaert B, Muller NL. Subacute and chronic bird breeder hypersensitivity pneumonitis: sequential evaluation with CT and correlation with lung function tests and bronchoalveolar lavage. *Radiology* 1993; 189: 111–118.

7. Vourlekis JS, Schwarz MI, Cherniack RM, *et al.* The effect of pulmonary fibrosis on survival in patients with hypersensitivity pneumonitis. *Am J Med* 2004; 116: 662–668.

8. Perez-Padilla R, Salas J, Chapela R, *et al.* Mortality in Mexican patients with chronic pigeon breeder's lung compared with those with usual interstitial pneumonia. *Am Rev Respir Dis* 1993; 148: 49–53.

9. Ohtani Y, Saiki S, Kitaichi M, *et al.* Chronic bird fancier's lung: histopathological and clinical correlation. *Thorax* 2005; 60: 665–671.

10. Ohtani Y, Saiki S, Sumi Y, *et al.* Clinical features of recurrent and insidious chronic bird fancier's lung. *Ann Allergy Asthma Immunol* 2003; 90: 604–610.

11. Reyes CN, Wenzel FJ, Lawton BR, Emmanuel DA. The pulmonary pathology of farmer's lung disease. *Chest* 1982; 81: 142–146.

12. Vourlekis JS, Schwarz MI, Cool CD, Tuder RM, King TE, Brown KK. Nonspecific interstitial pneumonitis as the sole histologic expression of hypersensitivity pneumonitis. *Am J Med* 2002; 112: 490–493.

13. Seal RM, Hapke EJ, Thomas GO, Meek JC, Hayes M. The pathology of the acute and chronic stages of farmer's lung. *Thorax* 1968; 23: 469–489.

14. Churg A, Muller NL, Flint J, Wright JL. Chronic hypersensitivity pneumonitis. *Am J Surg Pathol* 2006; 30: 201–208.

15. Lynch DA, Newell JD, Logan PM, King TE Jr, Muller NL. Can CT distinguish hypersensitivity pneumonitis from idiopathic pulmonary fibrosis? *AJR Am J Roentgenol* 1995; 165: 807–811.

16. Hartman TE, Swensen SJ, Hansell DM, *et al.* Nonspecific interstitial pneumonia: variable appearance at high-resolution chest CT. *Radiology* 2000; 217: 701–705.

17. Coleman A, Colby TV. Histologic diagnosis of extrinsic allergic alveolitis. *Am J Surg Pathol* 1988; 12: 514–518.

18. Lacasse Y, Selman M, Costabel U, *et al.* Clinical diagnosis of hypersensitivity pneumonitis. *Am J Respir Crit Care Med* 2003; 168: 952–995.

19. Katzenstein AL, Fiorelli RF. Nonspecific interstitial pneumonia/fibrosis. Histologic features and clinical significance. *Am J Surg Pathol* 1994; 18: 136–147.

20. Churg A, Myers J, Suarez T, *et al.* Airway centered interstitial fibrosis: a distinct form of aggressive diffuse lung disease. *Am J Surg Pathol* 2004; 28: 62–68.

21. Yousem SA, Dacic S. Idiopathic bronchiolocentric interstitial pneumonia. *Mod Pathol* 2002; 15: 1148–1153.

22. Fukuoka J, Franks TJ, Colby TV, *et al.* Peribronchiolar metaplasia: a common histologic lesion in diffuse lung disease and a rare cause of interstitial lung disease: clinicopathologic features of 15 cases. *Am J Surg Pathol* 2005; 29: 948–954.

23. King TE Jr. Clinical advances in the diagnosis and therapy of the interstitial lung diseases. *Am J Respir Crit Care Med* 2005; 172: 268–279.

CHAPTER 10

Pathology of pulmonary involvement in inflammatory bowel disease

T.V. Colby*, P. Camus#

*Dept of Pathology, Mayo Clinic College of Medicine, Mayo Clinic Arizona, Scottsdale, AZ, USA. #Dept of Respiratory Medicine, University Medical Center and Medical School, Dijon, France.

Correspondence: T.V. Colby, Dept of Pathology, Mayo Clinic Arizona, 13400 East Shea Boulevard, Scottsdale, AZ 85259, USA. Fax: 1 4803018372; E-mail: colby.thomas@mayo.edu

Background

Determining an association between two diseases is plagued by the problem of a coincidental *versus* a real association. This issue certainly arises in patients with inflammatory bowel disease (IBD) who develop pulmonary disease, particularly for the rare lesions. The conditions discussed in this chapter represent those which the current authors believe show a more than coincidental association with IBD, although there is no rigorous statistical or epidemiological proof of such an association [1, 2]. In this discussion, both ulcerative colitis (UC) and Crohn's disease (CD) are included. Patients with IBD who develop pleuropulmonary diseases may fall into one of three groups (table 1).

Table 1. – Lung disease in patients with inflammatory bowel disease (IBD)

Pulmonary disease associated with IBD
Pulmonary disease appears to be a primary process in airways or lung parenchyma
Pulmonary disease is secondary (for example, lung abscesses related to fistulae from Crohn's disease, *etc.*)
Pulmonary disease associated with therapy for IBD (direct toxic/idiosyncratic drug reactions, opportunistic infections
related to the immunosuppressive or other effects of the drug, *etc.*)
Unrelated, coincidental pulmonary disease

Pulmonary disease in patients with IBD

A recent study by STORCH *et al.* [3] outlines the broad approach primary-care physicians must take with patients with IBD and pulmonary disease. The major patterns of pulmonary disease in IBD are included in table 2.

Table 2. – Major patterns of lung disease in patients with inflammatory bowel disease

Drug-induced lung disease (including opportunistic infections)
Anatomic disease, including colobronchial and oesophagopulmonary fistulae
Overlap syndromes
Autoimmune disease
Thrombo-embolic disease
Subclinical pulmonary function abnormalities
Other pulmonary manifestations (including airway disease, airspace and interstitial disease, necrobiotic nodules, pleuritis)

Modified from [3].

Eur Respir Mon, 2007, 39, 199–207. Printed in UK - all rights reserved. Copyright ERS Journals Ltd 2007; European Respiratory Monograph; ISSN 1025-448x.

The study by STORCH *et al.* [3] includes a number of abnormalities that are not often mentioned in studies of lung disease in IBD patients. Fistulae in patients with CD are typically intra-abdominal, but rare cases of bronchocenteric fistulae and oesophago-pulmonary fistulae have been reported. STORCH *et al.* [3] use the term "overlap syndromes" to include the reported rare cases of concomitant sarcoidosis and IBD. While such an association may exist, from the pathologist's point of view, there is very little histological overlap in lung tissue. Overlap syndrome is also used to refer to a rarely described association between α_1-antitrypsin deficiency and IBD. Again, this has had relatively little impact on the pathological analysis.

Thrombo-embolic disease represents an important differential in IBD patients who have dyspnoea, and arterial or venous thrombotic events and hypercoagulable states are known to occur in IBD patients, mostly in patients with active disease.

Analogous to patients with collagen vascular diseases, a much larger percentage of patients with IBD are found to have pulmonary function abnormalities than clinically significant disease [3–5]. In several studies reviewed by STORCH *et al.* [3], >50% of patients with UC were found to have abnormal pulmonary function tests compared with controls. The most commonly described abnormality was a decrease in the diffusing capacity, and there is greater likelihood of changes in patients with active bowel disease. Clinically manifested pulmonary function abnormalities are common with conditions mentioned below.

In previous publications [2, 3], the clinicopathological characteristics of pulmonary disease in patients with IBD have been reviewed, and most of the lesions discussed have been included in the "other pulmonary manifestations" section in table 2. The clinico-pathological groups and their approximate frequency is shown in table 3. The International Registry of Bowel and Lung Disorders, maintained by P. Camus, now includes >120 cases and the disease frequency has remained relatively stable. The frequency of lesions seen histologically does not represent the overall frequency seen by the clinician. Thus, cases of bronchiolitis and interstitial lung disease (ILD) may be disproportionately represented in pathological series. Patients with UC develop airway disease more often, and the onset of clinical/pathological manifestations may follow the onset of UC by months to years. Airway disease may also develop years after colectomy. Infiltrative/ILD is more common in patients with CD, especially in those receiving drugs. For those patients on bowel disease-modifying drugs, cessation of exposure to the agent does not always translate into clinical improvement.

Table 3. – Pulmonary involvement in inflammatory disease

Primary site affected	Approx. cases %	Symptoms/clinical pattern	Imaging patterns
Subglottic region including trachea	7	Inflammation/stenosis, cough, dyspnoea, stridor, haemoptysis	Narrowing
Bronchi	50	Bronchitis, bronchial distention, mucoid impaction, bronchial suppuration, bronchiectasis, cough, wheeze, sputum production	Normal, distention, narrowing, bronchial wall thickening
Bronchioles	4	Bronchiolitis, bronchiolitis obliterans, cough, dyspnoea, sputum production, airflow obstruction	Tree in bud/centrilobular nodules, mosaic pattern
Parenchyma Infiltrative/interstitial	33	Interstitial lung disease, pulmonary infiltrates with eosinophilia, dyspnoea, fever	Patchy or diffuse infiltrates/opacities
Parenchymal nodules	6	Dyspnoea, chest pain, associated skin pyoderma	Lung nodules/consolidation $\pm$ cavitation

Approx.: approximately. Modified from [2].

Pathological findings

Large airways/bronchi

Large airway involvement was one of the first recognised forms of pulmonary manifestation of IBD and remains significant [1–3, 6–10]. The histological findings are nonspecific. Patients whose primary manifestation is simply chronic bronchitis may show minimal submucosal chronic inflammation under an intact mucosa without metaplastic change. Patients with (severe) chronic bronchial suppuration and/or bronchiectasis typically show marked band-like chronic inflammatory infiltrate in the submucosa and the overlying mucosa may be ulcerated or show metaplastic change (fig. 1). Acute

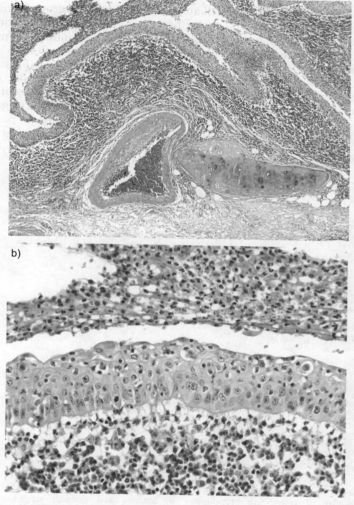

Fig. 1. – Bronchiectasis in chronic ulcerative colitis. a) The large airways show marked submucosal inflammation and some distortion of the mucosa. b) At higher power, the luminal exudates of neutrophils and metaplastic mucosal epithelium in the bronchi are apparent.

inflammation may also be prominent. Granulomas are not seen and this clinical pattern primarily affects patients with UC.

In cases of established bronchiectasis, the histological changes are more pronounced and bronchial structural changes are also present; secondary changes may also be present in the distal parenchyma, including recurrent pneumonias, abscess formation, *etc.*

Bronchiolar pathology

The spectrum of pathological changes in the small airways correlates with those seen on high-resolution computed tomography [1, 2, 8, 9, 11]. Thus, cases with prominent cellular infiltrates along airways and luminal exudates may show centrilobular nodules and "tree in bud" pattern, whereas those dominated by constrictive bronchiolitis show predominantly mosaic pattern.

The pathological findings in the small airways can be broadly grouped into those that are primarily cellular infiltrates and those that show predominantly scarring, although there is considerable overlap and patients with cellular infiltrates may develop progressive luminal narrowing and features of constrictive bronchiolitis (fig. 2). The cellular infiltrates in IBD are often marked and include varying degrees of acute inflammatory cells in the lumen and chronic inflammation in the walls, descriptively acute and chronic cellular bronchiolitis. Acute inflammation is not present in all cases. These cellular infiltrates are associated with a variable degree of scarring that can be subepithelial and narrow the lumen (constrictive bronchiolitis), transmural or peribronchiolar. Those cases associated with appreciable luminal narrowing (constrictive bronchiolitis) will show features of constrictive bronchiolitis radiologically.

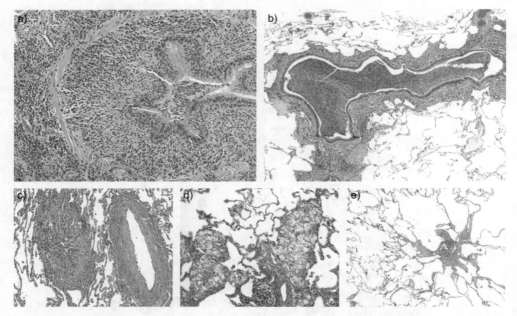

Fig. 2. – Bronchiolitis in chronic ulcerative colitis. a) Cellular infiltration with submucosal fibrosis and luminal compromise indicative of constrictive bronchiolitis. b) Scarring and purulent secretions in the lumen. c) Constrictive bronchiolitis (with airflow obstruction) and marked loss of bronchiolar lumens. d) Some cases of inflammatory bowel disease-associated bronchiolitis have prominent interstitial foam cells, similar to diffuse panbronchiolitis. e) Bronchiolar and peribronchiolar scarring.

In some bronchiolitis cases, the acute inflammatory exudate is suppurative and necrotising, and necrotic nodular foci (culture negative) develop and merge with the necrobiotic nodules described below.

One distinctive form of cellular bronchiolitis encountered in IBD is histologically indistinguishable from diffuse panbronchiolitis (DPB) as described in the Japanese population [1, 11]. These cases show an acute inflammatory reaction in the lumen with chronic inflammation in the airway wall and a marked prominent accumulation of interstitial foam cells (fig. 2d). It is this last feature (interstitial foam cells) that is so distinctive and the one feature that is indistinguishable from DPB, as originally described in Japan.

Cellular bronchiolitis (primarily chronic) with associated granulomas (fig. 3) has been described in CD [12, 13]. Typically, these are scattered non-necrotising granulomas and these cases do not show the typical coalescence of granulomas with associated fibrosis as encountered in sarcoidosis.

Parenchymal lesions

Infiltrative/interstitial lung disease. While rare progressive fibrosing interstitial pneumonias have been encountered in patients with IBD, the majority of infiltrative/ ILD cases fall into the spectrum of nonfibrotic processes showing the histological patterns currently termed: 1) nonspecific interstitial pneumonia (NSIP); 2) organising pneumonia (OP; formerly bronchiolitis obliterans organising pneumonia); and 3) eosinophilic pneumonia/eosinophil infiltrates [1–3, 13–20]. Among these groups, there is considerable overlap (figs 4 and 5) and distinguishing an NSIP pattern that may contain occasional foci of OP from an OP pattern may be somewhat academic; most patients will respond to oral/ parenteral corticosteroid administration. Granulomatous interstitial pneumonias and desquamative interstitial pneumonia have also been described but are quite rare.

Parenchymal nodules. As noted previously, some necrobiotic parenchymal nodules are seen in association with (and probably arise from) a purulent necrotising

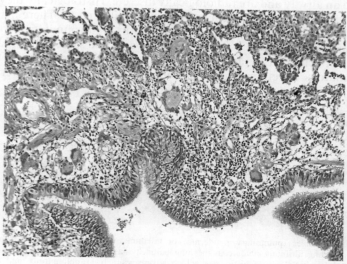

Fig. 3. – Granulomatous bronchiolitis in Crohn's disease. There are loose epithelioid cell granulomas in the bronchiolar submucosa.

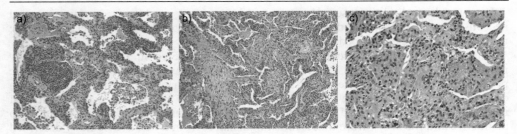

Fig. 4. – Interstitial lung disease in inflammatory bowel disease. While most cases tend to show one dominant pattern there are occasional cases that show mixed patterns. The case illustrated shows a) foci of cellular nonspecific interstitial pneumonia, b) foci of organising pneumonia, and c) foci with appreciable eosinophils suggesting eosinophilic pneumonia.

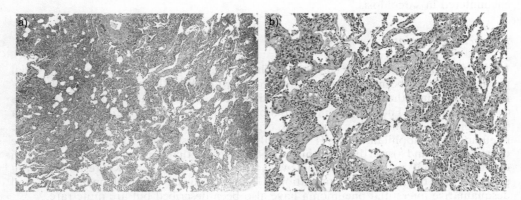

Fig. 5. – Interstitial pneumonia in Crohn's disease. There are mononuclear interstitial infiltrates and the pattern is cellular nonspecific interstitial pneumonia. Granulomas were not present. b) An enlarged view of a).

bronchiolitis [1–3]. Fully developed necrobiotic nodules typically show no anatomical relationship to an airway and are radiologically discrete. Histologically they show central necrosis and large numbers of degenerating neutrophils (fig. 6). There may be a rim of palisaded histiocytes peripherally and associated fibrin in surrounding airspaces but well-developed granulomatous features, including giant cells and sarcoid-like granulomas, are lacking. This distinct lack of granulomatous features helps to distinguish these nodules from granulomatous infections and Wegener's granulomatosis. However, appropriate

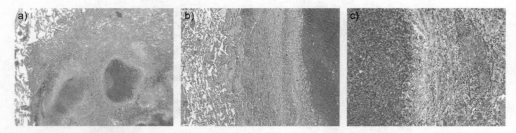

Fig. 6. – Necrobiotic nodules (pulmonary pyoderma) in inflammatory bowel disease. a) Irregular regions of necrosis with surrounding fibrinous exudate in the lung parenchyma. Two cases (b and c) show there is central necrosis of neutrophils with a rim of histiocytes, which is only vaguely granulomatous, and there is a lack of giant cells and sarcoid-like granulomas. Organising pneumonia (b) and airspace fibrin (c) are apparent in the viable tissue around the necrotic foci.

stains are required to rule out any infectious disease that may be amenable to specific treatment. They should also be distinguished from rheumatoid nodules; the latter tend to occur in a subpleural or septal location to show more fibrinoid change, better developed palisaded histiocytes and chronic inflammatory reaction in the periphery.

Vasculitis, including Wegener's granulomatosis, has been described in patients with IBD [21], but a true association is uncertain. To date, well-documented cases have not been encountered. It is well known that Wegener's granulomatosis may primarily involve the bowel and such cases may bear a considerable resemblance to CD.

Histopathological approach

In a patient with IBD and pulmonary disease, which has resulted in lung biopsy for interpretation by the pathologist, considerations should include those described in table 1. Any patient who has been immunosuppressed or who has been on a drug known to be associated with the development of infection (*e.g.* viral infections in patients on methotrexate or tuberculosis in patients on infliximab) should lead to exclusion of infection and performance of appropriate special stains and cultures. Toxic/idiosyncratic drug reactions may result in histological patterns (NSIP, OP, eosinophilic pneumonia, *etc.*) that are indistinguishable from their idiopathic counterparts and identical to cases secondary to IBD (fig. 7). In such cases the histological findings are nonspecific and the pathologist should simply report the pattern encountered and raise the various possible aetiologies, including drugs.

Management and prognosis

Details of clinical evaluation, management and prognosis for this group of patients are beyond the scope of this chapter. In general, patients with inflammatory disease of the airways who have not developed chronic bronchial suppuration or bronchiectasis have a favourable long-term outcome, often with inhaled steroids [1, 2]. Patients with established structural abnormalities, particularly bronchiectasis, may show considerable response to steroids but have persistent impairment.

IBD-associated bronchiolitis is generally treated with inhaled or oral steroids and

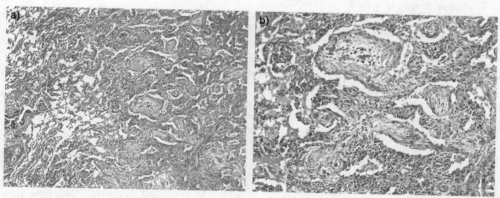

Fig. 7. – Drug-related interstitial pneumonia in a patient with inflammatory bowel disease (IBD). The histology is typical of organising pneumonia and as such could be a pattern encountered in IBD. In this case, it was linked to sulpha drug therapy. b) An enlarged view of a).

while the outlook for granulomatous bronchiolitis may be favourable, the outlook for patients with other forms of bronchiolitis, particularly those with constrictive bronchiolitis, is much less favourable [1, 2]. Patients with infiltrative/ILD generally receive oral steroids and have a favourable outcome [1, 2]. Similarly, the parenchymal necrobiotic nodules are also steroid responsive and have a favourable outcome despite the ominous histology with extensive acute inflammation and sterile abscess formation [1, 2].

Summary

The pulmonary pathology associated with inflammatory bowel disease is reviewed in the current chapter. Lung disease in this setting may be directly related to inflammatory bowel disease (IBD), secondary to other complications of IBD, or associated with therapy given for IBD. Cases that reach pathological evaluation include examples of inflammatory lesions of the subglottic region, trachea and large airways, inflammatory and obstructive lesions of the bronchioles, a variety of patterns of diffuse interstitial lung disease, and necrobiotic parenchymal nodules.

Keywords: Bronchiolitis, bronchitis, inflammatory bowel disease, interstitial lung disease, necrobiotic nodules, pathology.

References

1. Camus P, Piard F, Ashcroft T, Gal A, Colby TV. The lung in inflammatory bowel disease. *Medicine (Baltimore)* 1993; 72: 151–180.
2. Camus P, Colby TV. The lung in inflammatory bowel disease. *Eur Respir J* 2000; 15: 5–10.
3. Storch I, Sachar D, Katz S. Pulmonary manifestations of inflammatory bowel disease. *Inflamm Bowel Dis* 2003; 9: 104–115.
4. Tzanakis N, Samiou M, Bouros D, Mouzas J, Kouroumalis E, Siafakas NM. Small airways function in patients with inflammatory bowel disease. *Am J Respir Crit Care Med* 1998; 157: 382–386.
5. Tzanakis N, Bouros D, Samiou M, *et al.* Lung function in patients with inflammatory bowel disease. *Respir Med* 1998; 92: 516–522.
6. Butland RJA, Cole P, Citron KM, Turner-Warwick M. Chronic bronchial suppuration and inflammatory bowel disease. *Q J Med* 1981; 50: 63–75.
7. Moles KW, Varghese G, Hayes JR. Pulmonary involvement in ulcerative colitis. *Br J Dis Chest* 1988; 82: 79–83.
8. Garg K, Lynch DA, Newell JD. Inflammatory airways disease in ulcerative colitis: CT and high-resolution CT features. *J Thorac Imag* 1993; 8: 159–163.
9. Mahadeva R, Walsh G, Flower CD, Shneerson JM. Clincial and radiological characteristics of lung disease in inflammatory bowel disease. *Eur Respir J* 2000; 15: 41–48.
10. Vasishta S, Wood JB, McGinty F. Ulcerative tracheobronchitis years after colectomy for ulcerative colitis. *Chest* 1994; 106: 1279–1281.
11. Desai SJ, Gephardt GN, Stoller JK. Diffuse panbronchiolitis preceding ulcerative colitis. *Chest* 1989; 45: 1342–1344.
12. Vandenplas O, Casel S, Delos M, Triqaux JP, Melange M, Marchand E. Granulomatous bronchiolitis associated with Crohn's disease. *Am J Respir Crit Care Med* 1998; 158: 1676–1679.
13. Casey MB, Tazelaar HD, Myers JL, *et al.* Noninfectious lung pathology in patients with Crohn's disease. *Am J Surg Pathol* 2003; 27: 213–219.

14. Case records of the Massachusetts General Hospital. Weekly clinicopathology exercises Case 46–180. *N Engl J Med* 1980; 303: 1218–1225.
15. Swinburn CR, Jackson GJ, Cobden I, Ashcroft T, Morritt GN, Corris PA. Bronchiolitis obliterans organising pneumonia in a patient with ulcerative colitis. *Thorax* 1988; 43: 735–736.
16. Case records of the Massachusetts General Hospital. Case 12-1993. *N Engl J Med* 1980; 328: 869–876.
17. Dawson A, Gibbs AR, Anderson G. An unusual perilobular pattern of pulmonary interstitial fibrosis associated with Crohn's disease. *Histopathology* 1993; 23: 553–556.
18. Hotermans G, Benard A, Guenanen H, Demarcq-Delerue G, Malart T, Wallaert B. Non-granulomatous interstitial lung disease in Crohn's disease. *Eur Respir J* 1996; 9: 380–382.
19. Hoffmann RM, Kruis W. Rare extraintestinal manifestations of inflammatory bowel disease. *Inflamm Bowel Dis* 2004; 10: 140–147.
20. Omori H, Asahi H, Inoue Y, Irinoda T, Saito K. Pulmonary involvement in Crohn's disease report of a case and review of the literature. *Inflamm Bowel Dis* 2004; 10: 129–134.
21. Kedziora JA, Wolff M, Chang J. Limited form of Wegener's granulomatosis in ulcerative colitis. *Am J Roentgenol Radium Ther Nucl Med* 1975; 125: 127–133.

Previously published in the European Respiratory Monograph Series:

Monographs may be purchased from:

Publications Sales Department, Maney Publishing, Suite 1C, Joseph's Well, Hanover Walk, Leeds, LS3 1AB, UK.

Tel: 44 (0)113 2432800; Fax: 44 (0)113 3868178; E-mail: books@maney.co.uk; www.maney.co.uk

Customers in the Americas should contact: Old City Publishing Inc., 628 North 2nd Street, Philadelphia PA 19123, USA. Tel: 1 215 925 4390; Fax: 1 215 925 4371; E-mail: info@oldcitypublishing.com

EUROPEAN RESPIRATORY MONOGRAPH

Instructions to Authors

The European Respiratory Monograph is an official publication of the European Respiratory Society, which publishes "state of the art" review articles, only by invitation, under the co-ordination of a Guest Editor(s). All manuscripts should be sent in electronic format to: monograph@ersj.org.uk

Offers or queries regarding future content should be directed to the Editor in Chief: K. Larsson, Unit of Lung and Allergy Research, Division of Physiology, National Institute of Environmental Medicine, IMM, SE17177 Stockholm, Sweden. Fax: 46 8300619. E-mail: Kjell.Larsson@ki.se

INSTRUCTIONS FOR THE PREPARATION OF MANUSCRIPTS

Presentation

The manuscript should be accompanied by a presentation letter and a title page, with the name of the authors and their affiliation, the full mailing address, fax number and e-mail address of the corresponding author, and any source of support. A short running head should be given and not more than 6 keywords. The length of a chapter, in typescript form, should be approximately 20–30 pages of double-spaced type including text, figures, tables and references.

Text

Experimental paper format is not required, and should not include sections on methods, results and discussion. Headings and subheadings should be used to facilitate the readers. The Monograph aims to be educational. Clear distinction should be made between strong information (*i.e.* based on random, controlled clinical trials) and soft information (*i.e.* suggestive but inconclusive data). The text should start with an introduction and finish with a 10–15 line conclusion. A brief summary (no more than 300 words) is required with the typescript which should recapitulate the key points, rather than introducing the subjects to be discussed.

Tables and illustrations

Please include all tables and figures with your typescript. Each chapter must include at least one table or illustration. Every table and illustration must be cited in the text. The source of reproduction must be acknowledged (from [Ref. No.] with permission). See copyright information below.

Tables

Each table should be typed on a separate page and should have a short title. Other information should appear as footnotes to the table, indicated by superscript symbols. Large tables are difficult to read and print, and should be avoided.

Illustrations

Where a figure can replace or reduce a text passage, the figure is preferred. Figures should be named and numbered. Line drawings can be supplied as .jpeg, .gif, .tif or .btmp, and will be redrawn into house style. All photographic images should be provided with a minimum of 300 dots per inch (dpi) and should preferably be supplied in .jpeg, .tif or .eps format. Photomicrographs must have internal scale markers (linear scale). Please provide a clear legend for each figure which should be brief and nonrepetitive of information given in the text, all abbreviations should be expanded in the legend.

References

The author is free to decide on how many references he/she will use. References to original work are preferred to references or quotations from other chapters in the Monograph. However, the author is free to decide on what he/she will quote. Number references consecutively in the order in which they are first mentioned in the text, including those mentioned in tables and figures. Type the references in square brackets. Cite personal communications and unpublished work in the text only, giving the name and initials of the authors and the year of writing. Follow the style of the *European Respiratory Journal* (Vancouver style).

Copyright

You must obtain from the copyright holder (usually the publisher of the work) permission to reproduce figures, tables and extended quotations. The source of any such reproduction must always be acknowledged. **The original document should be included with your manuscript to the Editor in Chief.**

For any further details please refer to the instructions to the authors of the *European Respiratory Journal*.